Neurolaryngology

Christian Sittel
Orlando Guntinas-Lichius
Editors

Neurolaryngology

Springer

Editors
Christian Sittel
Department of Otorhinolaryngology/
Head and Neck Surgery
Clinical Centre Stuttgart
Stuttgart
Germany

Orlando Guntinas-Lichius
Department of Otorhinolaryngology and
Institute of Phoniatry and
Pedaudiology
Jena University Hospital
Jena
Germany

The volume Editors gratefully acknowledge the contribution offered by MedEl to the creation of some of the illustrations included in the book

ISBN 978-3-319-61722-0 ISBN 978-3-319-61724-4 (eBook)
https://doi.org/10.1007/978-3-319-61724-4

Library of Congress Control Number: 2017956142

Printed on acid-free paper

This Springer imprint is published by Springer Nature
The registered company is Springer International Publishing AG
The registered company address is: Gewerbestrasse 11, 6330 Cham, Switzerland

Foreword

The larynx acts as a switch between the trachea and the oesophagus, separating the airway from the alimentary tract. An additional and phylogenetically younger laryngeal function is phonation. Since these different tasks of the larynx require sensory detection, respiration, deglutition and phonatory stimuli to the laryngeal structures and motor control of muscular activity, it is obvious that central and peripheral neural control is essential for physiological laryngeal function. However, until some forty years ago, laryngologists were used to mainly deal with disorders of laryngeal structure, such as trauma, neoplastic lesions or inflammatory alterations.

Until the 1980s, there was a general lack of interest and knowledge in neurological disorders of the larynx. During the past four decades, much of the applied and basic research in neurolaryngology has been conducted in Japan and the United States, establishing the framework for further research work and clinical application of this discipline.

European laryngologists have eagerly anticipated these new directions for improved understanding of phonatory, respiratory and swallowing disorders in recent years and have taken an active and original role in many aspects of neurolaryngology.

This textbook brings together many of the leading neurolaryngologists from Europe and some of those from the United States who inspired the laryngeal community round two highly reputed and experienced editors to give a comprehensive approach to current clinical and experimental topics in the field. Much of the work presented here has been initialized during meetings and workshops of the European Laryngological Society and was inspired by landmark work set up by the American Laryngological Society and the American Broncho-Esophagological Association. Therefore, this volume witnesses the vibrant progress in neurology related to the larynx and testifies the fertility of transnational work, both in Europc, in Asia and Australia, and on a transatlantic scale.

The book is a comprehensive guide to key topics in neurolaryngology. It features detailed information on laryngeal paresis, laryngeal dystonia, upper motor neuron disorders, imaging and clinical assessment, laryngeal electromyography, functional therapy, botulinum toxin injection, phonosurgery, laryngeal reinnervation and laryngeal transplantation.

All those interested in functional laryngology, phonatory disorders, swallowing impairment and laryngeal airway issues will value this work and constantly refer to the resources compiled by the authors of this textbook.

Hans Edmund Eckel
President, Confederation of European
Otorhinolaryngology - Head and Neck
Surgery (CEORL) and Consultant ENT Surgeon
Klagenfurt General Hospital
Klagenfurt, Austria

Preface

The term neurolaryngology has been coined well over 30 years ago, but has not become as popular and naturally used as it is the case for its siblings like neurotology. In this subspecialty, the "neuro-" aspect is less obvious and often requires a closer look. However, neurolaryngology is covering a broad spectrum of conditions involving neurogenic dysfunction of the larynx and pharynx, including central and peripheral disorders. With the main focus on functional management, surgical interventions are primarily reconstructive and rehabilitative.

Neurolaryngology has been stimulated greatly from collaborations between laryngologists and neurologists who recognized that neurologic disorders could impair laryngeal function and that neurogenic etiology could be discerned frequently for seemingly idiopathic hoarseness and dysphagia.

In the last years, neurolaryngology has developed rapidly in response to the advances in the diagnosis and treatment of laryngeal disorders. Diagnostic procedures include many technical innovations that have expanded the armamentarium for treatment of benign and malignant disease. The goal of this book is to provide the reader with advanced experience in diagnosis and treatment of laryngeal disorders with specific focus on neurolaryngology. We hope that we can stimulate the reader to implement neurolaryngology in daily clinical routine or to broaden the perspective toward this field.

This book will provide the newest and comprehensive insights for clinical experience and surgery based on basic research in neurolaryngology. The reader will acquire experience in the diagnosis of neurolaryngological disorders and gain experience in a variety of surgical procedures. Because there is a substantial backlog demand, the book starts with special chapters on electrophysiological and pulmonological investigations, followed by a block of chapters dealing with all modern aspects of vocal cord immobility. Intraoperative nerve monitoring has become an indispensable tool to protect the recurrent laryngeal nerve. Therefore, a chapter is dedicated to this topic. Dystonia and other neurological diseases are domains for nonsurgical treatment, which is reflected by a sequence of chapters on these aspects. This is followed by a large block of chapters dealing with all contemporary, mainly minimally invasive, aspects of neurolaryngological surgery. All endoscopic surgeries, framework surgery, the new field of laryngeal pacing, and the rediscovered field of reinnervation surgery are described in detail. Finally, an outlook on future clinical research as perceived by some leading neurolaryngologists concludes the book.

We are greatly indebted to all contributors who were so kind to shoulder the extra burden of writing a chapter. In particular we would like to thank Sonja Burger, our outstanding scientific illustrator. Her distinctive and graphic style is present in the illustration of nearly all chapters. This book would not have been possible without the European Laryngological Society (ELS). The idea for this book came up during a meeting of the committee on neurolaryngology of the ELS, and many of the authors are involved in the ELS and this committee. Special thanks go to MED-EL for sponsoring the illustrations and moreover for passionately supporting emerging applications in the field of neurolaryngology.

Jena, Germany Orlando Guntinas-Lichius
Stuttgart, Germany Christian Sittel

Contents

Contributors

Mohammed I. Almohizea Department of Otolaryngology, Head and Neck Surgery, King Abdulaziz University Hospital, King Saud University, Riyadh, Saudi Arabia

Christoph Arens Department of Otorhinolaryngology, Head and Neck Surgery, University Hospital, Otto-von-Guericke-University Magdeburg, Magdeburg, Germany

Gauthier Desuter ENT Head & Neck Surgery, Cliniques Universitaires Saint-Luc, Université Catholique de Louvain, Brussels, Belgium

Frederik G. Dikkers Department of Otorhinolaryngology, Head and Neck Surgery, University Medical Center Groningen, University of Groningen, Groningen, The Netherlands

Susanne Fleischer Department of Voice, Speech and Hearing Disorders, University Medical Center Hamburg-Eppendorf, Hamburg, Germany

Carmen Górriz Gil Otolaryngology Head and Neck Surgery, Hospital Puerta de Hierro Majadahonda, Madrid, Spain

Orlando Guntinas-Lichius Department of Otorhinolaryngology, Institute of Phoniatry/Pedaudiology, Jena University Hospital, Jena, Germanyw

Kate Heathcote Otolaryngology, Poole Hospital NHS Trust, Poole, Dorset, UK

Felix J.F. Herth Pneumology and Critical Care Medicine, Thoraxklinik, University of Heidelberg, Heidelberg, Germany

Markus M. Hess Deutsche Stimmklinik, Hamburg, Germany

Rebecca J. Howell Otolaryngology, Head and Neck Surgery, University of Cincinnati, Cincinnati, OH, USA

Robert R. Lorenz Head and Neck Institute, Cleveland Clinic, Cleveland, OH, USA

David G. Lott Department of Otolaryngology Head and Neck Surgery, Mayo Clinic Arizona, Phoenix, AZ, USA

Lyndsay L. Madden Department of Otolaryngology, University of Pittsburgh Voice Center, Pittsburgh, PA, USA

Jean-Paul Marie Otorhinolaryngology, Head and Neck Surgery, University Hospital of Rouen, Rouen, Normandy, France

Andreas H. Mueller Otorhinolaryngology/Plastic Surgery, SRH Wald-Klinikum Gera, Gera, Germany

Iain J. Nixon Otorhinolaryngology/Head and Neck Surgery, NHS Lothian/Edinburgh University, Edinburgh, UK

Enyinnaya Ofo Advanced Head and Neck Surgery & Robotics Fellow, Royal Adelaide Hospital, Adelaide, SA, Australia

Gregory N. Postma Otolaryngology, Medical College of Georgia at Augusta University, Augusta, GA, USA

Vyas M.N. Prasad Department of Otolaryngology-Head and Neck Surgery, NG Teng Fong General Hospital Singapore, Singapore, Singapore

Marc Remacle Department of ORL-Head and Neck Surgery, CHL-Eich, Luxembourg, Luxembourg

Clark A. Rosen Department of Otolaryngology, University of Pittsburgh Voice Center, Pittsburgh, PA, USA

Ricard Simo Otorhinolaryngology Head and Neck Surgery, Guy's and St Thomas' Hospital NHS Foundation Trust, Guy's Hospital, London, UK

Christian Sittel Department of Otorhinolaryngology/Head and Neck Surgery, Clinical Centre Stuttgart, Stuttgart, Germany

Susanne Voigt-Zimmermann Department of Otorhinolaryngology, Head and Neck Surgery, University Hospital, Otto-von-Guericke-University Magdeburg, Magdeburg, Germany

Gerd Fabian Volk Department of Otorhinolaryngology, Jena University Hospital, Jena, Germany

Claus Wittekindt Department of Otorhinolaryngology, University of Gissen, Gissen, Germany

Electrophysiological Assessment 1

Gerd Fabian Volk and Orlando Guntinas-Lichius

Abstract

An electrophysiological examination normally includes the direct assessment of the nerve of interest and of its target muscles. Electrodiagnostics for the larynx are only well established for the investigation of the laryngeal muscles by laryngeal electromyography (LEMG). So far, techniques to investigate the nerves innervating the laryngeal muscles directly, for instance, by electric or magnetic stimulation of the recurrent nerve, do not produce reliable results or are only established in a few centers. Therefore, the focus of this chapter lies on LEMG. Although LEMG was established more than 60 years ago, many laryngologists do not routinely use even LEMG. Until recently, this was may be due to the continuous lack of agreement on methodology, interpretation, validity, and clinical application of LEMG. As a consequence, the American Academy of Otolaryngology—Head and Neck Surgery Neurolaryngology—and the working group on Neurolaryngology of the European Laryngological Society have published lately guidelines for the use of LEMG. The presentation of LEMG in this chapter is following these guidelines as it presents an update of the guideline of the European Laryngological Society. Furthermore, the basics and limitations of other electrodiagnostic tools are presented. The chapter concludes with an outlook on future perspectives of electrophysiological assessment of neurolaryngological disorders.

1.1 Introduction

The electrophysiological assessment is considered of use in the diagnosis of peripheral and central neurologic disorders affecting laryngeal function and differentiating neurolaryngological disorders from other disorders causing changes in laryngeal function, for instance, cricoarytenoid joint fixation [1]. Optimally, an electrophysiological

G.F. Volk
Department of Otorhinolaryngology,
Jena University Hospital, Jena, Germany

O. Guntinas-Lichius (✉)
Department of Otorhinolaryngology,
Institute of Phoniatry/Pedaudiology,
Jena University Hospital, Jena, Germany
e-mail: orlando.guntinas@med.uni-jena.de

C. Sittel, O. Guntinas-Lichius (eds.), *Neurolaryngology*,
https://doi.org/10.1007/978-3-319-61724-4_1

assessment includes both a direct examination of the nerve of interest and an examination of the related target muscles. In contrast to large nerves in the extremities, for instance, the median nerve, a direct stimulation or recording of laryngeal nerves is not possible, respectively, the length of the accessible regions of the recurrent nerve, of the superior laryngeal nerve, or of the vagal nerve is too short to allow the measurement of nerve conduction velocity. For these reasons, the electrophysiological assessment of the larynx is restricted in most departments to an examination of the laryngeal muscles by laryngeal electromyography (LEMG). Because of this, this chapter will present a detailed description of LEMG and will give some basic insight into other methods for a laryngeal electrophysiological assessment.

1.2 Indication for LEMG

When abduction or adduction of the true vocal fold as observed by laryngeal examination is reduced or absent, the preliminary diagnosis is respiratory immobility of the vocal fold. The most frequent cause is laryngeal paralysis but other possible causes also have to be considered. LEMG is an important diagnostic tool for this purpose [2–4]. Normal electrical activity patterns of the LEMG support a diagnosis of arytenoid fixation [5], whereas abnormal electrical activity patterns, including patterns of denervation or reinnervation, support the diagnosis of vocal fold paralysis [6]. An important limitation of LEMG has to be mentioned: Signs for a denervation due to axonal lesion can only be detected 10–14 days after the onset of vocal fold immobility. This time is needed until the degeneration of the nerve has reached the target muscles.

1.3 Equipment for LEMG

1.3.1 Electromyography (EMG) Electrodes

In EMG, potential differences (voltage potentials) are measured between electrodes, which are usually made of metal or polymers providing sufficient electrical conduction. In electromyography, surface and indwelling electrodes are used. Surface electrodes are placed on the skin or mucosa and do not penetrate the surface. For recording sum potentials through the mucosa, circularly or cylindrically shaped electrodes on nonconductive applicators are used. They are noninvasive but the least selective electrode type. In studies focusing on nerve conduction velocity and neuromuscular transmission, or in intraoperative monitoring of the thyroarytenoid muscle during thyroid surgery, surface electrodes are used. For this second purpose, surface electrodes are attached to the laryngeal tube above the cuff to ensure direct contact to the vocal folds. They can also be used as reference electrodes for monopolar needle electrodes or as common ground electrodes.

The recorded potential represents the weighted sum of all the individual potentials produced by the activated muscle, each divided by its respective distance from the electrode. As this creates a hemisphere of recording below the surface electrode which has fuzzy limits, these electrodes are not suitable for recording details or electrical events associated with individual motor units.

1.3.2 Needle Electrodes

There are several types of indwelling electrodes, of which needle electrodes are the most versatile: they occur as monopolar, concentric, bipolar concentric, and single-fiber needle electrodes. The monopolar needle electrode is a stainless steel needle fully insulated with a thin insulating coating, except for the tip. Solid needles are used for diagnostic purposes; for EMG-guided injection of botulinum toxin, the needle is hollow (Fig. 1.1). The recording area of this electrode is spherical. The reference electrode is placed at a myoelectric inactive location of the body and may be a surface electrode. For LEMG, a suitable place for the reference electrode is the skin over the manubrium sterni. The concentric needle electrode (Fig. 1.2) consists of a hollow steel needle with a steel, silver, or platinum wire running through the needle, which is fully insulated except for the tip. The

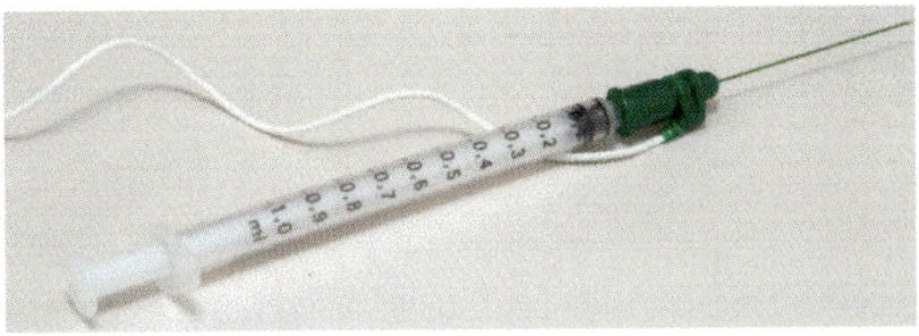

Fig. 1.1 For EMG-guided injection of botulinum toxin, the needle has to be hollow. The shaft of the needle is insulated except the tip. For a bipolar recording, the reference electrode (often a surface electrode) should be placed at a myoelectric inactive location of the body, e.g., the manubrium sterni

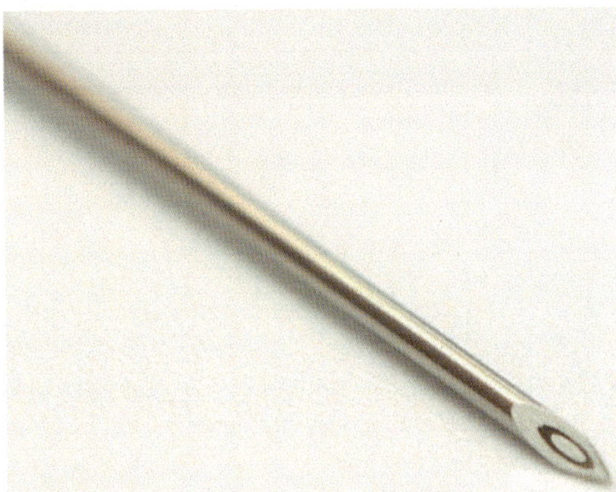

Fig. 1.2 The concentric needle electrode consists of a hollow steel needle with a steel, silver, or platinum wire running through the needle, which is fully insulated except for the tip

potential difference between the outer shaft of the needle and the tip of the wire is measured by connecting each of these to one port of the differential amplifier. Since the electrode cannula acts as a shield, the electrode has directional recording characteristics controlled by the angle and position of the bevel.

Comparing monopolar with concentric needle electrodes, potentials recorded by monopolar needle electrodes tend to be larger and longer with more phases than those recorded with concentric needle electrodes. This difference is based on the existence of more muscle fibers within the zone of detection, as well as on fewer cancelations due to potentials being recorded from the cannula of the electrode. The bipolar concentric electrode is sometimes called bifilar or double concentric. It is a hollow needle containing two platinum wires, each of which is insulated except for its tip. The outer shaft is grounded, and the two internal wires are each connected to one side of the differential amplifier, so that the potential difference between the two wires is measured. The recording range of the bipolar concentric electrode is restricted to the area between the two tips of the wires within the shaft, which makes it too small for many routine clinical purposes. The potentials are shorter and lower in the voltage than those recorded with concentric needle electrodes [7]. For single-fiber EMG, a fine wire capable of recording a single muscle fiber action potential is embedded at the tip of the needle shaft acting as reference.

1.3.3 Hooked-Wire Electrodes

The other common type of indwelling electrodes used in LEMG is the hooked-wire electrode (Fig. 1.3a). This electrode consists of two separate fully isolated fine wires except of the hooks, each with a maximum diameter of 50 μm often made of platinum. They are inserted into the muscle after having been threaded through a hollow-core needle [8]. For reaching the larynx, a curved (Fig. 1.3b) and a strait application tool (Fig. 1.3c) is available, depending if the patient is awake in a sitting position or lying during a suspension laryngoscopy. When the needle is withdrawn, the hooks on the end of the wires act as a barb, stabilizing the position of the electrodes within the muscle. These electrodes cannot be repositioned once placed but, as they bend easily, can be removed smoothly. The field of recording can vary during measurement, depending on the distance between the bared wires in the moving muscle [8]. The advantage of hooked-wire electrodes is that they are well tolerated after correct placement, so that they can be left in place for longer periods of time than needle electrodes.

1.3.4 Selection of Electrode Type

For comparative or quantitative evaluation, the same electrode type must be used when obtaining reference values, due to the previously mentioned

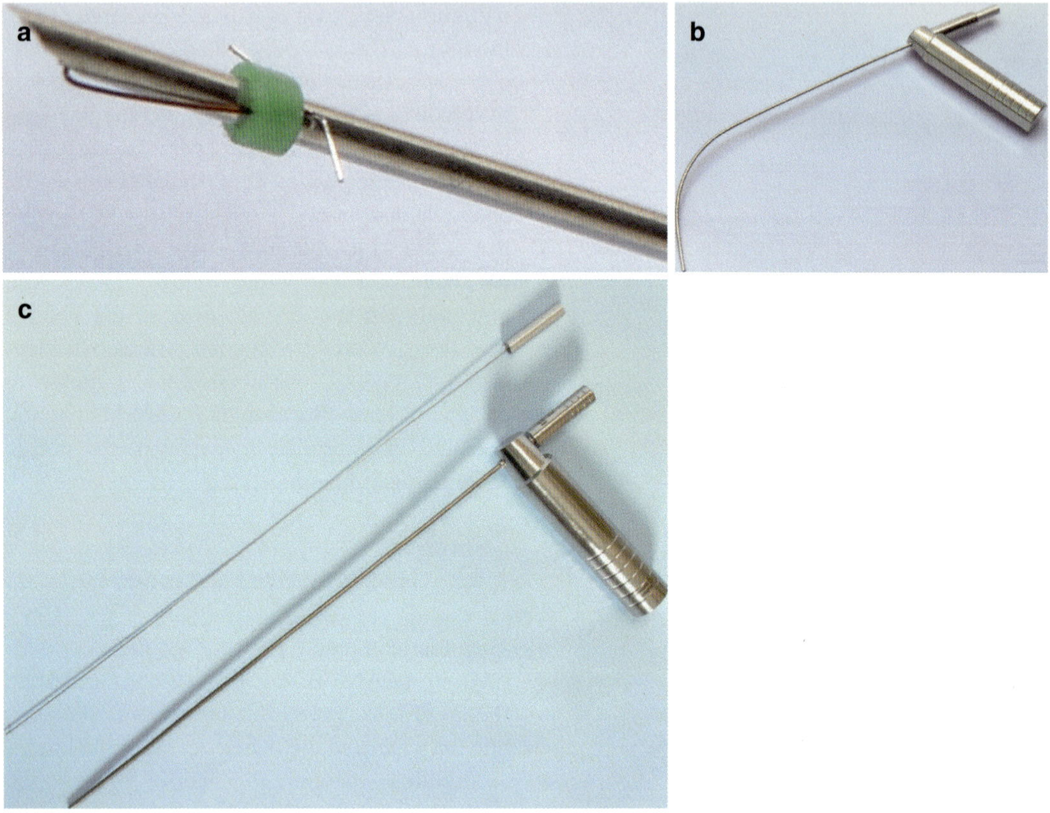

Fig. 1.3 (**a**) Hooked-wire electrodes are indwelling electrodes often used in LEMG. These electrodes consist of two separate fully isolated fine wires except of the hooks, each with a maximum diameter of 50 micrometers often made of platinum. They are inserted into the muscle after having been threaded through a hollow-core needle. The green rubber band holds back the hooks only for transport. (**b**) For reaching the larynx in an awake patient in a sitting position, a curved application tool is useful. (**c**) For reaching the larynx during a suspension laryngoscopy, a strait application tool is ideal

differences between electrode types. Filter settings must also be consistent. In general, monopolar electrodes pick up potentials from a larger spherical region than concentric electrodes [9].

For the transcutaneous approach to the laryngeal muscles, it is recommended to use concentric needle electrodes, providing a uniform field for motor unit action potential (MUAP) waveform analysis. They should have a length of 50 mm in order to reach even the posterior cricoarytenoid muscle in all patients and a thickness of at least 0.45 mm to provide rigidity for precise maneuvers behind the cricothyroid ligament [10]. The transoral approach with bipolar hooked wires allows an exact endoscopic controlled positioning into the target muscles and is useful for recording over a longer period of time or for recording multiple muscles simultaneously while the patient performs different tasks [11].

1.3.5 EMG Amplifier

Most clinical EMG amplifiers can be used with the differential configuration to obtain a cleaner signal: Two active electrode contacts are placed on the muscles being examined. Furthermore, a reference electrode is placed on the body. To reduce the risk of electrical injury, the patient must be grounded. The signal of interest is amplified as the difference of potentials (voltage) between each active electrode and the reference electrode. The frequencies of a muscle action potential range between 2 Hz and 10,000 Hz, and the frequency band of the electromyography machine is typically set from 10 Hz to 10,000 Hz.

In most settings, the electrodiagnostic signal can be heard in real time on a loudspeaker. Connected computers can then display the signals on-screen, as well as process, analyze, and store them on hard disks. In addition, electrical stimulators are incorporated into the system so that it cannot only record the electric activity of muscles but also stimulate muscles or nerves depending on the chosen parameters. For basic examinations of LEMG, a one-channel EMG amplifier is suitable. If the activity of several muscles is to be compared in synchrony, a multichannel EMG amplifier is required. Not only EMG activity of muscles can be recorded on additional channels but also behaviorally or physiologically relevant signals like voice production or respiration activity. This is essential for offline interpreting stored data afterward.

1.3.6 Microphone

When a microphone is connected to a channel of a multichannel EMG amplifier, a synchronic voice recording is possible. This allows a comparison of myoelectric activity with the patient's sound production (Fig. 1.4). Additionally, the recorded instructions and comments of the examiner can be helpful for interpretation of the stored data. The upper filter cutoff frequency of the microphone should be set to half the sampling rate of the system.

1.3.7 Thermistor and Piezoelectric Thorax Expansion Belt

Respiration is another fundamental parameter of voice production. It can be measured by placing a thermistor in front of a patient's nose or mouth. A thermistor detects the changes of air temperature caused by every breath and can thus be used to record respiration activity. Alternatively, the movement of the chest wall and/or the upper abdominal wall can be monitored by using thorax and/or abdomen expansion belts with piezoelectric sensors. This movement is related to effort and produces a low-frequency sinusoidal waveform as the patient inhales and exhales. For both the piezoelectric expansion belt and for the thermistor, the lower cutoff frequency should be set to 0.01 Hz (eliminating a possible drift of the signal) and the higher frequency from 10 Hz to 30 Hz for smoothing the signal.

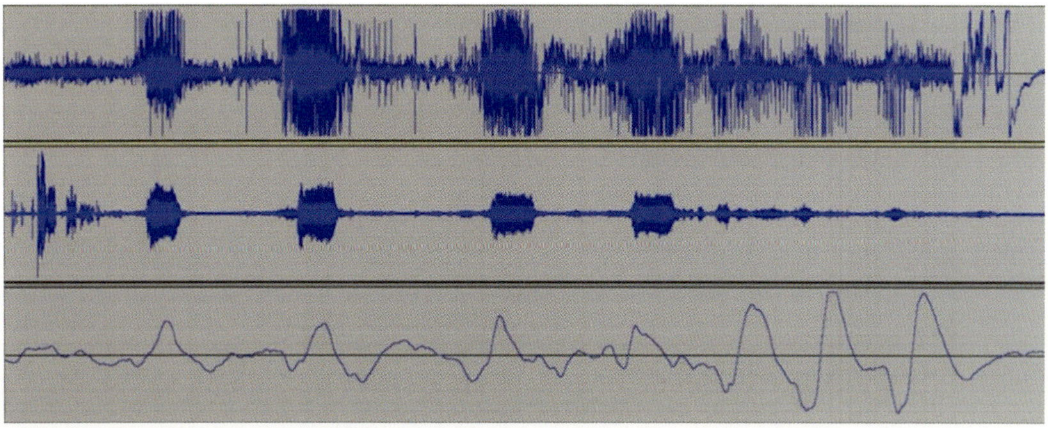

Fig. 1.4 Three-channel synchronic recording of TA activity by needle EMG, phonation by microphone, and respiration by the thorax belt. During phonation, good to detect in channel 2 via microphone, there is strong EMG activity in channel 1 recorded in the thyroarytenoid muscle. [Courtesy of Dr. med. Gerd Fabian Volk and www.lemg.org]

1.3.8 Indirect Laryngoscopy

The vocal fold motion status can be determined before, during, and after the LEMG with transnasal flexible laryngoscopy. Thus, potential swellings or bleedings can be detected in time. The use of a rigid laryngoscope with magnification is recommended for placing hooked-wire electrodes.

1.4 EMG Monitoring and Documentation

Recording an EMG from the laryngeal muscles is technically difficult, even though suitable methods are well described in literature since the 1970s [12]. Although otolaryngologists who regularly inject botulinum toxin into thyroarytenoid muscles for the treatment of laryngeal dystonia/spasmodic dysphonia are skilled in performing LEMG, only few have had training in interpreting MUAP signals. And because of the neurophysiological differences between the EMG of big muscles and of muscles of the larynx, even well-trained neurophysiologists can have difficulties in interpreting LEMG. Thus, we recommend that a laryngologist and an experienced user with clinical neurophysiology training should work as a team to gain experience with the specific attributes of laryngeal muscles.

1.5 Requirements and Preparations for LEMG

Laryngeal electromyography is a medical procedure requiring active cooperation by the patient. Thus, not only oral consent but also a detailed explanation of the intended procedure and expected responses is required. The patient's ability and willingness to cooperate has to be considered when planning an LEMG examination.

In addition, a detailed examination of the head and neck, including indirect or fiberoptic laryngoscopy and/or videostroboscopy, is important to detect altered anatomy, previous operations, or acute infections—conditions which can potentially hinder the electrode placement. Bleeding disorders caused, for example, by coagulopathy, warfarin, or acetylsalicylic acid are relative contraindications. Due to these rare but possible complications, emergency equipment including a cricothyrotomy set must be readily available. As with most medical procedures, LEMG should be carried out only if the medical information expected to be gained justifies the low risk of complications.

Special caution must be exercised in patients with narrow glottic gap due to bilateral vocal cord paralysis. In these cases, LEMG of the vocalis muscle should be performed only on one side at a time. During this test, the respiratory function of the patient must be monitored constantly to prevent breathing problems due to the LEMG. Electric stimulation studies should not be performed on patients with pacemakers without previous and subsequent cardiologic consultation.

For the LEMG, the patient is asked to adopt a comfortable position with a slightly reclined head. If necessary, the larynx can be anaesthetized locally with lidocaine, either applied transorally to the mucosal surface or with a transcutaneous intraluminal injection. For transcutaneous insertion with a concentric needle, the patient can be either sitting or supine, depending on the patient's needs and the examiner's experience. Hooked-wire electrodes are inserted transorally under visual control with an indirect laryngoscope. Thus, a sitting position of the patient is recommended. A detailed comparison between a transcutaneous and a transoral LEMG can be found in Table 1.1.

Table 1.1 Comparison between transcutaneous and transoral LEMG

Transcutaneous	Transoral
Inexpensive needles; one needle can be used for several muscles in one patient	Expensive hooked-wire electrodes; one electrode can be inserted only once in one muscle
Constant signal quality	Variable signal quality because tips of hooked-wire electrodes can move inside the muscle during activation
Position of needle can be corrected	Position of hooked-wire electrodes cannot be changed after insertion
Simultaneous measurements of several muscles are difficult due to the same approach of the needles to the laryngeal muscles	Multichannel measurements of several muscles possible
Placing the electrodes is guided by palpation, acoustic, and visual EMG feedback. Visual control with an endoscopy is possible, but only rarely necessary, e.g., when controlling the mucosal penetration or the transluminal PCA EMG to test stimulation. Transcutaneous EMG in combination with endoscopy is often stressful for the patient	Placing the electrodes occurs under direct visual control, but assessment of signal quality is possible only after removal of the application device. Thus, correction is only possible by discarding the electrodes and reinserting another pair

1.6 Insertion into the Laryngeal Muscles

1.6.1 Transcutaneous Insertion of the Needle Electrodes

At the beginning of the examination, main structures of the anterior neck are palpated to identify the midline, the cricoid cartilage, the lower border of the thyroid cartilage, the thyroid notch, and the hyoid bone. Figure 1.5 is a schematic drawing of the laryngeal cartilage, the laryngeal muscles, landmarks, and virtual planes of orientation between the landmarks. In obese patients or after neck surgery, palpating these landmarks can be difficult. With ultrasound, the landmarks can be localized and marked with a felt pen. If local anesthesia is used, excessive injections should be avoided to allow continued palpation of structures after injection. If the patient has a tracheotomy, it is usually necessary to remove the tracheotomy tube to be able to place the needle. If the patient does not tolerate a short-term removal, a nasal speculum may dilate the tracheostomy and maintain the airway open during the examination.

It is recommended to begin the LEMG with the thyroarytenoid muscle (TA) (Fig. 1.6), followed by an examination of the posterior cricoarytenoid (PCA) muscle (Fig. 1.7) if there is a good level of tolerance. Both muscles are innervated by the inferior recurrent laryngeal nerve (ILN). Finally, the needle should be inserted into the cricothyroid muscle (CT) (Fig. 1.8) (Table 1.2) to examine the function of the superior laryngeal nerve (SLN).

1.6.2 Transcutaneous Thyroarytenoid Muscle Recording

The cricothyroid notch, also known as cricothyroid space or cricothyroid membrane region, is the anatomic reference for the needle insertion. First, the needle pierces the skin in midline in sagittal direction and will be placed directly under the lower border of the thyroid cartilage (N). Second, the needle tip will be angled laterally (30° to [Sigma]) and superiorly (15° to [Pi]) and penetrates through the cricothyroid ligament without entering the airway (Fig. 1.6). It is also possible to place the needle tip around 5 mm

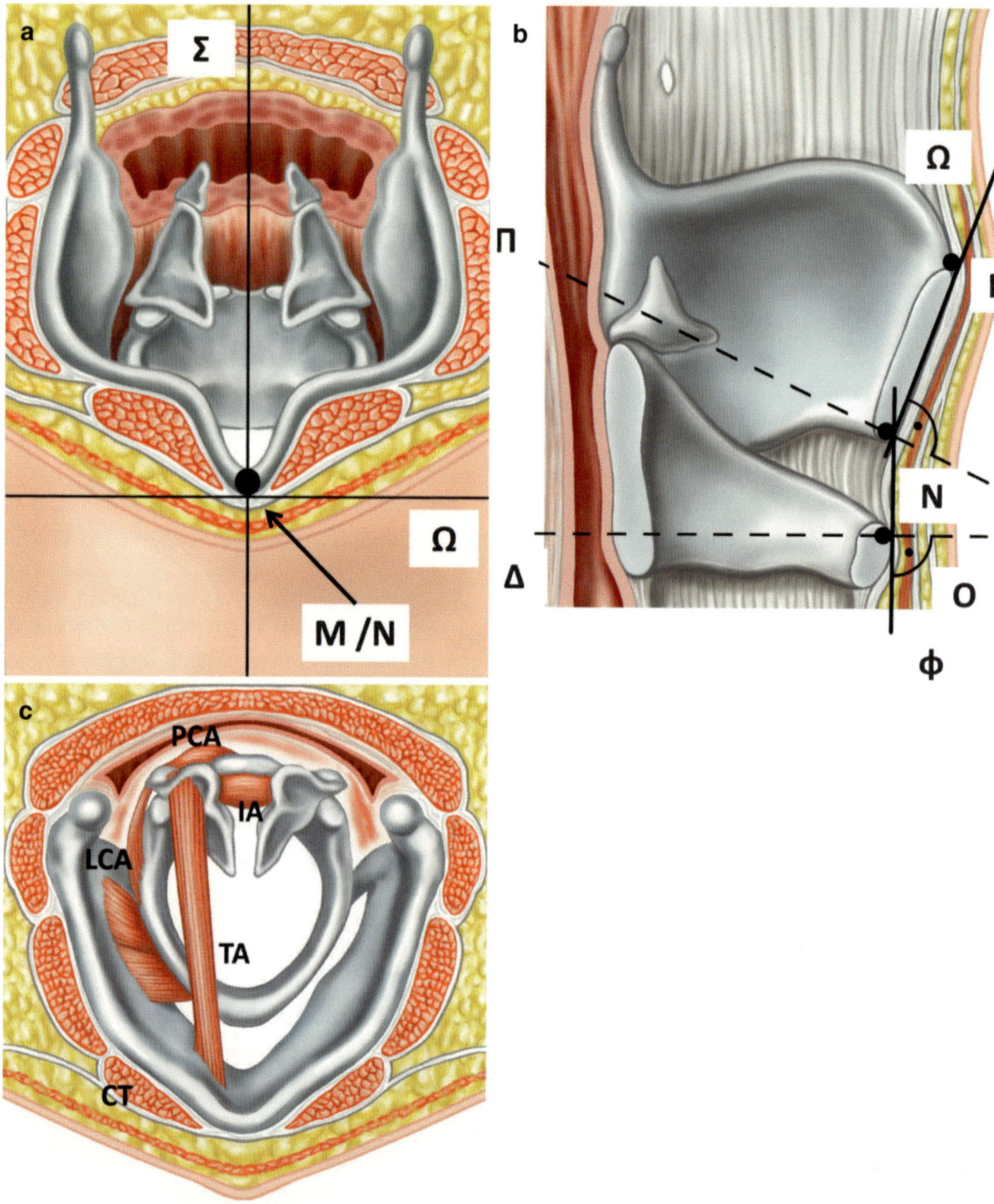

Fig. 1.5 Schematic representation of the laryngeal cartilage, laryngeal muscles, landmarks, and virtual planes of orientation. (**a**) Fronto-superior view; (**b**) inner view of the left hemilarynx: M, thyroid notch; N, center of inferior border of the thyroid cartilage; O, center of the anterior arc of the cricoid cartilage; [Sigma], midsagittal plane containing M, N, and O; [Omega], plane lying at right angle to [Sigma] containing M and N; [Phi], plane lying at right angle to [Sigma] containing N and O; [Pi], plane perpendicular to [Omega] and [Sigma]; [Delta], plane perpendicular to [Phi] and [Sigma]. (**c**) Superior view with laryngeal muscles: CT, right cricothyroid muscle; TA, right thyroarytenoid muscle; IA, right and left interarytenoid muscles (the muscles of the two sides intertwine); LCA, right lateral cricoarytenoid muscle; PCA, right posterior cricoarytenoid muscle

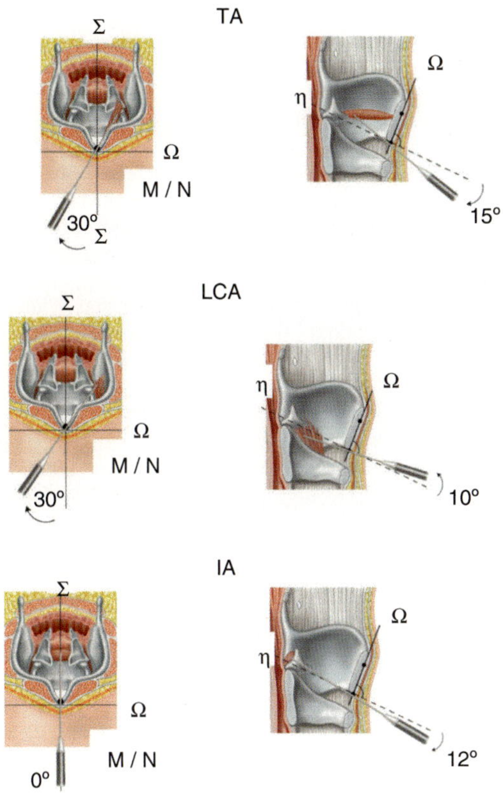

Fig. 1.6 EMG approaches to TA, LCA, and IA. Left fronto-superior view, right inner view of left hemilarynx

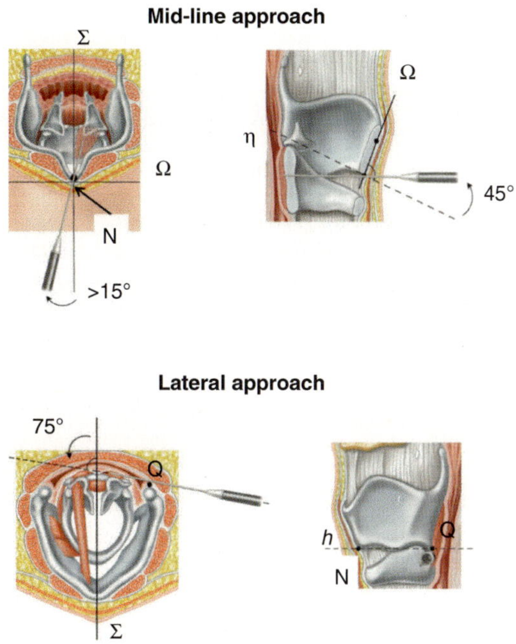

Fig. 1.7 EMG approaches to PCA. Upper row midline approach, left fronto-superior view, right inner view of left hemilarynx, lower row lateral approach, left superior view, right left lateral view

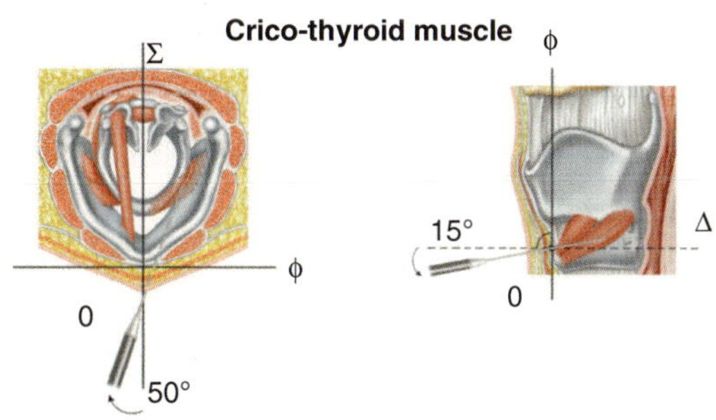

Fig. 1.8 EMG approach to CT. Left superior view, right lateral view of left cricoid

laterally of the midline. In this case, the needle should be angled 20° laterally and 15° superiorly. Depending on the thickness of the neck and the entry angle, the thyroarytenoid muscle should be reached after pushing the needle 15 mm through the ligament. Coughing of the patient generally indicates that the needle has penetrated the airway and is causing irritation of the mucosa. A burst of sine waves modulated by phonation also indicates that the electrode tip has entered the airway. In both cases, the needle should be withdrawn to the cricothyroid ligament and reinserted more laterally.

The position of the needle is confirmed by asking the patient to say /a:/ ("aa") or holding his breath by a glottal stop (Table 1.3). During both procedures, EMG activity sharply and sustainably increases. Also swallowing causes a short strong thyroarytenoid activity during the glottal stop. While deeply breathing in and out, the resting activity drops periodically during expiration. If the needle is placed too laterally and records the activity of the lateral cricoarytenoid muscle (LCA) (Fig. 1.6), EMG activity increases and rapidly drops during phonation (Table 1.3). Viewed from the cricothyroid space, the TA and LCA are nearly on the same axis and in direct contact to each other. It is thus not always possible to reliably differentiate between these two muscles. However, this is not necessary for most clinical questions.

Table 1.2 Implementation of laryngeal EMG

Muscle	Transcutaneous needle EMG	Transoral EMG	Identification
Thyroarytenoid (TA) innervated by the inferior recurrent laryngeal nerve (ILN)	Pierce the skin in midline in sagittal direction. Penetrate the cricothyroid ligament directly under the lower border of the thyroid cartilage in an angle of 30° laterally and 15° superiorly. Alternatively, to reduce the risk of entering the airway, the cricothyroid ligament can be penetrated around 5 mm laterally to the side to be examined. In this case, the needle should be angled 20° laterally and 15° superiorly. After 15 mm behind the ligament, the thyroarytenoid muscle should be reached	Spray lidocaine transorally onto the mucosa of the soft palate, the pharynx, and the larynx to decrease the pharyngeal reflex. Inject glycopyrrolate i.v. to reduce salivation. Visual control of insertion by flexible fiberoptic or rigid laryngoscopy or directly in the operating room. Hooked-wire electrodes are inserted laterally to the free edge of the vocal fold by using the curved application device by INOMED©. If the needle is placed too laterally, recording the activity of the lateral cricoarytenoid muscle (LCA), EMG activity increases and drops rapidly during phonation	Validation of position by phonating */a:/* or holding breath in a glottal stop. Both procedures increase EMG activity strongly and sustainably. Swallowing causes a short, strong thyroarytenoid activity during the glottal stop. While breathing deeply in and out, the resting activity drops periodically during expiration. If the needle is placed too laterally and records the activity of the lateral cricoarytenoid muscle (LCA), EMG activity increases and rapidly drops during phonation
Posterior cricoarytenoid (PCA) innervated by the inferior recurrent laryngeal nerve (ILN)	Midline approach: Pass a needle posteriorly through the cricothyroid membrane, airway, and cricoid cartilage. Only possible in non-ossified larynges. Insertion of the electrode too cranially is a common reason for difficulties in locating the PCA. Pierce the skin and penetrate the cricothyroid ligament in midline in sagittal direction. A burst of sine waves modulated by phonation indicates that the electrode tip is vibrating freely in the airway. Approximately 5–10 mm lateral to the midline, the posterior mucosa of the airway is penetrated. After drilling through the lamina of the cricoid cartilage by slowly rotating the needle, the tip of the needle should be right in the muscle. Pushing any further will cause a penetration of the cricopharyngeal muscle Lateral approach: Rotate the larynx manually and pass the electrode posterior to the thyroid lamina. This requires a good mobilization of the whole larynx during the procedure, which can cause discomfort to the patient	Spray lidocaine transorally onto the mucosa of the soft palate, the pharynx, and the larynx to decrease the pharyngeal reflex. Inject glycopyrrolate i.v. to reduce salivation. Visual control of insertion by flexible fiberoptic or rigid laryngoscopy or direct laryngoscopy in the operating room. Insert the hooked-wire electrodes from the pharyngeal side 10 mm caudally to the interarytenoid area by using the curved application device by INOMED©. If the electrode is inserted too cranially, the arytenoid muscle instead of the cricoarytenoid muscle will be recorded. If the needle is placed too caudally, the activity of the cricopharyngeal muscle will be recorded	Position is confirmed through detection of increased EMG activity during sniffing and with a considerably weaker EMG activity during swallowing and phonation of the sound */a:/*. If the needle is placed too dorsally (by transcutaneous insertion) or too caudally (by transoral insertion), the activity of the cricopharyngeus muscle is recorded. The strong constant EMG activity of the cricopharyngeus muscle will decrease during swallowing

Table 1.2 (continued)

Muscle	Transcutaneous needle EMG	Transoral EMG	Identification
Cricothyroid (CT) innervated by the superior laryngeal nerve (SLN)	5 mm insertion lateral to the midline on level of the cricothyroid notch. Movement tangential to the cricothyroid membrane (around 50°) until the electrode enters the muscle after 15–20 mm. If no activity is recorded, the needle must be withdrawn a few millimeters and aimed more laterally. Too laterally, the needle will pierce the sternohyoid muscle	Not possible	To validate the position of the electrode, the patient is asked to phonate /a:/ at a low pitch and then to raise the pitch. If the electrode is in a normal cricothyroid muscle, the EMG activity will increase sharply. The activity of the sternohyoid muscle can be tested by raising the head of the lying patient or pressing your fingers against his forehead if patient is sitting

Table 1.3 Identification of laryngeal muscles

Muscle	Physiological reaction/identification features
Thyroarytenoid (TA)	– Patient phonates */a:/*: a sudden sustained increase in EMG activity while phonating – Forced sniffing inspiration: decrease in EMG activity – Swallowing: during swallowing, short maximal activity with decrease in activity at the end of the swallowing
Posterior cricoarytenoid (PCA)	– Forced sniffing inspiration: increase in EMG activity – Patient phonates /a:/: a decrease in EMG activity while phonating – Swallowing: during swallowing, short maximal activity with decrease in activity at the end of the swallowing
Lateral cricoarytenoid (LCA)	– Patient phonates /a:/: a short initial increase in EMG activity followed by a decrease while phonating – Swallowing: during swallowing short maximal activity with decrease in activity at the end of the swallowing
Cricothyroid (CT)	– Patient phonates a low note on /a:/ and then increases pitch: with increasing pitch, the interference patterns become dense
Cricopharyngeal part of inferior pharyngeal constrictor	– Constant resting tone; during swallowing decrease in activity; no respiration-dependent activity

Using a fiberoptic scope, moving the needle within the substance of the thyroarytenoid muscle and observing the vocal fold movement confirms the position of the electrode. This procedure may cause the patient to swallow or cough.

1.6.3 Transcutaneous Posterior Cricoarytenoid Muscle Recording

The posterior cricoarytenoid (PCA) muscle can be accessed by passing a needle posteriorly through the cricothyroid membrane, airway, and cricoid cartilage or by rotating the larynx manually and passing the electrode posteriorly to the thyroid lamina (Fig. 1.7) (Table 1.2). The lateral approach requires a good mobilization of the whole larynx during the procedure, which can cause discomfort to the patient. The midline approach is only successful in not totally ossified cricoids. However, even in older patients, the cricoid cartilage is rarely completely ossified. Insertion of the electrode too cranially is a common reason for difficulties in locating the PCA. This is often due to the fact that the posterior cricoarytenoid muscle lies more caudally than assumed by many physicians.

For the midline approach, again, the cricothyroid notch (N) is the anatomic reference for the needle insertion. The needle pierces the skin and penetrates the cricothyroid ligament in the midline in a sagittal direction (45° below [Pi]). A burst of sine waves modulated by phonation indicates that the electrode tip is vibrating freely in the airway. After entering the airway, irritation of the mucosa may cause the patient to cough. To avoid further trauma while coughing, a short interruption without needle movement while the patient is breathing slowly should help the patient to adapt to the sensation. Approximately 5–10 mm laterally to the midline (or 15° laterally from [Sigma]), the posterior mucosa of the airway is penetrated. By slowly rotating the needle, it is drilled through the lamina of the cricoid cartilage. Having penetrated the whole cartilage, the tip of the needle should be right in the PCA muscle. Pushing any further will cause a penetration of the cricopharyngeal muscle.

The correct position is confirmed by detecting increased EMG activity during sniffing and considerably weaker EMG activity during swallowing and phonation of the sound /a:/. If the needle is placed too deeply, recording the activity of the cricopharyngeal muscle, a strong constant EMG activity will be observable, decreasing during swallowing (Table 1.3).

Penetrating the cricoid cartilage bears the theoretically risk of a local infection of the bradytrophic cartilage. If the patient shows any post-interventional signs of infection, a systemic antibiosis should be started.

1.6.4 Transcutaneous Posterior Cricothyroid Muscle Recording

The cricothyroid notch (N) is the anatomic reference for the needle insertion. The needle pierces the skin 5 mm laterally to the midline, on the level of the center of the cricothyroid notch at an angle of around 50° to the midline [Sigma] (Fig. 1.8). After insertion, the needle should be moved tangentially to the cricothyroid membrane until entering the muscle after 15–20 mm [10]. If no activity is recorded, the needle should be withdrawn a few millimeters and aimed more laterally. If the needle is inserted too laterally, the needle will pierce the sternohyoid muscle. To confirm the position of the electrode, the patient is asked to phonate /a:/ at a low pitch and then to raise the pitch. If the electrode is in a normal cricothyroid muscle, the EMG activity will increase sharply (Tables 1.2 and 1.3). The activity of the sternohyoid muscle can be tested asking the patient to push his/her forehead against the examiners' fingers.

1.7 Transoral Insertion of the Needle Electrodes

The thyroarytenoid, posterior cricoarytenoid, lateral cricoarytenoid, and interarytenoid muscles (Fig. 1.5) can also be examined by using hooked-wire electrodes positioned indirectly under optic guidance or directly in the operating room.

The examination begins after topical application of lidocaine transorally onto the mucosa of the soft palate, the pharynx, and the larynx, in order to decrease the pharyngeal reflex. Additionally, the systemic application of glycopyrrolate is possible to decrease the salivation.

The use of either a flexible fiberoptic laryngoscope through the nose or a rigid laryngoscope through the mouth is essential depending on the need of the patient and the experience of the physician.

It is recommended to begin the LEMG with the thyroarytenoid muscle (TA), followed by an examination of the posterior cricoarytenoid (PCA) muscle if there is a good level of tolerance (Table 1.2). A transoral EMG of the cricothyroid muscle (CT) is not possible.

1.7.1 Transoral Thyroarytenoid Muscle Recording

The hooked-wire electrodes are inserted laterally to the free edge of the vocal fold to avoid any harm to phonation (Table 1.2). The position of the electrodes is confirmed by asking the patient to phonate /a:/ or to hold his breath in a glottal stop (Table 1.3). During both procedures, the EMG activity sharply and sustainably increases, and swallowing causes a short strong thyroarytenoid activity during the glottal stop. While breathing deeply in and out, the resting activity drops periodically during expiration. If the needle is placed too laterally, recording the activity of the lateral cricoarytenoid muscle (LCA), EMG activity increases and drops rapidly during phonation (Table 1.3).

1.7.2 Posterior Cricoarytenoid Muscle Recording

The posterior cricoarytenoid (PCA) muscle can be accessed by inserting the hooked-wire electrodes from the pharyngeal side 10 mm caudally to the interarytenoid area (Table 1.2).

If the electrode is inserted too cranially, the interarytenoid muscle will be recorded instead of the posterior cricoarytenoid muscle. If the needle is placed too caudally, recording the activity of the cricopharyngeal muscle, a strong constant EMG activity will be observable, decreasing during swallowing (Table 1.2). The correct position is confirmed through the detection of increased EMG activity during sniffing and with considerably weaker EMG activity during swallowing (in differentiation to the cricopharyngeal muscle) and phonation of the sound /a:/ (in differentiation to the interarytenoid muscle; Table 1.3).

1.8 Functional Electrical Stimulation of the PCA

For the differential diagnoses of recurrent laryngeal nerve paralysis and other causes of vocal fold immobility, e.g., cricoarytenoid joint ankylosis or luxation, a combination of laryngeal electromy ography and temporary electrical stimulation of the PCA has been found useful [13].

For this purpose, the PCA—the only abductor muscle—is electrically stimulated via the same electrode (EMG needles of platinum or hooked-wire certified for electrostimulation) used for the EMG examination of this muscle. This can be done with every EMG machine equipped with an internal stimulator, usually available for evoked potential examinations. Stimulation parameters should be set at 0.3 ms–0.5 ms pulse duration and 2 mA–3 mA amplitude, starting with lower values (stimulation effect depending on innervation status and electrode position). Three Hertz is the optimal frequency parameter for position testing as it causes muscle twitching, and 30 Hz is the optimal frequency parameter for testing maximal vocal cord abduction. A simultaneous endoscopy must be performed in order to detect the effect of the electrical stimulus on vocal cord movement.

As known from previous studies, the PCA is best stimulated where the branches of the recurrent laryngeal nerve (RLN) reach motor end plates. These precise "hot spots" are the optimal contact points to stimulate with biphasic electrical pulses, in order to provoke a subsequent abduction of the vocal folds. They vary in position between individual patients and stimulation sides [14].

The positioning of the needle for stimulation is similar to the procedure described above for transcutaneous EMG of the PCA muscle. However, repeated repositioning of the needle may be required to locate the "hot spot." By using a noninvasive surface electrode (Fig. 1.9), the investigator can safely search for the "hot spot" without risking permanent damage to the RLN. However, the necessary stimulation current will be larger compared to the direct stimulation

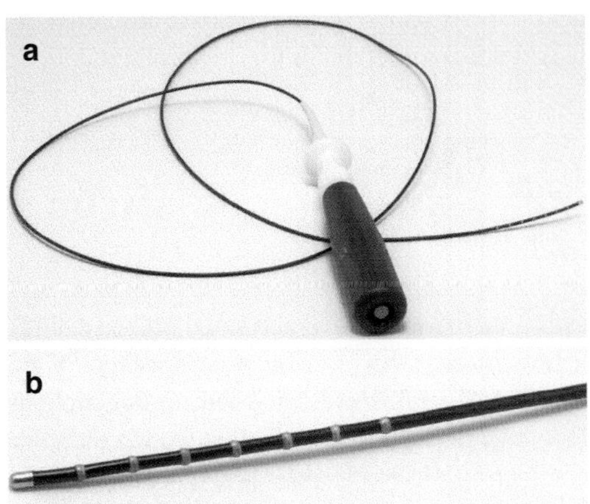

Fig. 1.9 Electrostimulation equipment. (**a**) Osypka "hot-spot" finder with eight contact electrodes. (**b**) Magnification of the tip of the Osypka "hot-spot" finder

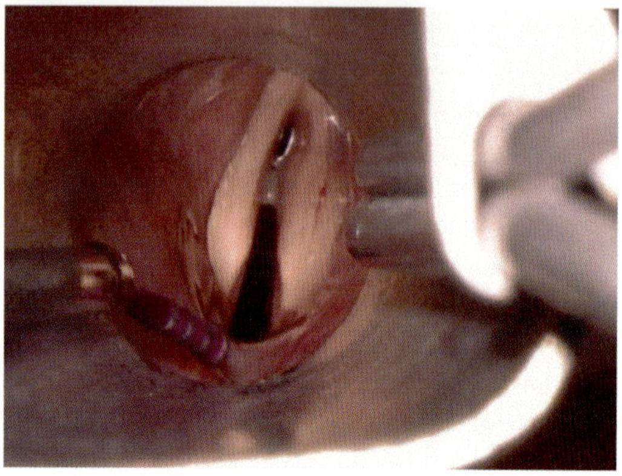

Fig. 1.10 Microscopic view onto the larynx of a patient with jet ventilation: the Osypka "hot-spot" finder (purple electrode) will be inserted into the retropharyngeal space to stimulate the cricoarytenoid muscle. (For the video, go to www.lemg.org)

using a needle electrode, leading to potentially unpleasant sensations during stimulation. In addition, positioning of the surface electrode into the postcricoid region in awaken patients is difficult. Experience so far shows that the procedure is most successful during rigid endoscopy under general anesthesia without muscle relaxation (Fig. 1.10).

With the described parameters of stimulation, it is not possible to stimulate the muscle itself but only the small demyelinated branches of the nerve only micrometers before they reach the motor end plates. Thus, only innervated muscles can be detected. Atrophic or denervated muscle fibers would not contract under this electrostimulation.

1.9 Interpretation and Documentation of LEMG

An EMG examination should be performed and evaluated in a structured and standardized examination process. In a widely used scheme, the EMG in general is evaluated during insertion, at rest, and during different strength of voluntary contraction. These standards cannot be simply transferred to laryngeal EMG, because the voluntary activation of an individual laryngeal muscle is not possible. When activated, the laryngeal muscles perform complex movements, always involving multiple muscles. In order to distinguish between different levels and sites of physiological and pathological muscle function, the patient may be asked to breathe deeply, to phonate, or to perform specific maneuvers of tight laryngeal closure. These strategies and the expected electrophysiological findings are described in the following:

During the insertion of the needle into the muscle, an insertion activity should occur. Typically, the insertion of the needle causes bursts of electrical activity. These should last no longer than several hundred milliseconds. They are caused by the fact that the needle itself contains some electrical energy, which, when placed near the muscle membrane, causes a relative change in the surrounding electrical energy. If the electrical charges surrounding the muscle membrane are unstable, e.g., during early nerve and muscle injuries, the insertional activity is prolonged. Healing of nerve and muscle injuries sometimes results in the replacement of normal muscle with scar tissue or fat, which insulates the remaining muscle fibers and causes a decrease in insertion activity. The muscle activity triggered by inserting the needles into the TA, CT, and PCA can be graded as follows:

1. No activity
2. Normal activity (<300 ms)
3. Increased activity
4. Strongly increased activity

In contrast to skeletal muscles, where electric silence can be observed during relaxation of the target muscle, it is hardly possible for a healthy and awake person to reach complete relaxation of the larynx. The maximal rest of the small muscles of the larynx can be observed during quiet breathing. This physiological background activity makes it hard to interpret muscle activity triggered by inserting the needle. Equally, detecting pathological spontaneous activity is much more difficult in laryngeal than in most other muscles. At the same time, a lesion of the nerve also reduces the background activity and thus often makes the interpretation easier than in physiologically innervated laryngeal muscles.

In a resting muscle and a non-moving electrode, the examiner should check for pathological spontaneous activity. Under normal conditions, no spontaneous electrical activity should be present during rest. However, a severely denervated muscle can show some such activity in the form of unstable electrical charges. Such spontaneous activity implies that the muscle is degenerating or that the nerve has been injured and that the injury is ongoing. Spontaneous activity can include fibrillation potentials (Fig. 1.11), increased insertional fibrillations (insertional activity), myotonic discharges, complex repetitive discharges (Fig. 1.12), fasciculations (Fig. 1.13), and positive sharp waves (Fig. 1.14). Specifically, fibrillation potentials are defined as low-amplitude, short-duration units generated by a single muscle fiber, indicating axonal degeneration. However, this symptom may occur only 10–14 days after the injury, since it takes some time for the nerve to degenerate to such a degree that the release of the neurotransmitter acetylcholine into the neuromuscular junction is completely fatigued and no more depolarization of the muscle will occur any longer. This degree of denervation occurs only in severe nerve injury. Spontaneous activity indicates a poor prognosis for recovery. Once regeneration begins, the muscle receives electrical impulses from the regenerated nerve and the spontaneous activity ceases.

Spontaneous activity should be recorded and classified as:

1. No reproducible pathologic spontaneous activity (detectable in max. one location)
2. Low pathologic spontaneous activity (detectable in multiple locations)
3. Moderate pathologic spontaneous activity (detectable in many locations or long lasting in one location)
4. Significant pathologic spontaneous activity (detectable in many locations and long lasting, screen filling)

Neural and muscular lesion may result in a reduced number of normal motor unit action potentials and a reduced recruitment during volitional activity. Recruitment is defined as the activation of motor units with increasing strength of voluntary muscle contraction. It reflects the number of motor unit action potentials identifiable during increasing activation when performing tasks like voicing. Preferentially, individual action potentials are evaluated in correspondence with minimal activation. In theory, the interference pattern during maximal activation of the muscle should be recorded and graded. But in laryngeal electromyography, maximal activation means often a dislocation of the needle and discomfort for the patient. So a phonation on /a:/ on a conformable level of loudness and a forced sniffing inspiration are more feasible for getting a good recoding of the laryngeal muscles. The volitional activity, differentiated in agonistic and antagonistic maneuvers, should be graded as follows:

1. No activity (Fig. 1.15)
2. Single-fiber activity (Fig. 1.16) and single-fiber pattern (Fig. 1.17)
3. Moderately decreased recruitment pattern (Fig. 1.18)
4. Mildly decreased recruitment pattern (Fig. 1.19)
5. Normal/dense recruitment pattern (Fig. 1.20)

In order to reveal synkinesis, the patient is asked to perform agonistic and antagonistic maneuvers while recording LEMG to provoke physiologic and synkinetic activity. The results are evaluated as follows (for documentation, see Table 1.4): The TA is analyzed (a) during phonation (agonistic maneuver), (b) glottal stop (agonistic maneuver), (c) forced sniffing inspiration (antagonistic maneuver), and (d) deep expiration (antagonistic maneuver). The PCA is analyzed during (c) forced sniffing inspiration (agonistic maneuver), (f) deep expiration (agonistic maneuver), (g) phonation (antagonistic maneuver), and (h) glottal stop (antagonistic maneuver).

A laryngeal muscle can be expected to be synkinetic misdirected reinnervated when the muscle shows similar activity both during agonistic and antagonistic maneuvers. For the TA/LCA complex, Statham had propagated a ratio greater than 0.65 of antagonistic mean peak-to-peak

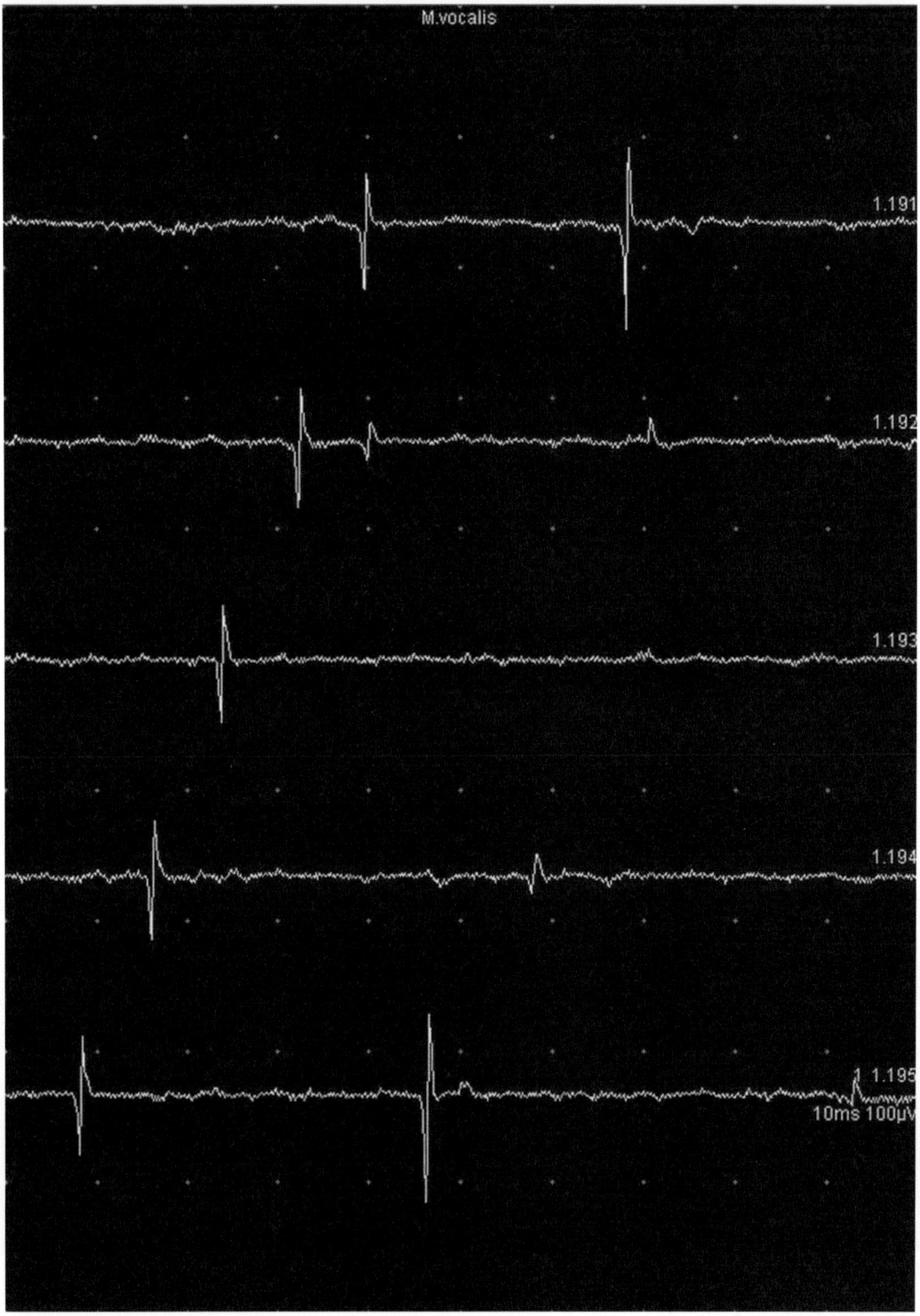

Fig. 1.11 LEMG of the thyroarytenoid muscle with fibrillation potentials as a form of pathological spontaneous activity. The fibrillation potentials (fibs) have an amplitude of around 100 µV. (For the video, go to www.lemg.org)

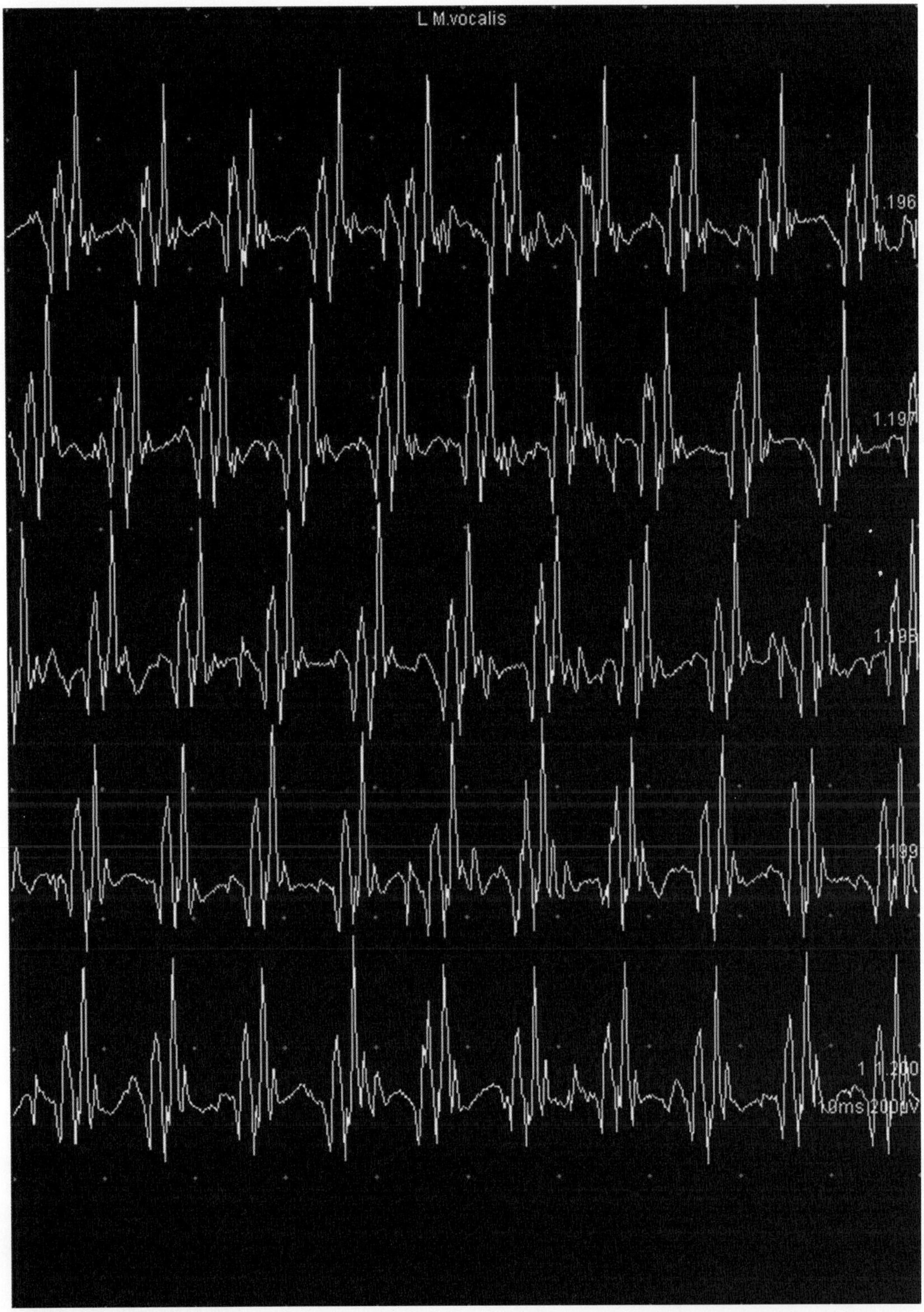

Fig. 1.12 Recording of the thyroarytenoid muscle with complex repetitive discharges as a form of pathologic spontaneous activity. Complex repetitive discharges are polyphasic or serrated formations, having uniform amplitude and frequency and an abrupt beginning and ending. (For the video, go to www.lemg.org)

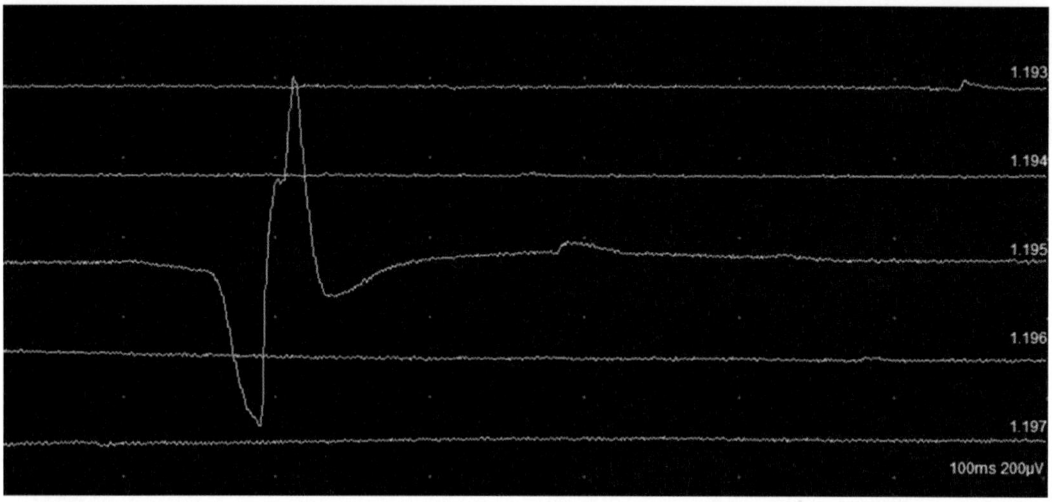

Fig. 1.13 A fasciculation potential as an example for spontaneous activity can be observed in a severely denervated muscle. Fasciculation potentials are the result of the spontaneous discharge of a motor unit, are commonly benign in origin, but may be seen with other EMG abnormalities in diseases such as ALS. Such spontaneous activity implies that the muscle is degenerating or that the nerve has been injured and that the injury is ongoing. The presented picture is recorded in a big muscle of the extremities

amplitude compared with the agonistic maneuvers [15]. For the PCA, no threshold is published yet.

But to improve the accuracy of this electrophysiologic-based diagnosis, additional clinical facts should be considered:

- Signs of auto-paralyses of the vocal folds in the laryngoscopy
- A medical history that offers the possibility of reinnervation (trauma and/or enough time for reinnervation)

The CT is not expected to show any synkinesis, since it is innervated by the superior laryngeal nerve. In this muscle, action potentials and maximal activation are identified by asking the subject to phonate with a sliding increase in pitch. In a physiological situation, activation increases with pitch.

For routine clinical use, it is convenient to classify electrophysiological findings according to Seddon [16] into neurapraxia, axonotmesis, or neurotmesis. For neurapraxia, the diagnostic criterion in LEMG is the detection of a rarified recruitment pattern or of single action potentials, during voluntary contraction without pathological spontaneous activity (e.g., positive sharp waves or fibrillation activity). Axonotmesis should be suspected if spontaneous activity, indicating neural degeneration, is detected. This may be the case 10–14 days after the onset of paralysis. This classification includes a certain level of prognosis on recovery, since neurapraxia is most likely to recover completely within 8–12 weeks, whereas axonotmesis is thought to have only a poor chance of recovery to a functional level [17]. If reinnervation occurs following axonotmesis, it is usually associated with sequelae, such as synkinesis, due to neuronal misdirection [18–20]. The result is a simultaneous activation of both the abducting and adducting intrinsic laryngeal muscles. This kind of dysfunction following reinnervation is called "autoparalytic syndrome" in facial nerve disorders [21]. Neurotmesis, i.e., the complete destruction of the whole nerve structure across its entire diameter, is assumed never to recover unless the damaged nerve endings have direct contact.

Waveform morphology refers to the shape, amplitude, and duration of the motor unit potentials, which are the electrical signals captured by the EMG. Although it is strongly dependent on the

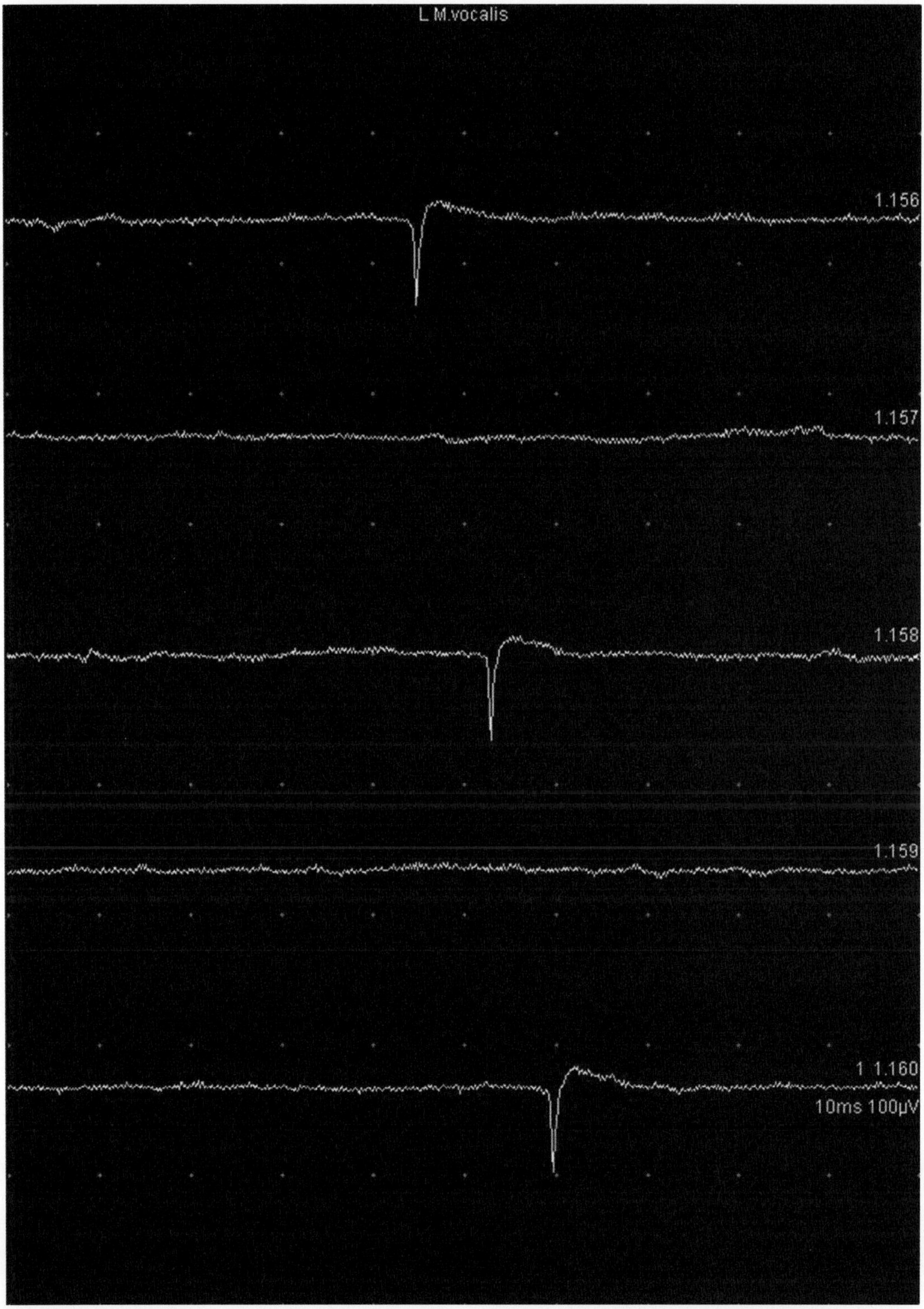

Fig. 1.14 Positive sharp waves are characterized by a constant rhythm. They first appear 10–14 days after the injury, since it takes some time for the nerve to degenerate. Metabolic change within the muscle after denervation or the result of increased postsynaptic receptor sensitivity to acetylcholine after denervation is postulated as explanation. These examples of pathologic spontaneous activity are recorded in a since 2-month complete denervated larynx. So the potentials could be recorded without the physiological background activity typical for the larynx. (For the video, go to www.lemg.org)

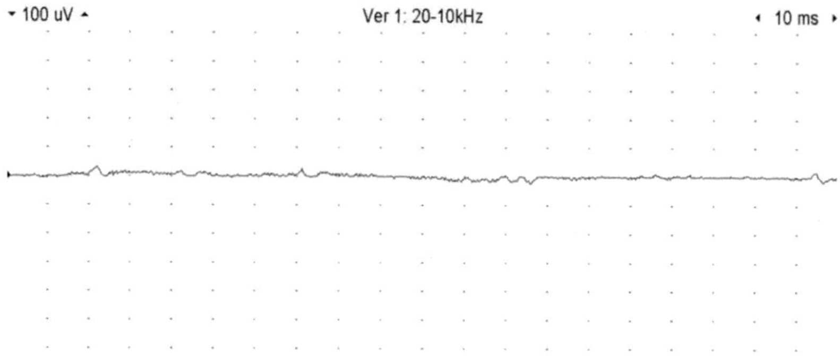

Fig. 1.15 Examples of activation (interference patterns) of the thyroarytenoid muscle recorded with a concentric needle electrode 0.45 × 38 mm during phonation: no activity

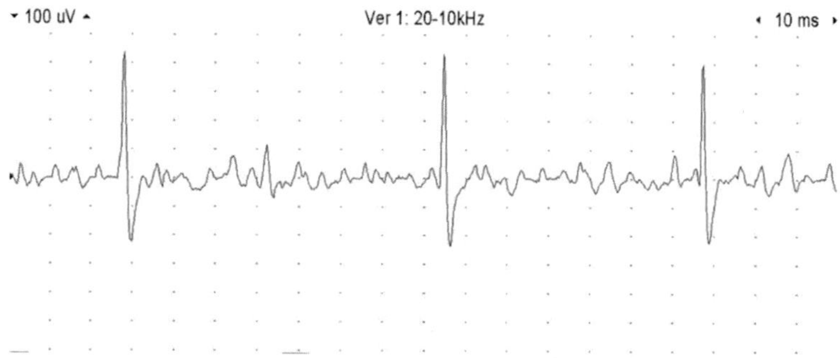

Fig. 1.16 Examples of activation (interference patterns) of the thyroarytenoid muscle recorded with a concentric needle electrode 0.45 × 38 mm during phonation: single-fiber activity, the minimal form of single-fiber patterns. Only one nerve fiber activates one motor unit in the recording area of the EMG needle

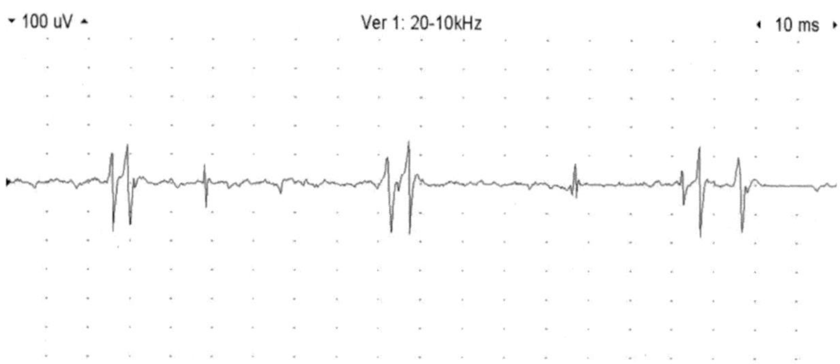

Fig. 1.17 Examples of activation (interference patterns) of the thyroarytenoid muscle recorded with a concentric needle electrode 0.45 × 38 mm during phonation: single-fiber pattern, with at least tree motor units of different morphology firing. In contrast to single-fiber activity, more than one motor unit is active in the recording area of the EMG needle

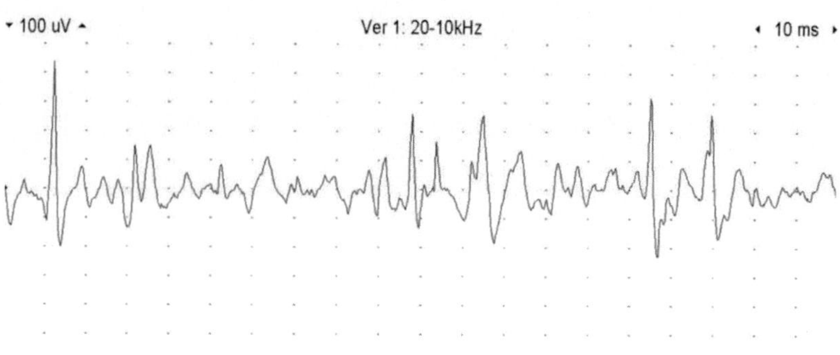

Fig. 1.18 Examples of activation (interference patterns) of the thyroarytenoid muscle recorded with a concentric needle electrode 0.45 × 38 mm during phonation: strongly decreased recruitment pattern

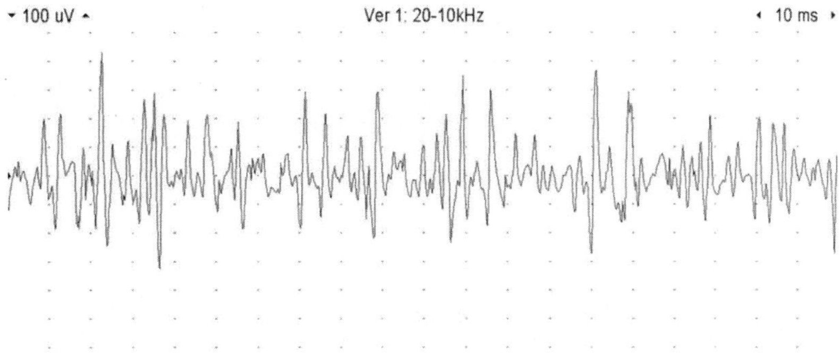

Fig. 1.19 Examples of activation (interference patterns) of the thyroarytenoid muscle recorded with a concentric needle electrode 0.45 × 38 mm during phonation: mildly decreased recruitment pattern

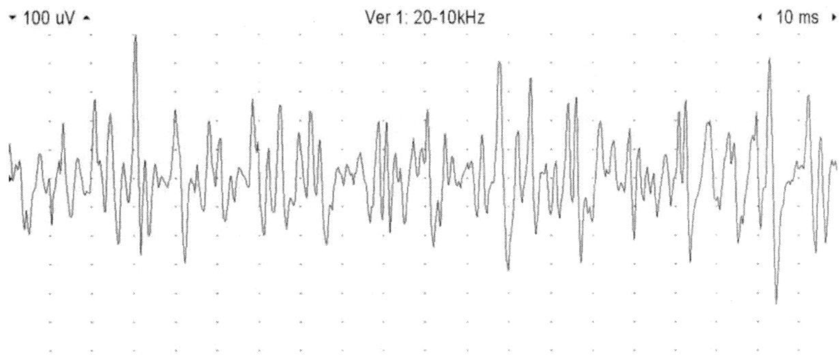

Fig. 1.20 Examples of activation (interference patterns) of the thyroarytenoid muscle recorded with a concentric needle electrode 0.45 × 38 mm during phonation: normal/dense recruitment pattern

needle used for recording, it usually has an amplitude of 200–500 mV and lasts about 5–6 ms [22].

Most of the reference data in general electromyography are obtained from the examination of big skeletal muscles. This cannot be applied without reservation to the small muscles in general and to the small muscles of the larynx in particular. These do not bear weight and have motor units with a high innervation ratio. This means that every nerve fiber supplies only a smaller number of muscle fibers. This situation affects the parameters of the MUAPs of the laryngeal muscles, making them rather short in duration and small in amplitude compared to MUAPs from big muscles. If one considers only the duration of the MUAP, this may mean that neurogenic lesions of the laryngeal muscle are missed. For example, MUAP duration of 7 ms may be normal for big skeletal muscles, for which the MUAP can last up to 12 ms. But for a laryngeal MUAP, a duration of 7 ms should be considered rather long and can point to a neurogenic lesion. Similar considerations should be taken regarding the mean amplitude of the MUAP.

The amplitude of the motor unit potential reflects the number and the strength of the muscle fibers innervated by one nerve ending, while the duration depends on the velocity of the neural input, which in turn is influenced by the insulation of the nerve. Nerves that are well insulated and have an intact and functioning sheath are able to transmit electrical impulses faster, because electrical impulses are transmitted from one node of Ranvier to another, the so-called saltatory conduction. The shape of the motor unit potential reflects changes in the electrical activity of the muscle membrane. Normally measured in a certain distance to the motor end plates, it has a biphasic pattern with an upward positive spike and a downward negative spike. Motor unit action potentials recorded close to motor end plates appear often polyphasic. In the small laryngeal muscles, it is hard to avoid. Nevertheless, the waveform morphology of the motor unit potential provides along with other information regarding the phase of recovery. After injury, the nerve goes through a process of denervation, followed by regeneration. During denervation, there is no neural input into the muscle, and, thus, no

Table 1.4 Documentation of LEMG

Muscle	Not done	Not tolerated	Not found	Activity upon insertion and spontaneous activity at rest							
				Insertion activity				Pathological spontaneous activity (PSA)			
				None	Normal	Increased	Strongly increased	None	Low	Moderate	Dense
TA right	☐	☐	☐	☐	☐	☐	☐	☐	☐	☐	☐
TA left	☐	☐	☐	☐	☐	☐	☐	☐	☐	☐	☐
PCA right	☐	☐	☐	☐	☐	☐	☐	☐	☐	☐	☐
PCA left	☐	☐	☐	☐	☐	☐	☐	☐	☐	☐	☐
CT right	☐	☐	☐	☐	☐	☐	☐	☐	☐	☐	☐
CT left	☐	☐	☐	☐	☐	☐	☐	☐	☐	☐	☐

Volitional Activity

Muscle	Pattern of agonistic maneuvers					Pattern of antagonistic maneuvers				
	None	Single fiber pattern	Strongly decreased	Mildly decreased	Normal	None	Single fiber pattern	Strongly decreased	Mildly decreased	Normal
TA right	☐	☐	☐	☐	☐	☐	☐	☐	☐	☐
TA left	☐	☐	☐	☐	☐	☐	☐	☐	☐	☐
PCA right	☐	☐	☐	☐	☐	☐	☐	☐	☐	☐
PCA left	☐	☐	☐	☐	☐	☐	☐	☐	☐	☐
CT right	☐	☐	☐	☐	☐	☐	☐	☐	☐	☐
CT left	☐	☐	☐	☐	☐	☐	☐	☐	☐	☐

Synkinesis

Muscle	None	Low	Clear	Comments:
TA right	☐	☐	☐	
TA left	☐	☐	☐	
PCA right	☐	☐	☐	
PCA left	☐	☐	☐	

Morphology

Muscle	Normal biphasic MU Potential	Early Reinnervation Potentials (low amplitude; long duration)	Giant polyphasic reinnervation potentials (high amplitude; long duration)	Myogenic polyphasic potentials (low amplitude; normal duration)
TA right	☐	☐	☐	☐
TA left	☐	☐	☐	☐
PCA right	☐	☐	☐	☐
PCA left	☐	☐	☐	☐
CT right	☐	☐	☐	☐
CT left	☐	☐	☐	☐

abnormal waveforms are produced. Abnormal motor unit potential morphologies are produced during the period of regeneration. During the early phases of regeneration, tiny nerves return to the muscles, atrophied during the time of denervation. Early in the regrowth process, the insulation of the nerve is decreased. The combination of the tiny, minimally insulated nerves and the weak muscle fibers produces electrical signals on the LEMG that are seen as motor unit potentials with small amplitudes, long durations, and polyphasic shapes. These waveforms are sometimes referred to as nascent units and imply the presence of a recent nerve injury. During regeneration, the nerves become healthier and better insulated through regrowth of their sheaths (Fig. 1.21). The muscle fibers become stronger and gain mass. However, not all nerve fibers regenerate. Fibers that do regenerate usually branch more extensively than they did before the injury, and they spread to innervate as many denervated muscle fibers as possible. The motor unit potentials that are produced as a result of this ongoing regeneration have greater amplitudes than normal. These motor unit potentials have a prolonged duration and are often described as giant polyphasic potentials. Previous nerve injury can be inferred from their presence.

If the nerve is not injured but the muscle is damaged, the morphology of the motor unit potential is different. The intact nerve functions well, and the duration of the motor unit potential is normal. Instead, the electrical charges in the muscle membrane are abnormal, resulting in a polyphasic shape. The decreased amplitude reflects the decreased muscle mass and force of contraction. As mentioned above, detecting these criteria in LEMG is complicated by the physiological background activity and the physiological appearance of polyphasic MUAPs caused by the small distance to the motor end plates. The different archetypal waveform morphology can be classified as described in detail in Table 1.5. The important waveforms are:

1. Normal biphasic motor unit potential
2. Early (sometimes polyphasic) reinnervation potentials with low amplitude and long duration
3. Giant polyphasic reinnervation potentials with high amplitude and long duration
4. Myogenic polyphasic potentials with low amplitude but normal duration

1.10 LEMG in Children

LEMG is also a safe and easy-to-use method for the assessment of children [23]. Typical questions are to determine the likelihood of recurrent laryngeal nerve function return in children who have undergone patent ductus arteriosus ligation, in children with centrally correctable lesions, and in children with idiopathic vocal fold immobility. There is no age limit; even in children <1 year of age, a measurement is possible. The investigation is normally performed in general anesthesia. In older children, an investigation of the alert patient is preferable (see above). Principally, the investigation is not different from LEMG assessment in adults under general anesthesia: The patient is placed in suspension using a laryngoscope. Anesthesia is lightened until the child is breathing regularly and spontaneously. Needle electrodes are placed endoscopically directly into the laryngeal muscle of interest, mostly the TA of each vocal fold. Intraoperative LEMG is then recorded during spontaneous respiration. The LEMGs are analyzed for the presence of normal-appearing motor unit action potentials (MUAPs), abnormal appearing MUAPs, and overall comparison between both laryngeal sides. The timing of the MUAPs in relation to the respiratory cycle has to be analyzed [24]. This comparison of both sides (in cases of unilateral disease) is very important when only a recording in general anesthesia is feasible because no data of a voluntary-evoked LEMG is available in such cases.

1.11 Magnetic Stimulation

One shortcoming of LEMG is the dependence on cooperation of the patient and the variability to evoke a muscle response. Maximal stimulation and consistent responses by an evoked stimulation of the laryngeal nerves would be optimal to ensure that all motor units comprising the target

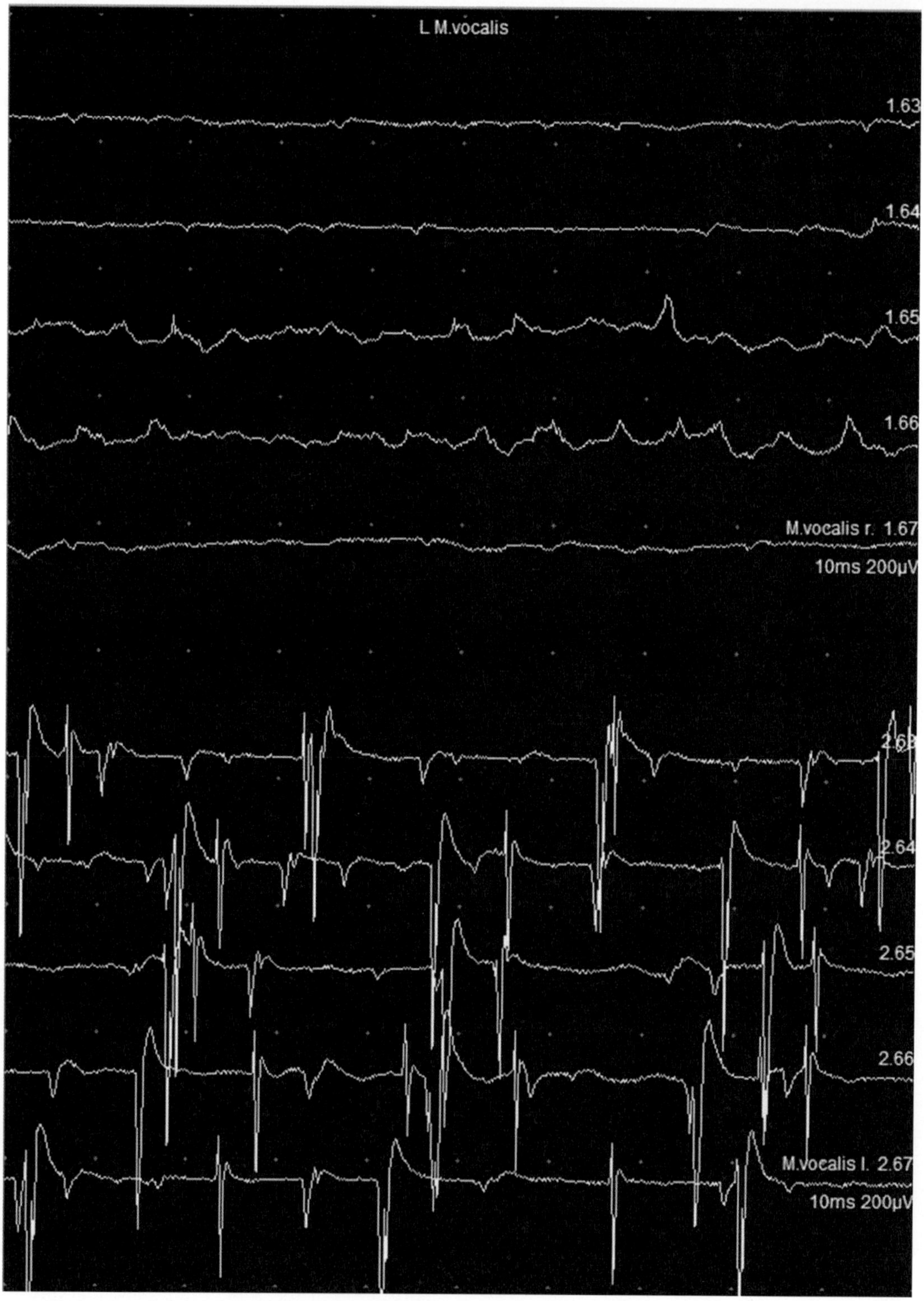

Fig. 1.21 Two-channel LEMG recording of two pairs of hooked-wire electrodes, placed into each vocal fold to record simultaneous voluntary activity of the right and the left thyroarytenoid muscles: track 1.63–1.67 no activity of the right thyroarytenoid muscle; track 2.63–2.67 single-fiber pattern with polyphasic reinnervation potentials of the left thyroarytenoid muscle

Table 1.5 Physiologic and synkinetic activity

Maneuver	TA	PCA
Phonation	Physiological activity	Synkinetic activity
		Few □···moderate □···strong □···very strong □
Glottal stop	Physiological activity	Synkinetic activity
		Few □···moderate □···strong □···very strong □
Forced sniffing inspiration	Synkinetic activity	Physiological activity
	Few □···moderate □···strong □···very strong □	
During deep expiration	Synkinetic activity	Physiological activity
	Few □···moderate □···strong □···very strong □	

muscle would be activated. Principally, an electrical or magnetic stimulation of the laryngeal nerves is possible. Whereas magnetic stimulation is established, transcutaneous or transmucosal stimulation still is experimental or only performed in individual centers. Therefore, electrically evoked LEMG is presented later in "Transcutaneous Insertion of the Needle Electrodes" about future perspectives.

Magnetic stimulation has an advantage over electrical stimulation in that the nerve response can be obtained even when the exact location of the nerve is not known or not accessible [25]. This is the case for the laryngeal nerves in the neck. Moreover, magnetic stimulation is painless. Theoretically, three different stimulations are possible with magnetic stimulation: a cranial stimulation of the contralateral motor cortex, an ipsilateral stimulation of motoneurons in the related brainstem nucleus, and an ipsilateral peripheral stimulation of the related nerve. In case of laryngeal stimulation, normally a cranial and/or peripheral stimulation is performed. The brainstem stimulation is not reliable, because the hot spot for stimulation is difficult to find, and often it cannot be ruled out that by bypass also a cranial and/or peripheral stimulation is performed.

1.11.1 Cranial and Peripheral Laryngeal Magnetic Stimulation

A commercially available 1.5 T stimulator with a flat figure-of-eight coil (typically 9 cm outer diameter) should be used. The subject is seated. To determine the cranial stimulation area, a flexible thin plastic grid with coordinates marked 1 cm apart from each other is attached to the scalp. The cranial zone (CZ) is determined according to the international 10–20 system [26]. The point of optimal excitability for the activation of the contralateral laryngeal muscles has to be determined in both hemispheres [27]. This point existed at a position approximately 8 cm lateral and 1 cm anterior to the CZ.

The midpoint of the central section of the tangentially held coil is placed on the scalp at the point of optimal excitability. Stimulation is done with an initial intensity of 50–60%. Depending upon the response, the stimulus intensity is gradually increased to 100% until the highest potential response was obtained. This maximal potential is recorded (recording technique, see below) for both contralateral and ipsilateral laryngeal muscles. For peripheral stimulations the center of the coil is positioned at the tip of the mastoid bone to stimulate the vagus nerve proximal to its exit from the skull at the jugular foramen using a stimulus intensity of 50–60%. Like for central stimulation, the hot spot with the maximal potential is defined.

1.11.2 Laryngeal Magnetic Stimulation Recording and Analysis

Normally, concentric needle electrodes or hooked-wire electrodes are used for the recording like for LEMG (see above). Recording from the TA, PCA, and CT is possible. Reliable reference data is available for the TA and CT [27]. Responses (MUAPs) from a series of at least five stimulations from each site of stimulation are recorded. The highest compound muscle action potential is taken as measure. The contralateral and ipsilateral compound muscle action potential cortical and/or peripheral latencies for each muscle are measured. The latency of a muscle response is measured in milliseconds from the trigger onset to the beginning of a first deflection after the stimulus artifact.

1.12 Future Perspectives

One novel technique discussed in the chapter (see "Functional Electrical Stimulation of the PCA") is the use of electrostimulation to activate laryngeal muscles. Electrostimulation is routinely used in other areas like facial nerve stimulation during parotid surgery. In the larynx, electrostimulation provides additional information about the functional status of the target muscles in conditions of chronic denervation or synkinetic reinnervation. Prospective studies will reveal whether this new technique is worth integrating into clinical routine when performing LEMGs.

Up to now, the interpretation and classifications of LEMG results are mostly descriptive or at best semiquantitative. Automatic algorithms providing criteria for interference pattern density like turns and amplitudes or the automated analysis of synkinetic activity are promising but not yet well established for LEMG in clinical routine in different centers [15, 28, 29].

As discussed in detail in "Magnetic Stimulation," one important shortcoming of LEMG is the dependence on cooperation of the patient and the variability to evoke a muscle response. Direct stimulation of laryngeal nerves is so far only established in some centers by magnetic stimulation. A novel technique is to use an irritative stimulation of the laryngeal mucosa (laryngeal closure reflex) as stimulus for an assessment of laryngeal nerve conduction [30]. Reflex responses of the laryngeal adductor muscles can be recorded. The characterization of abnormal reflex responses in patients awaits further study.

Another interesting future area might be the LEMG from the vestibular fold [31]. The vestibular fold is composed of loose connective tissue consisting of elastic fibers containing fatty cells with muscle fibers from TA [32]. After cordectomy and laryngeal reconstruction, TA fibers are present in the vestibular fold, with motor unit recruitment during sound emission fold [31]. Here, LEMG might help in the future to improve reconstruction techniques after cordectomy.

References

1. Blitzer A, Crumley RL, Dailey SH, Ford CN, Floeter MK, Hillel AD, et al. Recommendations of the neurolaryngology study group on laryngeal electromyography. Otolaryngol Head Neck Surg. 2009;140(6):782–93.
2. Volk GF, Hagen R, Pototschnig C, Friedrich G, Nawka T, Arens C, et al. Laryngeal electromyography: a proposal for guidelines of the European laryngological society. Eur Arch Otorhinolaryngol. 2012;269(10):2227–45.
3. Rickert SM, Childs LF, Carey BT, Murry T, Sulica L. Laryngeal electromyography for prognosis of vocal fold palsy: a meta-analysis. Laryngoscope. 2012 Jan;122(1):158–61.
4. Ingle JW, Young VN, Smith LJ, Munin MC, Rosen CA. Prospective evaluation of the clinical utility of laryngeal electromyography. Laryngoscope. 2014;124(12):2745–9.
5. Rontal E, Rontal M, Silverman B, Kileny PR. The clinical differentiation between vocal cord paralysis and vocal cord fixation using electromyography. Laryngoscope. 1993;103(2):133–7.
6. Koufman JA, Postma GN, Whang CS, Rees CJ, Amin MR, Belafsky PC, et al. Diagnostic laryngeal electromyography: the wake Forest experience 1995–1999. Otolaryngol Head Neck Surg. 2001;124(6):603–6.
7. Guld C, Rosenfalck A, Willison RG. Technical factors in recording electrical activity of muscle and nerve in man. Electroencephalogr Clin Neurophysiol. 1970;28(4):399–413.
8. Basmajian JV. Electromyography in normal intact mammals before and after birth. Rev Can Biol. 1962;21:259–65.
9. Gitter AJ, Stolov WC. AAEM minimonograph #16: instrumentation and measurement in electrodiagnostic medicine--part I. Muscle Nerve. 1995;18(8):799–811.
10. Storck C, Gehrer R, Hofer M, Neumayer B, Stollberger R, Schumacher R, et al. Laryngeal electromyography: electrode guidance based on 3-dimensional magnetic resonance tomography images of the larynx. J Voice. 2012;26(1):110–6.
11. Hillel AD. The study of laryngeal muscle activity in normal human subjects and in patients with laryngeal dystonia using multiple fine-wire electromyography. Laryngoscope. 2001;111(4 Pt 2 Suppl 97):1–47.
12. Hirano M. Recent advance in laryngeal electromyography in human. Kurume Med J. 1969;16(3):119–26.
13. Forster G, Arnold D, Bischoff SJ, Schubert H, Scholle HC, Muller AH. Laryngeal pacing in minipigs:

in vivo test of a new minimal invasive transcricoidal electrode insertion method for functional electrical stimulation of the PCA. Eur Arch Otorhinolaryngol. 2013;270(1):225–31.
14. Zealear DL, Rainey CL, Jerles ML, Tanabe T, Herzon GD. Technical approach for reanimation of the chronically denervated larynx by means of functional electrical stimulation. Ann Otol Rhinol Laryngol. 1994;103(9):705–12.
15. Statham MM, Rosen CA, Smith LJ, Munin MC. Electromyographic laryngeal synkinesis alters prognosis in vocal fold paralysis. Laryngoscope. 2010;120(2):285–90.
16. Seddon H. Three types of nerve injury. Brain. 1943;66:237–88.
17. Sittel C, Stennert E, Thumfart WF, Dapunt U, Eckel HE. Prognostic value of laryngeal electromyography in vocal fold paralysis. Arch Otolaryngol Head Neck Surg. 2001;127(2):155–60.
18. Blitzer A, Jahn AF, Keidar A. Semon's law revisited: an electromyographic analysis of laryngeal synkinesis. Ann Otol Rhinol Laryngol. 1996;105(10):764–9.
19. Kirchner JA. Semon's law a century later. J Laryngol Otol. 1982;96:645–57.
20. Sasaki CT, Horiuchi M, Ikari T, Kirchner JA. Vocal cord positioning by selective denervation. Old territory revisited. Ann Otol Rhinol Laryngol. 1980;89(6 Pt 1):541–6.
21. Stennert E. Why does the frontalis muscle "never come back"? Functional organization of the mimic musculature. Eur Arch Otorhinolaryngol. 1994:S91–S5.
22. Heman-Ackah YD, Mandel S, Manon-Espaillat R, Abaza MM, Sataloff RT. Laryngeal electromyography. Otolaryngol Clin N Am. 2007;40(5):1003–23. vi-vii
23. Maturo SC, Braun N, Brown DJ, Chong PS, Kerschner JE, Hartnick CJ. Intraoperative laryngeal electromyography in children with vocal fold immobility: results of a multicenter longitudinal study. Arch Otolaryngol Head Neck Surg. 2011;137(12):1251–7.
24. AlQudehy Z, Norton J, El-Hakim H. Electromyography in children's laryngeal mobility disorders: a proposed grading system. Arch Otolaryngol Head Neck Surg. 2012;138(10):936–41.
25. Barker AT, Freeston IL, Jalinous R, Jarratt JA. Magnetic stimulation of the human brain and peripheral nervous system: an introduction and the results of an initial clinical evaluation. Neurosurgery. 1987;20(1):100–9.
26. Jasper HH. Report of committee on methods of clinical exam in EEG. Electroencephalogr Clin Neurophysiol Suppl. 1958;10:370–5.
27. Khedr EM, Aref EE. Electrophysiological study of vocal-fold mobility disorders using a magnetic stimulator. Eur J Neurol. 2002;9(3):259–67.
28. Statham MM, Rosen CA, Nandedkar SD, Munin MC. Quantitative laryngeal electromyography: turns and amplitude analysis. Laryngoscope. 2010;120(10):2036–41.
29. Smith LJ, Rosen CA, Niyonkuru C, Munin MC. Quantitative electromyography improves prediction in vocal fold paralysis. Laryngoscope. 2012;122(4):854–9.
30. Sulica L, Carey B, Branski RC. A novel technique for clinical assessment of laryngeal nerve conduction: normal and abnormal results. Laryngoscope. 2013;123(9):2202–8.
31. Ricz H, Bastos P, Aguiar-Ricz L, Marques W Jr, Mamede RC. Electrophysiologic activity of the vestibular fold. Arch Otolaryngol Head Neck Surg. 2010;136(6):616–20.
32. Reidenbach MM. The muscular tissue of the vestibular folds of the larynx. Eur Arch Otorhinolaryngol. 1998;255(7):365–7.

2 Pulmonological Assessment

Felix J.F. Herth

Abstract

Patients with acute asthmatic symptoms or chronic cough, seen by a pulmonologist, are often diagnosed as asthma patients. Most of the classical asthma patients are reporting improved symptoms after using inhalers. Especially in patients with uncontrolled asthma, differential diagnosis of diseases of the larynx and the vocal cords has to be discussed. Therefore, a dedicated analysis of the history, lung function as well as examination of the vocal cords/larynx is recommended.

2.1 Introduction

Patients seen by a pulmologist, which may have to be considered a differential diagnosis for laryngeal or vocal cord disorders, are patients with asthma or chronic cough. The history of those patients may sound very similar to an asthmatic patient with reports of shortness of breath, wheezing and cough with exposure to exercise or a number of irritants. Most patients will have been given a diagnosis and have received frequent prednisone bursts with only marginal or no responses [1]. The related dyspnoea is often characterised by sudden onset and short duration and is also mostly self-limited. Some patients seen by a pulmologist will report audible wheezing during inspiration and/or expiration.

2.2 History and Examination of Asthma Patients

Presented to a pulmonologist, the favourite diagnosis is an obstructive lung disease. Following the actual guidelines of the Global Initiative for Asthma (GINA), the patients are asked during the initial assessment for typical symptoms like wheeze, shortness of breath, chest tightness and cough. Most of the patients report more than one of these symptoms [2].

The symptoms occur variably over time and often are worse at night or/and triggered by exercise, laughter, allergens, cold air or viral infections. Possible questions should be directed to detecting the possible evidence of postnasal drip or gastro-oesophageal reflux. The reported presence of allergies, nasal congestion, throat

F.J.F. Herth
Pneumology and Critical Care Medicine, Thoraxklinik, University of Heidelberg, Röntgenstr. 1, Heidelberg 69126, Germany
e-mail: felix.herth@med.uni-heidelberg.de

C. Sittel, O. Guntinas-Lichius (eds.), *Neurolaryngology*,
https://doi.org/10.1007/978-3-319-61724-4_2

clearing, hoarseness, chronic cough, headaches, heartburn, indigestion, water brash, throat burning, halitosis, increased cough lying flat and cough worse at night are all clues of postnasal drip and/or GER disease as likely contributing factors [1, 2].

The diagnosis is established by a lung function measurement, with a FEV1 below normal and a reduced FEV1/FVC ratio. As confirmation of reversible airflow limitation, spirometry with both inspiratory and expiratory loops, assessed following pre- and post-bronchodilator administration, should be obtained. In case of cough as the leading symptom, cough variant asthma is a possible diagnosis, characterised by cough and airway hyperresponsiveness, documenting variability in lung function [2].

Initially, most of the patients are treated with a combination of long-acting bronchodilators and inhaled corticosteroids. Once asthma has been diagnosed, lung function and symptoms should be controlled, and in case of an uncontrolled situation, the dosage of the inhalers should be increased. At the end that may lead to the start of oral corticosteroids, with the risk of significant systemic adverse effects, e.g. cataract, glaucoma, osteoporosis and adrenal suppression [1, 2].

2.3 Differential Diagnosis

If the patients are reporting a difficult-to-control situation, physicians should maintain scepticism regarding the diagnosis. Misdiagnosis of non-asthmatic conditions as uncontrolled asthma has been reported to be as high as 12–30% [1].

Various differential diagnoses to a classical asthma should be discussed by the chest physicians. Based on the region, vocal cord dysfunction and exercise-induced asthma are the major alternative diseases to think about. Also patients with a neurological disorder like Parkinson disease and stroke or rare diseases like Parkinsonism-plus syndromes, Wilson disease, post-polio syndrome, myasthenia gravis or myopathic disorders, seen by a pulmonologist, should be examined with regard to a disorder of the larynx.

Table 2.1 Stepwise fibre-optic examination by a pulmonologist

• Evaluation of the glottis at rest for tremor or paradoxical motion during quiet breathing
• Evaluation for pooling of secretions
• Evaluation of glottal closure pattern, vocal fold motion and supraglottic hyperfunction
• Evaluation of agility and fatigability of vocal folds
• Repeat vocal tasks during visualisation and included – "Sniff" manoeuvre alternates adduction with abduction and will emphasise movement abnormalities such as a subtle paresis

In all those cases, an evaluation should be redone starting with a careful history on asthma symptoms including dyspnoea cough, wheezing and nocturnal awakenings. In addition, information should be obtained on exacerbating triggers. Next to other tests, a fibre-optic examination is recommended. The procedure is described in Table 2.1.

2.4 Vocal Cord Dysfunction

Vocal cord dysfunction (VCD) is characterised by an intermittent extrathoracic airway obstruction mainly during inspiration; the leading symptom is dyspnoea of varying intensity. In Europe, otolaryngologists sometimes use the term VCD incorrectly to describe various voice disorders, such as spastic dysphonia.

The first case report was published in 1974 by Patterson [3] who demonstrated laryngoscopic evidence of VCD, which he named "Munchausen's stridor". Since the early studies, there has been increased awareness and interest in understanding this condition.

Until now, there exists no international definition of the disease; due to this, lack of uniformity studies of the incidence, prevalence and risk factors is problematic. There have been no prospective cohort studies to assess the development of new cases, so a true incidence is missing. Several studies, prospective as well as retrospective, reported a prevalence range from 2.5 to 22%. Dyspnoea is the leading symptom. It occurs in children as well and seems more common in females [4].

Regarding the pathogenesis of VCD, a lack of understanding still exists. VCD is often observed associated with GER, laryngopharyngeal reflux (LPR), postnasal drip, asthma and psychological factors [5].

Sensory receptors from the nose to the bronchi exist, detecting irritant stimuli, leading to glottic closure reflexes to protect the lungs from exogenous agents. The laryngopharynx coordinates the four basic physiologic functions of the upper aerodigestive tract: airway protection, breathing, swallowing and phonation. Given the role of the larynx to protect the lungs, it is understandable that chronic postnasal drip as well as GER (retrograde flow of gastric contents into the oesophagus) may lead to increased laryngeal sensitivity and consequent laryngeal hyperresponsiveness [4, 5].

Another discussed mechanism is pathological alterations of olfactory chemoreception. It is hypothesised that olfactory triggers may activate the glottic closure reflex and thereby trigger a VCD.

Other reports suggest that the larynx can become hypersensitive due to a sensory neuropathy. Some patients with VCD may have had primarily a functional disorder of the larynx.

2.4.1 Diagnostic Work Flow in Case of VCD

The typical dyspnoea is characterised by sudden onset, short duration and self-limitation. Most VCD patients will have been given a diagnosis of asthma as described before. Specific attention should be given to detecting the possible evidence of postnasal drip, GER and LPR. The reported presence of allergies, nasal congestion, throat clearing, hoarseness, chronic cough, heartburn, indigestion, throat burning and cough worse is reported. Psychological assessment should include a query regarding any history of psychological distress or any history of abuse [4].

Spirometry in-between attacks is mostly completely normal. During an attack, spirometry can show variable extrathoracic airway obstruction on the flow-volume loop. A maximal inspiratory flow at 50% of forced vital capacity (MIF50)/maximal expiratory flow at 50% of forced vital capacity (MEF50) ratio of <1 suggests a VCD-related problem (Figs. 2.1 and 2.2). The utility of this non-invasive measurement requires validation. Radiographic studies are generally useless in establishing the diagnosis.

Flexible fibre-optic examination of the larynx is the recommended test. Changes of

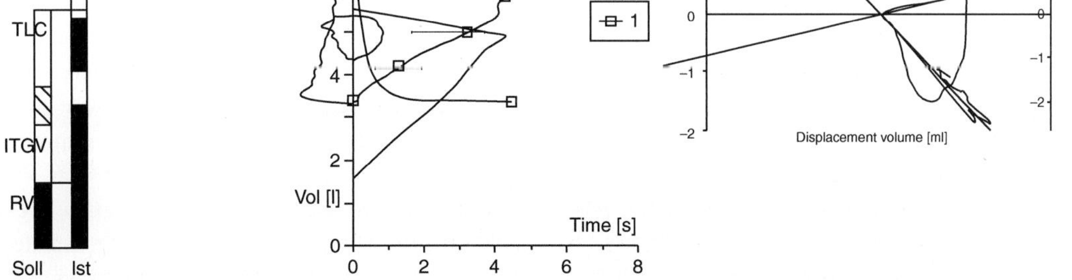

Fig. 2.1 Lung function of a VCD case (maximal inspiratory flow at 50% of forced vital capacity (MIF50) (– –)/maximal expiratory flow at 50% of forced vital capacity (MEF50) (–) <1)

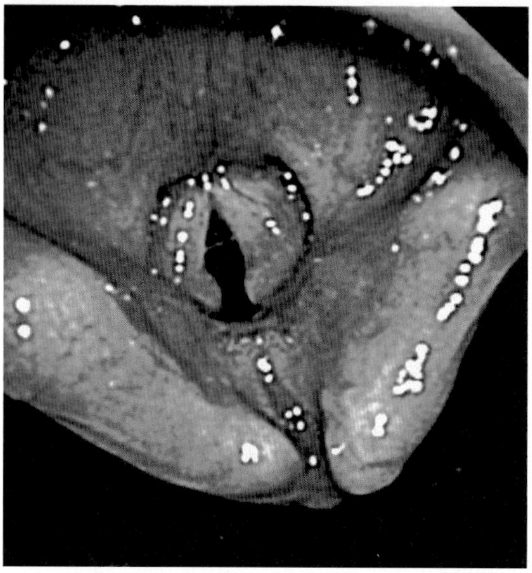

Fig. 2.2 Laryngoscopy of a VCD case (inspiratory)

chronic rhinitis and postnasal drip and chronic inflammation, with cobblestoning of the nasal turbinates and/or the posterior oropharynx, can been seen. During the examination, the patient should do a couple of manoeuvres to define their abnormalities. Typically, the patients are asked to say "EEE". This leads normally to symmetrical adduction of the vocal folds. Asking patients to breathe quietly in and out will sometimes lead to the paradoxical adduction of the vocal folds. Patients must be asked to do a forced vital capacity manoeuvre as well [4, 6].

2.4.2 Treatment of VCD

The treatment of VCD is adapted to the underlying medical and psychological factor problem. Understanding the complex nature of VCD, a multidisciplinary approach is recommended. Pulmonologists, otolaryngologists, allergists, speech therapists, psychosocial medicine, rehabilitation medicine and vocational counsellors should be interacting to find out the optimal management for those patients [7].

2.5 Exercise-Induced Asthma (EIA)

Another disease, sometimes misinterpreted as asthma, is EIA. Here symptoms and signs of asthma occur after intensive physical exercise or exercise-induced bronchoconstriction (EIB). EIA appears frequently in asthmatic children and adults without anti-inflammatory treatment and is also reported in 70–80% of untreated patients with asthma.

The possible differential diagnoses to EIA are exercise-induced VCD, exercise-induced hyperventilation and exercise-induced arterial hypoxemia (EIAH) [8].

The mechanisms of EIA are related to markedly increased ventilation during exercise. The activity leads to increased ventilation. The inhaled air must be heated up to body temperature and is fully saturated with water vapour on the way down to the lungs. The increased ventilation stimulated an increased water and heat loss via respiration. Cooling of the bronchial system causes parasympathetic nerve stimulation, which leads to bronchoconstriction, causing also reflex vasoconstriction of bronchial venules. At the end of increased ventilation, a vasodilatation occurs. This combination of smooth muscle constriction and mucosal oedema in patients leads to a reduced size of the bronchial lumen and an increased airway resistance. These mechanisms explain why EIA mostly occurs shortly after exercise and not during exercise, an important fact in the diagnosis of EIA [8, 9].

This effect can also happen on the level of the larynx, leading to an exercise-induced vocal cord dysfunction and the associated symptoms.

The diagnosis of EIA is made using standardised exercise test, like on a treadmill or on an exercise bicycle. The recommended exercise load should be high, preferably >95% of maximum exercise load. The test should also be standardised with regard to environmental temperature and humidity [8, 10].

According to the commonly used guidelines, mild forms should be treated with inhaled b2-agonists as needed. More severe forms also needed the use of inhaled steroids [8].

2.6 Final Conclusions

Patients with coughing and shortness of breath are often diagnosed with asthma. In some cases, the symptoms are related to disorders of the vocal cord and/or the larynx. Therefore, a critical assessment including a fibre-optic examination is crucial in those patients. Especially patients, presented as typical asthma candidates, but not responding to the typical treatment, should undergo a re-evaluation including all possible differential diagnoses.

References

1. Chung KF, Wenzel SE, Brozek JL, et al. ERS/ATS guidelines on definition, evaluation and treatment of severe asthma. Eur Respir J. 2014;43:343–73.
2. Global Initiative For Asthma: Pocket guide for asthma management and prevention. http://ginasthma.org/2016-pocket-guide-for-asthma-management-and-prevention/. Accessed 24 Aug 2016.
3. Patterson R, Schatz M, Horton M. Munchausen's stridor: non-organic laryngeal obstruction. Clin Allergy. 1974;4:307–10.
4. Kenn K, Balkissoon R. Vocal cord dysfunction: what do we know? Eur Respir J. 2011;37:194–20.
5. Morris MJ, Allan PF, Perkins PJ. Vocal cord dysfunction: aetiologies and treatment. Clin Pulm Med. 2006;13:73–86.
6. Bahrainwala AH, Simon MR. Wheezing and vocal cord dysfunction mimicking asthma. Curr Opin Pulm Med. 2001;7(1):8–13.
7. Haines J. Diagnosing and treating vocal cord dysfunction. Nurs Times. 2011;107(42):18–20.
8. Carlsen KH, Anderson SD, Bjermer L, et al. Exercise-induced asthma, respiratory and allergic disorders in elite athletes: epidemiology, mechanisms and diagnosis: part I of the report from the joint task force of the European Respiratory Society (ERS) and the European academy of allergy and clinical immunology (EAACI) in cooperation with GA2LEN. Allergy. 2008;63:387–403.
9. Stensrud T, Berntsen S, Carlsen KH. Humidity influences exercise capacity in subjects with exercise-induced bronchoconstriction (EIB). Respir Med. 2006;100:1633–41.
10. Bougault V, Turmel J, St-Laurent J, et al. Asthma, airway inflammation, and epithelial damage in swimmers and cold-air athletes. Eur Respir J. 2009;33:740–6.

Vocal Cord Immobility: Nomenclature

3

Frederik G. Dikkers

Abstract

The terms used to describe vocal fold motion impairment are confusing and not standardized. This results in a failure to communicate accurately and to major limitations of interpreting research studies involving vocal fold impairment. Here, standard nomenclature for reporting vocal fold impairment is proposed.

Overarching terms of vocal fold immobility and hypomobility are rigorously defined. This includes assessment techniques and inclusion and exclusion criteria for determining vocal fold immobility and hypomobility. In addition, criteria for use of the following terms have been outlined in detail: vocal fold paralysis, vocal fold paresis, vocal fold immobility/hypomobility associated with mechanical impairment of the cricoarytenoid joint, and vocal fold immobility/hypomobility related to laryngeal malignant disease.

This chapter represents the first rigorously defined vocal fold motion impairment nomenclature system. This chapter provides detailed definitions to the terms vocal fold paralysis and vocal fold paresis.

3.1 Introduction

Significant variability exists regarding the terminology used to describe vocal fold motion impairment (no or reduced motion) in the literature and among the medical community. Terms such as vocal fold palsy, vocal fold immobility, vocal fold paralysis, vocal fold paresis, and hemilaryngeal palsy are at times used interchangeably, or at other times, the same term is used to represent different findings among clinicians. This confusion is present for both unilateral vocal fold motion abnormalities and bilateral vocal fold motion problems. As a result of the lack of consensus on specific nomenclature, communication with patients and between clinicians is impaired. In addition, research findings from different institutions are difficult to interpret or compare due to this confusion in terms. The establishment of

F.G. Dikkers
Department of Otorhinolaryngology,
Academic Medical Center, University of Amsterdam,
P.O. box 22660, 1100 DD Amsterdam,
The Netherlands
e-mail: f.g.dikkers@amc.nl

C. Sittel, O. Guntinas-Lichius (eds.), *Neurolaryngology*,
https://doi.org/10.1007/978-3-319-61724-4_3

precise nomenclature to describe vocal fold motion impairment will lead to a better understanding of the patient's clinical picture and facilitate future research in the field of vocal fold motion impairment.

The authors recognize a need for a defined nomenclature to describe vocal fold motion abnormality. It is beyond the purview of this chapter to discuss the diagnostic criteria for each term in detail—details will be discussed in Chaps. 4, 5, and 6. This chapter will also not discuss the topics of inappropriate vocal fold motion that can occur in certain conditions, such as paradoxical vocal fold motion disorder or vocal cord dysfunction [1, 2]. In addition, this chapter will not discuss hyperkinetic vocal fold motion diseases such as spasmodic dysphonia or essential tremor of the larynx. Furthermore, the focus of this project is limited to the true vocal fold(s) and not supraglottic structures. What follows are definition of terms which we advocate to be used for description of vocal fold motion impairment: vocal fold immobility, vocal fold paralysis, vocal fold hypomobility, and vocal fold paresis. We provide definitions and descriptions for each of these terms.

3.2 Definition and Assessment of Vocal Fold Motion

Descriptions of vocal fold motion typically reflect motion of the full length of the vocal fold, rather than the individual components (i.e., cartilaginous vs. membranous). It is often best to focus one's attention on vocal fold motion at the location of the vocal process of the arytenoid cartilage during adductory or abductory tasks (phonation, cough, Valsalva, sniffing, inspiration, etc.). For this proposal, vocal fold motion also strictly refers to only motion of the vocal fold (level of the glottis) and, thus, does not include motion of any aspect of the supraglottis (false vocal fold, petiole nor supraglottic portion of the arytenoid cartilages).

In some cases of vocal fold immobility, the superior part of the arytenoids is tilted anteriorly making visualization of the vocal process difficult. In these situations, the movement (or lack thereof) of the posterior membranous vocal fold should be used to assess the vocal fold mobility status. Often the laryngeal examination can be recorded and reviewed to look at various details. If slight or minimal motion is only seen on moving image playback (frame-by-frame review), then it does not meet the definition of substantive or gross vocal fold motion. This proposal is based on seeing the presence (or determining the absence) of *purposeful* movement of the vocal fold. Specifically, the gross motion of the vocal fold should be task appropriate (abduction with sniff and respiration and/or adduction with cough, phonation, etc.). This definition does not involve the small movement of the vocal fold associated with respiration or the movement of the vocal fold from contralateral vocal fold contact.

Movement of the vocal fold is completely different from movement of the "mucosal wave" of the vocal fold. Thus, none of the terms discussed in this proposal pertain to mucosal vibration or pliability that is typically assessed with stroboscopy (or high-speed video). Misinterpretation of "vocal fold motion" can occur when the mucosa of the vocal fold is seen to "move" because of the Bernoulli effect during inhalation. This does not constitute substantive, purposeful vocal fold motion. Likewise, mucosal wave vibration seen during phonation (using stroboscopy) does not provide evidence of purposeful vocal fold motion.

Vocal fold motion determination can be made with a variety of laryngeal visualization methods (mirror, flexible, or rigid endoscopes) on awake individuals, not involving vocal fold palpation (i.e., direct laryngoscopy). Vocal fold motion determination can also be made during general anesthesia with the patient breathing spontaneously.

Determination of the vocal fold motion status should be done with the patient relaxed and comfortable (flexible endoscopy may be better than rigid or mirror endoscopy for this) and involves gross motion (visualization of purposeful vocal fold motion or an absence of such motion) seen during the actual exam. Flexible laryngoscopy has the vital benefit of allowing the patient to perform tasks of phonation and vegetative tasks (cough, laugh, respiration) in the most "natural" position. Peroral approaches to laryngeal visualization using an angled telescope can give greater magnification and excellent optical quality but involves a relatively "unnatural" position (tongue protrusion) which may or may not create an examination artifact. Proponents of the latter examination technique appropriately argue that if vocal fold motion is normal on a peroral examination, then no further examination is required. However, if there is any abnormality of vocal fold motion (speed or range of motion) seen on a rigid exam, then these findings should be confirmed or discarded by a transnasal flexible laryngoscopy evaluation. Often patients will display different degrees and/or patterns of motion with different tasks. Judgment of motion or amount of motion should be observed with a variety of tasks, especially with the patient performing tasks such as alternating between /i/ and sniff or vegetative tasks (cough, laugh, etc.). The best gross vocal fold motion that occurs consistently throughout the exam seen during any of the exam tasks should be used to make the final decision on motion (yes or no) and degree of motion impairment.

3.3 Vocal Fold Motion Impairment and Etiology

A vocal fold is immobile if there is no active or voluntary adduction or abduction on clinical examination. A hypomobile vocal fold has reduced range and/or speed of motion on either adductory or abductory tasks. These two terms describe the qualitative physical exam finding of vocal fold motion and makes no assumption of the etiology and thus the diagnosis for the impaired motion. The terms, vocal fold immobility and vocal fold hypomobility, should be used when a definitive etiology for the motion impairment has not been established. The use of this terminology does not imply an idiopathic status of the vocal fold motion impairment because its use informs the reader that all possible causes of the vocal fold motion impairment have not yet been fully evaluated. These terms are the ideal terms for description of the results of the physical examination of the vocal folds (preferably via flexible laryngoscopy). When vocal fold hypomobility is seen on flexible laryngoscopy, further description of degree of vocal fold hypomobility (mild, moderate, or severe), description of the speed of vocal fold motion (reduced, normal, etc.), and/or description of the range of motion assessed (decreased or normal) can be used as subjective descriptors of the examiner's physical exam findings. None of these descriptors have been validated to date, but they do play an important role in the clinical description of the vocal fold motion assessment.

The terms vocal fold paralysis and vocal fold paresis indicate a neurologic etiology of the vocal fold motion abnormality seen on physical examination.

3.3.1 Neurogenic Vocal Fold Motion Impairment

A very common cause of vocal fold motion impairment cases is due to a neurogenic etiology. The use of the term neurogenic implies an abnormality in either the central or peripheral nervous system. This abnormality can occur anywhere from the brain to the neuromuscular junction of the systems involved with vocal fold motion. A paralyzed vocal fold (vocal fold paralysis) is a vocal fold that is immobile due to a known or suspected neurogenic etiology (most commonly a recurrent laryngeal or vagus nerve injury). The paralyzed vocal fold shows absence of gross motion, although a small degree of arytenoid movement may be observed with contraction and release of the inter-arytenoid muscle during glottal tasks. The known or suspected neurogenic etiology can be established by clinical history, by other signs of vagal dysfunction like velopharyngeal insufficiency, and/or by other related cranial nerve deficits or electrodiagnostic testing (laryngeal electromyography). Clinical history that supports a neurogenic etiology for vocal fold paralysis includes but is not limited to:

- Onset of voice change coinciding with neck or chest surgery in the vicinity of the course of the ipsilateral recurrent laryngeal nerve (RLN) or vagus nerve or nonsurgical trauma to the same areas
- Onset of voice change coinciding with surgery or nonsurgical trauma to the skull base or brainstem
- Lateral medullary cerebrovascular accident (Wallenberg's stroke)
- Onset of voice change coinciding with intubation/general anesthesia
- Onset of voice change in the context of an upper respiratory infection (URI), where the voice remained poor after the other URI symptoms have resolved
- Radiographic evidence of a mass impinging on the RLN or vagus nerve

A patient who presents with an immobile vocal fold and has a related history of an appropriate antecedent event at the time of the voice change may be regarded to have a suspected vocal fold paralysis. The level of suspicion depends on the particular circumstance of the event (clinical history ± physical exam findings).

Electrodiagnostic testing via laryngeal electromyography (LEMG) can be used to confirm a neurogenic etiology for vocal fold paralysis and may provide important prognostic information and alter treatment plans [3, 4]. The precise role of LEMG in the assessment of vocal fold motion impairment and interpretation of LEMG findings are areas of active investigation and are beyond the scope of this chapter. When the vocal fold is immobile and the patient history is ambiguous, LEMG may be useful to distinguish between a mechanical and a neurogenic etiology. This situation is most common in the clinical scenario of sudden onset of dysphonia with an associated vocal fold immobility following orotracheal intubation (or use of a laryngeal mask airway) associated with non-head and neck or chest surgery [5, 6]. In this scenario, the vocal fold immobility could be due to a vocal fold paralysis from the ETT cuff or a mechanical injury to the cricoarytenoid joint associated with the intubation (see paragraph "Vocal fold motion impairment related to the mechanical impairment of the cricoarytenoid joint") [7, 8]. In this clinical situation, an LEMG can assist with determining the etiology for the immobile vocal fold (neurogenic vs. mechanical).

Vocal fold paresis involves partial motion impairment due to a known or suspected neurogenic etiology. It demonstrates some, but not normal, preservation of gross vocal fold mobility. A paretic vocal fold can have motion abnormalities in that either the range of motion or the speed of vocal fold motion is reduced. The most obvious cases are seen when the vocal fold motion abnormality is judged abnormal relative to that of the contralateral vocal fold.

We believe that a definition of vocal fold paresis based on impaired motion (including aspects of range of motion and speed of movement) is relatively straightforward and therefore clinically useful. This is frequently seen when upon follow-up of vocal fold paralysis patients, laryngeal examination reveals gross recovery of vocal fold motion but not completely normal in the areas of range of motion and/or speed of movement. Many other laryngeal exam findings have been proposed to be associated with vocal fold paresis, including those based on the static appearance of the vocal fold (e.g., bowed appearance or reduced bulk) or based on stroboscopy findings, e.g., phase asymmetry, adduction of the contralateral ventricular fold, decreased false vocal fold tone with related increased "exposure" of the laryngeal ventricle, petiole deviation, and global laryngeal movement (e.g., rotation), as well as evidence of reduced laryngeal sensation. Since these laryngeal findings have to date unproven specificity for vocal fold paresis, we propose that the definition of paresis be used based only on observed motion impairment (hypomobility) with the appropriate neurogenic etiology history. While LEMG may confirm a neurogenic cause for the hypomobility, it may not be possible to establish an LEMG diagnostic threshold that separates normal from abnormal, rendering an electromyographic definition for paresis less useful [9].

The term vocal fold palsy has been previously used variably to describe both vocal fold paralysis and paresis. Palsy is a term that can be used to encompass the entire spectrum of neurogenic vocal fold motion impairment; however, because of its lack of clarity, we do not endorse the use of palsy in the context of vocal fold motion impairment.

3.3.2 Vocal Fold Motion Impairment Related to the Mechanical Impairment of the Cricoarytenoid Joint

Mechanical causes of vocal fold motion impairment are far less common than neurogenic causes of vocal fold immobility (vocal fold paralysis) and typically involve a dysfunction of the cricoarytenoid (CA) joint. These can include dislocation/subluxation vs. fixation of the CA joint. These alterations of the CA joint may be related to trauma (both internal and external), neoplastic infiltration, extrinsic compression from large tumors, or inflammatory processes (such as CA joint arthritis/synovitis) [10–17]. Another cause of mechanical vocal fold motion impairment is scarring of the inter-arytenoid region (i.e., the soft tissue around the CA joint and the posterior commissure of the larynx) [18]. This condition may be related to internal or external trauma [19]. Comparable to arthrogenic motion impairment, the diagnosis of vocal fold motion impairment secondary to scarring of the inter-arytenoid region may be confirmed with the use of laryngeal electromyography (to rule out an underlying neurogenic etiology) and/or with palpation of the inter-arytenoid area [20–23]. Palpation of the inter-arytenoid area is best performed under either local anesthesia or general anesthesia without an endotracheal tube in place [21, 22].

3.3.3 Vocal Fold Motion Impairment Related to Laryngeal Malignant Disease

In esophageal, tracheal, and bronchogenic cancer, vocal fold motion impairment can be readily attributed to recurrent laryngeal nerve infiltration and is hence neurogenic (vocal fold paralysis). Controversy exists if vocal fold hypomobility in the face of malignant disease along the path of the vagus or recurrent laryngeal nerve is a vocal fold paresis or not. This issue is beyond the scope of this chapter and requires further investigation to include malignant invasion as an etiology of vocal fold paresis. Vocal fold impairment secondary to laryngeal cancer may result from infiltration of the cricoarytenoid joint, infiltration of intra-laryngeal nerve supply, or from tumor masses infiltrating laryngeal muscles [24].

A differentiation between these causative factors is usually neither feasible nor germane to clinical care. Therefore, it seems appropriate to classify these lesions as a different entity (vocal fold immobility due to laryngeal malignant disease). In laryngeal cancer staging, vocal fold mobility is a component used for the classification of the primary tumor for glottic, supraglottic, and subglottic carcinomas [25, 26]:

T1—tumors have normal mobility of the vocal cords.

T2—tumors present with impaired vocal cord mobility.

T3—tumors present with vocal cord fixation.

In this context, the terms "impaired mobility" and "fixation" have been poorly defined to date and leave room for interpretation. It would be reasonable to "update" the terminology of the staging systems by replacing "impaired vocal cord mobility" with vocal fold hypomobility and "vocal cord fixation" with vocal fold immobility.

3.4 Proposed Classification

This chapter proposes that patients with vocal fold motion impairment should be described and classified (unilateral or bilateral condition) using these rigorously defined terms: vocal fold immobility, vocal fold hypomobility, vocal fold paralysis, or vocal fold paresis. The terms of vocal fold immobility and hypomobility are global terms that are both physical exam descriptors and useful when the specific etiology of the vocal fold motion abnormality (neurogenic or mechanical) has not yet been determined. The terms vocal fold paralysis and vocal fold paresis denote a vocal fold motion abnormality (immobile and hypomobile, respectively) with a known or strongly suspected neurogenic etiology. In addition, the terms vocal fold immobility/hypomobility should be used when there is vocal fold abnormality in the context of a laryngeal malignancy (not malignancy along the path of the vagus or recurrent laryngeal nerve) and vocal fold impairment (immobility or hypomobility) related to malignant laryngeal disease.

Vocal fold immobility An immobile vocal fold due to either a neurogenic or mechanical limitation of the cricoarytenoid joint or laryngeal malignant disease.

Vocal fold hypomobility A vocal fold that has purposeful, gross motion but is not normal in terms of motion, range of motion, and/or speed. The etiology between neurogenic or mechanical or laryngeal malignant disease has not yet been determined.

Vocal fold paralysis An immobile vocal fold due to a neurogenic etiology. The cause can be either due to central nervous system pathology (i.e., lateral medullary infarct) or peripheral nervous system abnormality (vagus or recurrent laryngeal nerve).

Vocal fold paresis A hypomobile vocal fold due to a neurogenic etiology.

Vocal fold immobility/hypomobility related to the mechanical impairment of the cricoarytenoid joint Vocal fold motion impairment (immobile or hypomobile) due to either anatomic abnormality of cricoarytenoid joint (dislocation, fixation, etc.) or scar tissue of the soft tissues of the posterior commissure (posterior glottis stenosis).

Vocal fold motion immobility/hypomobility related to laryngeal malignant disease Vocal fold motion impairment (immobile or hypomobile) due malignant invasion of the intrinsic larynx (intra-laryngeal neural, muscle, or joint).

Conclusion

This chapter describes the first proposed system to provide detailed description and definitions of terms for vocal fold motion impairment. These terms now have a specific definition and can be used to facilitate physician education and research regarding patients with vocal fold motion impairment. This proposal is designed to be clinically useful and be appropriate to most but not all clinical scenarios. The proposed language will facilitate improved clinical and scientific communications in both oral and written descriptions of vocal fold motion impairment. We hope this proposal based on expert opinion will stimulate further discussion and research on this topic.

Acknowledgments This work was a joint effort of the US-based authors (Clark A. Rosen, Ted Mau, VyVy N. Young, Katherine C. Yung) and the Committee on Nomenclature of the European Laryngological Society (Marc Remacle, Markus Hess, Hans E. Eckel, Anastasios Hantzakos, Frederik G. Dikkers). It has been published as Rosen CA, Mau T, Remacle M, Hess M, Eckel HE, Young V, Hantzakos A, Yung KC, Dikkers FG. Nomenclature proposal to describe vocal fold motion impairment. Eur Arch Otorhinolaryngol 2016; 273(8):1995–9.

References

1. Matrka L. Paradoxic vocal fold movement disorder. Otolaryngol Clin N Am. 2014;47(1):135–46.
2. Morris MJ, Christopher KL. Diagnostic criteria for the classification of vocal cord dysfunction. Chest. 2010;138(5):1213–23.
3. Smith LJ, Rosen CA, Niyonkuru C, Munin MC. Quantitative electromyography improves prediction in vocal fold paralysis. Laryngoscope. 2012;122(4):854–9.
4. Ingle JW, Young VN, Smith LJ, Munin MC, Rosen CA. Prospective evaluation of the clinical utility of laryngeal electromyography. Laryngoscope. 2014;124(12):2745–9.
5. Wason R, Gupta P, Gogia AR. Bilateral adductor vocal cord paresis following endotracheal intubation for general anaesthesia. Anaesth Intensive Care. 2004;32(3):417–8.
6. Chan TV, Grillone G. Vocal cord paralysis after laryngeal mask airway ventilation. Laryngoscope. 2005;115(8):1436–9.
7. Rosenberg MK, Rontal E, Rontal M, Lebenbom-Mansour M. Arytenoid cartilage dislocation caused by a laryngeal mask airway treated with chemical splinting. Anesth Analg. 1996;83(6):1335–6.

8. Echternach M, Maurer CA, Mencke T, Schilling M, Verse T, Richter B. Laryngeal complications after thyroidectomy: is it always the surgeon? Arch Surg. 2009;144(2):149–53.
9. Sulica L. Vocal fold paresis: an evolving clinical concept. Curr Otorhinolaryngol Rep. 2013;1(3):158–62.
10. Sataloff RT, Bough ID Jr, Spiegel JR. Arytenoid dislocation: diagnosis and treatment. Laryngoscope. 1994;104(11 Pt 1):1353–61.
11. Dillon JP, Gallagher R, Smyth D. Arytenoid subluxation. Ir J Med Sci. 2003;172(4):206.
12. Niwa Y, Nakae A, Ogawa M, et al. Arytenoid dislocation after cardiac surgery. Acta Anaesthesiol Scand. 2007;51(10):1397–400.
13. Senoglu N, Oksuz H, Ugur N, Dogan Z, Kahraman A. Arytenoid dislocation related to an uneventful endotracheal intubation: a case report. Cases J. 2008;1(1):251.
14. Usui T, Saito S, Goto F. Arytenoid dislocation while using a McCoy laryngoscope. Anesth Analg. 2001;92(5):1347–8.
15. Paulsen FP, Rudert HH, Tillmann BN. New insights into the pathomechanism of postintubation arytenoid subluxation. Anesthesiology. 1999;91(3):659–66.
16. Miller FR, Wanamaker JR, Hicks DM, Tucker HM. Cricoarytenoid arthritis and ankylosing spondylitis. Arch Otolaryngol Head Neck Surg. 1994;120(2):214–6.
17. Peters JE, Burke CJ, Morris VH. Three cases of rheumatoid arthritis with laryngeal stridor. Clin Rheumatol. 2011;30(5):723–7.
18. Bogdasarian RS, Olson NR. Posterior glottic laryngeal stenosis. Otolaryngol Head Neck Surg. 1980;88(6):765–72.
19. Lichtenberger G. Endoscopic microsurgical management of scars in the posterior commissure and interarytenoid region resulting in vocal cord pseudoparalysis. Eur Arch Otorhinolaryngol. 1999;256(8):412–4.
20. Rosen CA, Amin MR, Sulica L, et al. Advances in office- based diagnosis and treatment in laryngology. Laryngoscope. 2009;119(Suppl 2):S185–212.
21. Anderson TD. In-office determination of cricoarytenoid joint mobility. Laryngoscope. 2006;116(4):670–1.
22. Krishna P, Rosen C. Office-based arytenoid palpation. Ear Nose Throat J. 2006;85(8):520–2.
23. Koufman JA, Postma GN, Whang CS, et al. Diagnostic laryngeal electromyography: the wake Forest experience 1995–1999. Otolaryngol Head Neck Surg. 2001;124(6):603–6.
24. Katilmis H, Ozturkcan S, Ozdemir I, et al. A clinicopathological study of laryngeal and hypopharyngeal carcinoma: correlation of cord-arytenoid mobility with histopathologic involvement. Otolaryngol Head Neck Surg. 2007;136(2):291–5.
25. Edge S, Byrd DR, Compton CC, Fritz AG, Greene FL, Trotti A. AJCC cancer staging manual. 7th ed. New York: Springer; 2010.
26. Sobin LH, Gospodarowicz MK, Wittekind C. TNM classification of malignant tumours. 7th ed. New York, NY: Wiley; 2009.

Unilateral Vocal Fold Immobility

4

Christoph Arens and Susanne Voigt-Zimmermann

Abstract

Immobility of the vocal folds may have different aetiologies and, consequently, may impact differently on voice function, swallowing and breathing.

Vocal fold immobility mostly occurs secondary to paralysis, paresis or palsy of the nerves innervating the larynx, tumours, scarring or pathological changes of the arycricothyroid joint and interarytenoid tissue. Additionally, functional and psychogenic reasons may coincide with vocal fold immobility. By definition, unilateral vocal fold immobility (ULVFI), as presented here, applies only to the mobility of the entire vocal fold and not to the so-called mucosal wave (phonatory immobility). The influence on the voice and the prognosis depend on the origin of the ULVFI, e.g. differences in type, fixation position and level of the possibly paralyzed vocal fold (slack or tense); the size of glottal gap; the mobility of the arytenoid cartilages; and/or the extent of tumours and scars.

In the case of a paralyzed vocal fold, symptoms can be improved by temporary augmentation (e.g. hyaluronic acid supplements) in combination with voice therapy to prevent muscle atrophy. Irreversible damage of recurrent or vagal nerve can be sufficiently compensated by phonosurgery (permanent injection laryngoplasty with polydimethylsiloxane particles as well as implantation, e.g. cartilage) in combination with voice therapy as well as with different types of thyroplasty. Less frequently applied, reinnervation of the larynx by end-to-end anastomosis, free nerve transplantation or use of neuromuscular pedicles are also published as surgical alternatives.

C. Arens (✉) • S. Voigt-Zimmermann
Department of Otorhinolaryngology, Head and Neck Surgery, University Hospital, Otto-von-Guericke-University Magdeburg, Leipziger Strasse, 44
Magdeburg, Germany
e-mail: christoph.arens@med.ovgu.de

C. Sittel, O. Guntinas-Lichius (eds.), *Neurolaryngology*,
https://doi.org/10.1007/978-3-319-61724-4_4

Office-based mobilization of luxated arytenoid cartilage, resection of tumours, surgical treatment of scars and interarytenoid mucosal bridges are further treatment options.

The success of these procedures depends on various factors, e.g. etiological and anatomical conditions, and especially on extraordinary surgical skills on the part of the surgeon.

4.1 Introduction

The types of ULVFI up to complete immobility are diverse, as are their origins. Immobility may be caused by a vocal fold pathology, impairment of neural control or damage of the surrounding tissue. As a result, mobility of the complete larynx, the arytenoids or the vocal cords may be impaired (Table 4.1).

The most common reason is unilateral vocal fold paralysis (ULVFP), predominantly an iatrogenic lesion caused by thyroid surgery as well as by other transcervical surgery approaches or tumour surgery on the neck or upper mediastinum.

Table 4.1 Causes of vocal fold immobility

Reasons for immobility of vocal folds	Comment
Palsy/paresis/paralysis	Most frequent reason
	Lesion of recurrent nerve
	Lesion of vagal nerve
Movement impairment of arytenoid cartilage/cricothyroid joint abnormalities/ankyloses	(Sub)luxation (e.g. after emergency intubation)
	Rheumatoid arthritis
	Long-term intubation
Interarytenoid tissue changes (fibrosis)	After trauma or surgery
	Interarytenoid mucosal bridge (mucosal and cartilage)
Tumours/scars in surrounding tissue	Hypopharyngeal and/or pharyngeal tumours
	Before resection by tumour infiltration
	After resection by scar formation

The key symptom is postoperative hoarseness with changes of vocal pitch, monotonous intonation, loss of range, voice fatigue, problems with loudness and shortness of breath. Most cases of ULVFP are reversible. Other reasons are movement impairment of arytenoid cartilage, interarytenoid tissue changes and tumours and scars in surrounding tissue.

In a patient population with immobility of the vocal folds (643 unilateral and 184 bilateral), Rosenthal et al. [1] detected that ULVFI was predominantly caused by surgical iatrogenic injury (Fig. 4.1). The inferior laryngeal nerve was mostly damaged by thyroid surgery. However, other surgical interventions such as carotid endarterectomy or spine surgery were increasing causes of paralysis of the inferior laryngeal nerve. Injuries in the motor cortex could also lead to neurogenic immobility. Additionally, in some cases the recurrent laryngeal nerve was also damaged at the jugular foramen up to the tracheoesophageal groove. However, functional aspects and psychological impairments might also lead to vocal fold immobility.

4.1.1 Symptoms of ULVFI

Vocal fold immobility usually becomes symptomatic through acute or gradual onset of hoarseness. Symptoms of unilateral vocal fold movement restrictions vary very heterogeneously and gradually. In vocal fold paresis, however, the voice sounds less breathy in comparison to laryngoscopic findings [2]. Phonatory immobility, different tension and position of the paralyzed vocal fold impair the mucosal wave and lead to a loss of the normal vibration pattern of vocal folds and to roughness and biphonation.

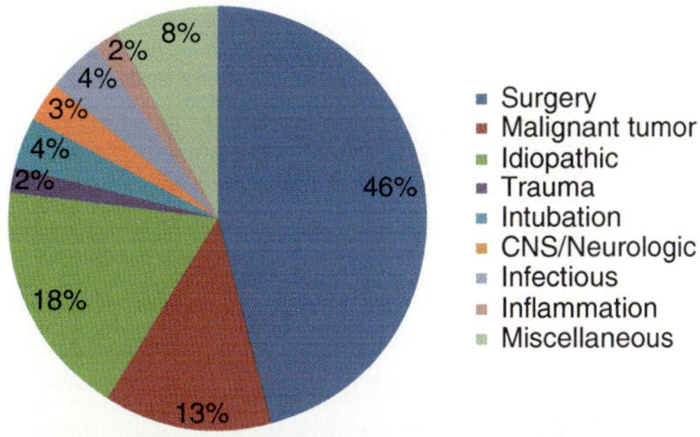

Fig. 4.1 Characteristic frequencies of the reasons of unilateral vocal fold immobility in retrospective hospital-based data sets

Impaired vocal folds may vibrate at different frequencies, resulting in rough voice as well as biphonation. A falsetto voice frequently develops secondary to remaining innervations of parts of the vocalis and the cricothyroid muscle [2].

ULVFI with different levels of the vocal folds and/or a glottal gap result in a breathy voice. Additional symptoms are swallowing difficulties or moderate breathing problems. These symptoms are important for differential diagnosis and indicate an underlying neurogenic disease. In unilateral vocal fold paralysis, about 60% of the patients complain of dysphagia and 75% of patients report difficulties in breathing (during speaking and physical activities) [3]. If a tumour is causative for VFI, in most cases the predominate symptom is a rough voice.

Vocal fold scars (Fig. 4.2) lead to hoarseness, an increase in fundamental frequency, a decrease of self-confidence in intonation and control of voice volume and furthermore to voice effort and vocal fatigue. If deeper layers are involved in vocal fold scars and substance is missing, vocal fold mobility may disappear. The voice is nearly aphonic.

The distinction between still mobile and totally immobile vocal folds, and between unilateral or bilateral immobility, is of crucial importance because of the impact that these factors have on the possible management of the voice disorder [1].

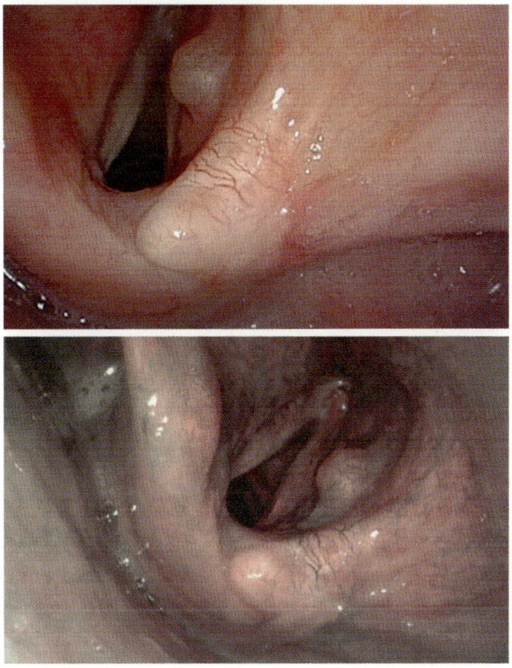

Fig. 4.2 Scar of the right aryepiglottic s and the arytenoid region secondary to laser resection of a hypopharyngeal cancer resulting in impairment of the vocal fold mobility. There is a cystic lesion of the right ventricular fold

4.1.2 Vocal Fold Paresis

Vocal fold paresis is the most common reason for immobility of the vocal folds. It can be complete (paralysis) or incomplete with diminished mobility, uni- or bilateral (more on bilateral immobility and paresis in Chap. 5). Unilateral vocal fold paresis/paralysis becomes postoperatively symptomatic through hoarseness and moderate dyspnea. 25% of patients with unilateral vocal fold paralysis also develop a swallowing disorder in combination with aspiration [4].

The most frequent cause of unilateral vocal fold paresis/paralysis is a peripheral lesion of the recurrent laryngeal nerve, but the superior laryngeal nerve may also be affected (Table 4.2). This leads to immobility of the arytenoid cartilage on the recurrent laryngeal nerve (RLN)-injured side [5]. It may be caused by iatrogenic or traumatic lesion, postoperatively, or by tumours or viral infection. It

Table 4.2 Aetiology of vocal fold paralysis [6]

Reason	Comment	Frequency
Iatrogenic/traumatic (24–79%)	Thyroidectomy	Temporary 9.8%
		Permanently 2.3%
	Thyroid gland carcinoma	3.2–7.2%
	Oesophagectomy	<1%
	Resection of bronchial carcinoma	7–36.2%
	Endarterectomy of the carotid artery/cardiac and vascular surgery	0.8–7.3%
	Mediastinoscopy	0.2–6%
	Surgery of spinal column with anterior cervical approach	Up to 10%
	Intubation	Unknown
Neoplastic	Thyroid gland carcinoma	0.9–1.6%
	Bronchial carcinoma	1.5–43%
	Other malignancies (e.g. neck metastasis)	Up to 19.8%
Systemic diseases	Sarcoidosis, neurotropic viruses, e.g. HSV, VZV, EBV	Unknown
Neurogenic	MS, ALS, apoplexy, poliomyelitis, polyneuropathies, brain tumours	Unknown
Idiopathic paralysis	No reason found after comprehensive diagnostic work-up	2–41%

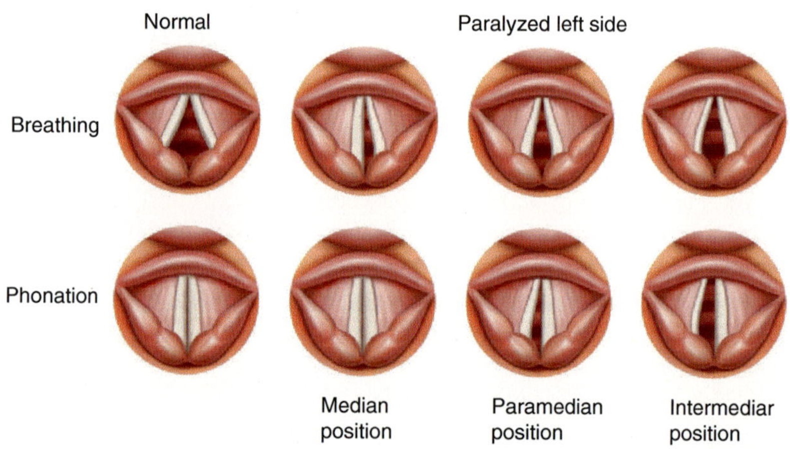

Fig. 4.3 Schematic representation of the normal and paralyzed left vocal fold

may have toxic (allergic, infectious), cerebrovascular, or neuropathic reasons, as result of radiation therapy, but it can also be idiopathic (Table 4.2).

The extent, degree and prognosis of paralysis and the shape of the resulting glottal gap depend on the underlying cause. In unilateral vocal fold paresis/paralysis, a large variability of vibration behaviour can be observed. Vocal fold paralysis is very different in terms of the position and impairment of the affected vocal folds.

The position of the paralyzed vocal fold determines the form of the glottal gap during phonation: median position (full circuit possible), paramedian position (even gap) and intermediate position (larger gap with bowed vocal fold due to impairment of the cricothyroid muscle) (Figs. 4.3 and 4.4). However, this classification is not sufficient and does not include the different levels of both vocal folds secondary to loss of tension at the affected side.

Rosato et al. [7] measured sequelae after thyroid surgery in nearly 15,000 patients in Italy: permanent paralysis of the laryngeal recurrent nerve (LRN) (1.0%), transient palsy (2.0%),

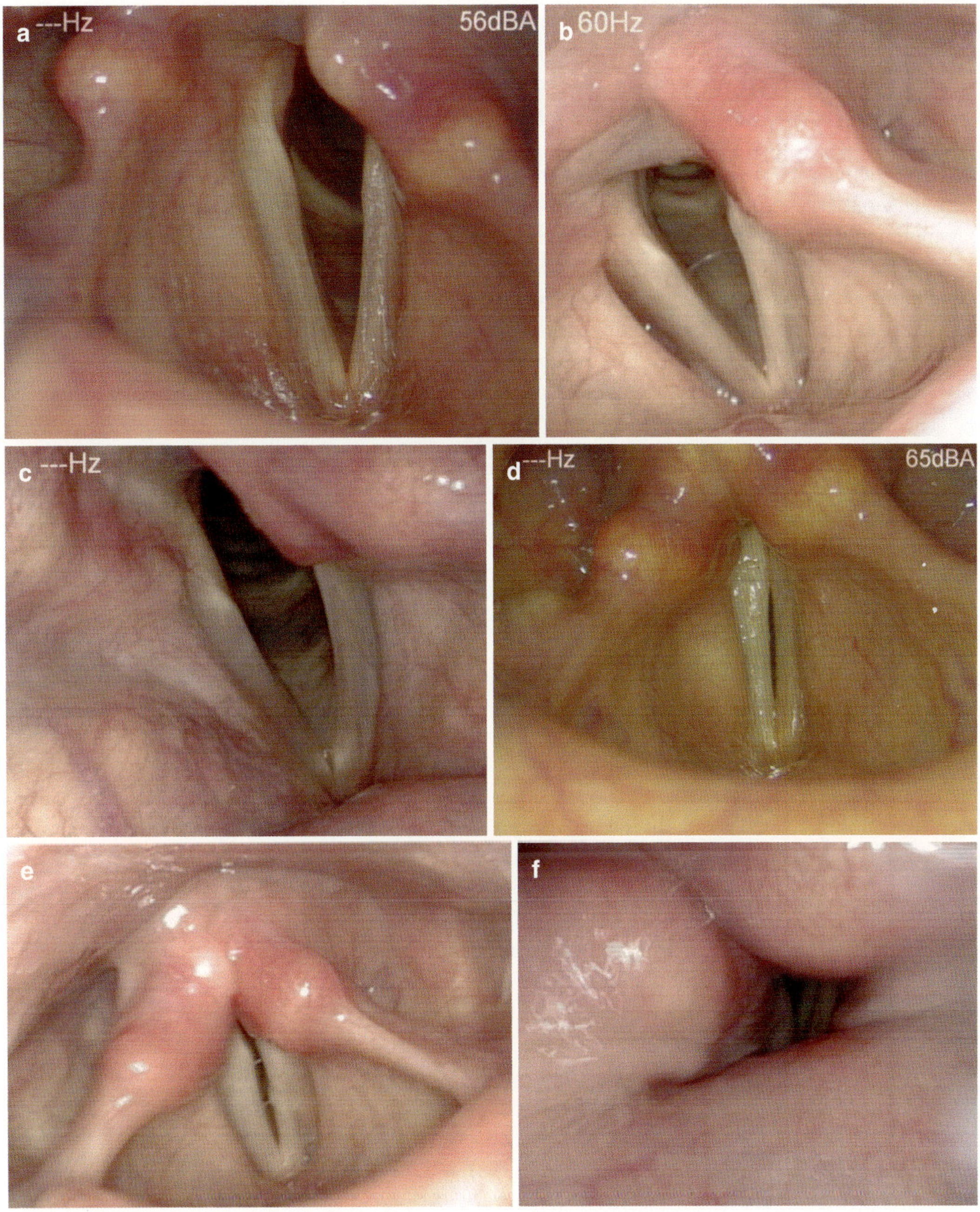

Fig. 4.4 Three cases of left sided unilateral vocal fold paralysis (ULVFP) in different positions, resulting in different glottal gaps during phonation. [(**a–c**) respiration and (**d–f**) phonation]. All ipsilateral arytenoid cartilages are tilted in an anterior-medial position. The degree of excavation and functional decompensation increases from cases 1 to 3

diplegia (0.4%), damaging of superior laryngeal nerve (3.7%), dysphagia (1.4%), haemorrhage (1.2%) and wound infection (0.3%).

In our own patient population (n = 156) in Magdeburg, Germany, from 1990 to 2011, we observed 76 cases (50 male and 26 female) of unilateral vocal fold paresis with an age peak of onset of 57 years on average. In ULVFI, dysphonia was the most common symptom; in bilateral VFI it was dyspnea. The predominant causes of ULVFI were thyroid surgery (37%), idiopathic origin (21%), further surgical intervention (7%) and viral infections (7%).

Damage of the vagal nerve affects the entire laryngeal muscles and the sensitivity of the laryngeal mucosa. Furthermore, pharyngeal and oesophageal muscles are involved. Impairment of all ipsilateral laryngeal muscles and a vocal fold predominantly fixed in a lateral position results in a large and three-dimensional glottal gap during phonation with severe breathiness. The affected arytenoid cartilage moves into a more anterior-medial position secondary to loss of muscle tension. Vagal damage is often combined with persistent dysphagia and hyperrhinolalia.

Neurogenic vocal fold paralysis is caused by cerebrovascular or inflammatory diseases, traumatic brain damage and degenerative diseases of the cerebellum (more on immobility of central origin in Chap. 6). Supranuclear disorders, for example, in Parkinson's disease or myasthenia gravis, may also be accompanied by vocal fold immobility. Occasionally, it may occur in amyotrophic lateral sclerosis. In most cases, voice changes are combined with articulation and swallowing disorders. These symptoms sometimes also occur in peripheral vocal fold paralysis, which is caused by lesions of the nucleus (e.g. Wallenberg's syndrome) or the infranuclear structure.

Rosenthal et al. [1] confirm that many patients with unilateral and bilateral immobility have spontaneous remissions, depending on the cause (Table 4.3). Inflammation, infection or iatrogenic strain of the recurrent laryngeal nerve may cause only temporary immobility. However, tumour invasion and iatrogenic dissection of the recurrent laryngeal nerve always result in permanent vocal fold paralysis. Jeannon et al. [8] report 9.8% temporary and 2.3% permanent vocal fold paralysis after thyroid surgery.

Table 4.3 Occurrence of hoarseness after thyroid surgery

Onset of hoarseness	Reason	Prognosis: return of mobility
Directly after surgery	Transection	Possible
	Ligation	
	Strain	Impossible
	Pressure on nerve	
	Contusion (tweezers, clamp)	
	Heat of the thermal cautery	
Few days after surgery and later	Scaring	Impossible
	Nerve swelling (oedema)	Possible

4.1.3 Impaired Mobility or Fixation of the Cricoarytenoid Joint

Immobility of the arytenoid cartilage may be caused by rheumatoid arthritis, granulomatosis with polyangiitis and inflammation (capsular scarring) or a result of intubation with luxation (Fig. 4.5) of the arytenoid cartilage [9–11]. Most intubation trauma is caused by emergency intubation. Typically the left arytenoid cartilage is affected due to the right-handed approach of the anesthesiologist. Rubin has stated that external laryngeal trauma is the second most common origin of luxation of the arytenoid cartilage. Arytenoid cartilage-related vocal fold immobility may range from minor impairments of mobility with minimal voice problems to ankylosis with complete immobility of the arytenoid cartilages.

In this context it is worth noting that different terms like subluxation, luxation and dislocation are used to describe the types of arytenoid cartilage displacement [12]. Luxation occurs when the joint surfaces are completely separated. In subluxation, there is still contact between the two joint surfaces.

In our opinion, the term dislocation is misleading in connection with impaired mobility even when intubation trauma may occur. As Wang [13] describes, considerable force is necessary to destroy structural supports leading to arytenoid dislocation. For this reason, luxation seems to us to be the most appropriate term.

Sataloff et al. [14] describe disruption of the cricoarytenoid joint as an uncommon disorder. In our opinion, disruption or dislocation of the arytenoid cartilage may just as easily be caused by sharp neck trauma and is not exclusively a result of intubation or endoscopy. The overall incidence

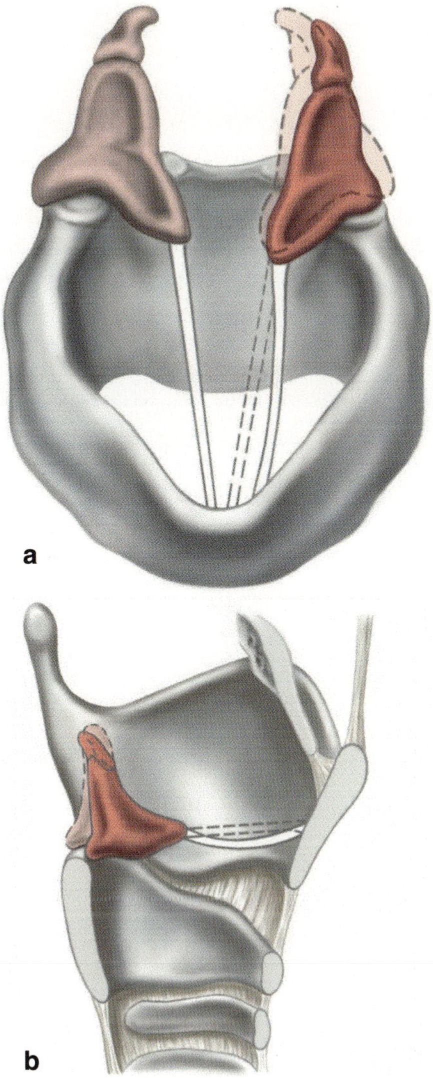

Fig. 4.5 (**a**) Frontal view: subluxation of the left arytenoid cartilage. (**b**) Lateral view: subluxation of the arytenoid cartilage and paradox posterior position of the upper pole leading to a bending of the vocal cord

of arytenoid dislocation is unclear but is reported [15] to occur in 0.1% of tracheal intubations.

Eckel et al. [10] point out that a fixation of the cricoarytenoid joint (arthrogenic dysphonia) is clinically similar to vocal fold immobility in the case of paralysis of the recurrent laryngeal nerve.

Intubation trauma leads to tearing of the joint capsule with secondary capsulitis and synovitis. Additionally, there may be hematoma in the joint space leading to impairment of the joint play.

Combined diagnosis with laryngoscopy, videostroboscopy, computed tomography (CT) and electromyography (EMG; see Chap. 1) is important for early diagnosis of arytenoid luxation. In agreement with Norris and Schweinfurth [16], we would like to point out that flexible laryngoscopy alone is not suitable for distinguishing arytenoid luxation from laryngeal nerve injury.

Ankylosis is a complete and irreversible fixation of the cricoarytenoid joint. It may be caused by laryngeal trauma and rheumatoid arthritis of the larynx. Already in 1959, Copeman et al. described an ankylosis of the cricoarytenoid joint. Postmortem it was completely obliterated and the site replaced by fibrofatty tissue with small collections of leucocytes [17].

4.1.4 Interarytenoid Scars and Bridges

On the one hand, prolonged endotracheal intubation with arytenoidal mucosal ulcerations may lead within hours to inflammation of the tissue, to ischemic ulcerations and, secondarily, to scars of the cricoarytenoid joints resulting in so-called postintubation phonatory insufficiency (PIPI) [18, 19].

On the other hand, it may result in decreased mobility of the arytenoid through the development of granuloma at the contact points and secondary scarring (Fig. 4.6). The pressure of the endotracheal tube on the posterior and medial portions of the glottis can be more than 100 mmHg. The ulceration leads to fibrosis (Fig. 4.7), to scarring and bridges (Fig. 4.8a,b) and thus to immobility of the vocal folds [12].

4.1.5 Immobility of the Vocal Folds Caused by Tumours and Scars

Predominantly malignant tumours may impair the mobility of the vocal folds because of their size, shape and/or localization. Tumours involving more than one fourth of the thyroarytenoid muscle lead to impairment of the

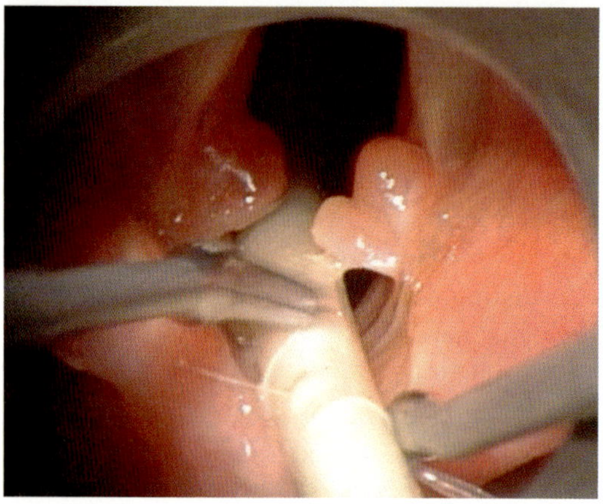

Fig. 4.6 Intubation granulomas after long-term intubation

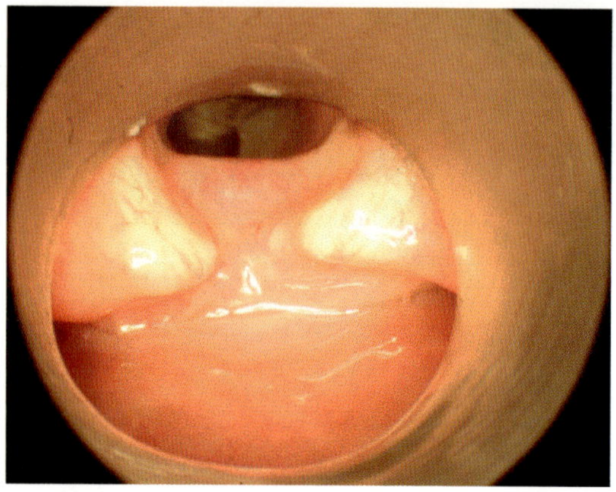

Fig. 4.7 Interarytenoid fibrosis after long-term intubation

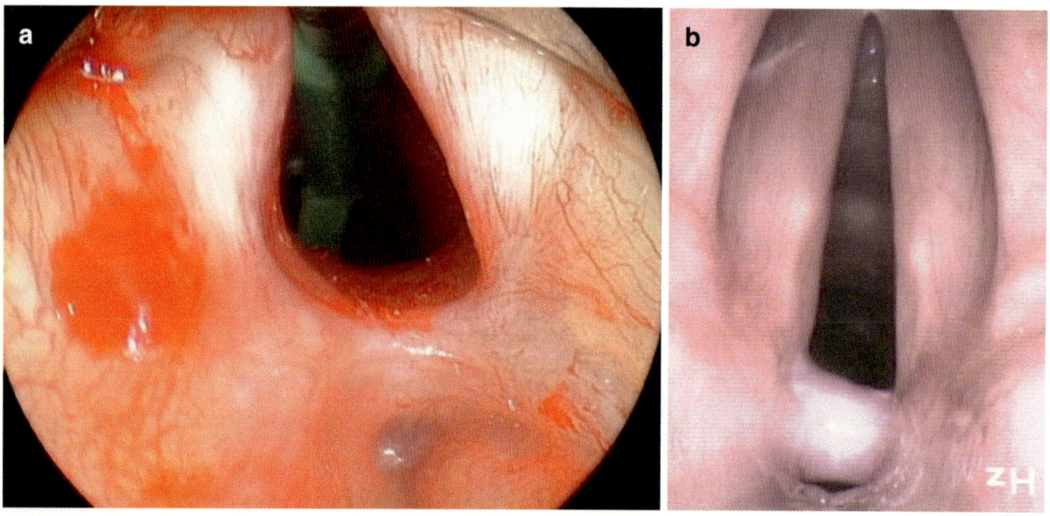

Fig. 4.8 Two cases of interarytenoid bridges: (**a**) fibrous and (**b**) bony

vocal fold. Especially tumours growing at the arytenoid cartilage may hinder the movement of the vocal fold by invading the joint capsule or the joint itself [20]. Brasnu et al. [21] describe the immobility of the vocal fold secondary to the weight of the tumour located at the top of the arytenoid cartilage without any tumour extension of the cricoarytenoid muscles. Fixation is a criteria of the TNM classification, which classifies tumours T3 or higher.

On the other hand, tumour resections of the larynx and/or hypopharynx involving the area of the arytenoid may lead to scar development resulting in restricted mobility of the vocal folds (Fig. 4.9).

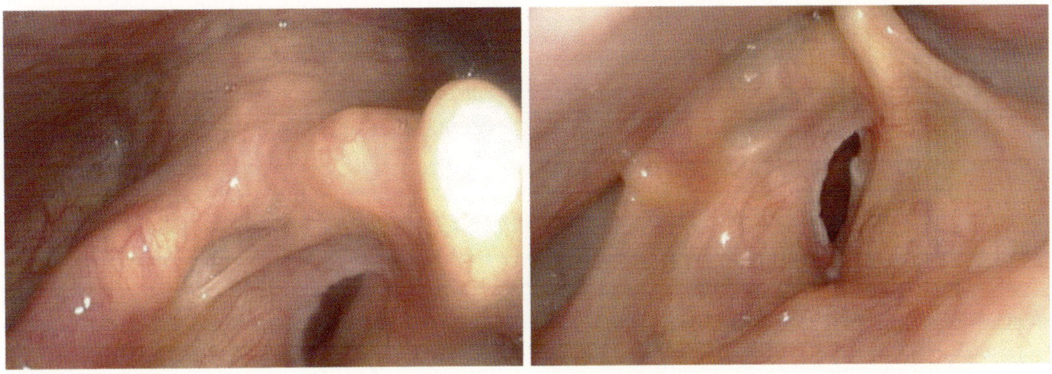

Fig. 4.9 A 47-year-old male with recurrent HPV-associated cancerization of both vocal folds after several microlaryngoscopies resulting in a posterior web formation occluding the glottic lumen and scar formation impairing the mobility of the right arytenoid cartilage

4.2 Diagnostics in ULVFI

Since the etiology and symptomatology of vocal fold immobility are heterogeneous, wide-ranging diagnostics have to be carried out based on the ELS basic protocol for voice diagnostics [22, 23]. Vocal performance, aerodynamic aspects and the individual voice handicap of patients has to be quantified.

Essential tools for the assessment of impaired movement, immobility of the vocal folds, are patient-reported symptoms, endoscopic and stroboscopic examination of the vocal folds and EMG assessment for establishing neural damage.

4.2.1 Patient-Reported Symptoms

Wide-ranging symptoms, many anamnestic details, functional and patient-related aspects like the individual impairment, social or occupational role of the voice and the overall health situation, as well as prognostic information all play a major role in the differential diagnosis and the development of treatment options.

The impaired movement of one vocal fold may be well compensated by the contralateral vocal fold (depending on origin and severity). Acute respiratory distress may lead to serious life-threatening situations, e.g. in the case of bilateral vocal fold paralysis. Thus, the main symptom of unilateral vocal fold immobility is hoarseness, not so much difficulties in breathing. Other complaints are problems with getting loud, monotone intonation, problems with singing and discomfort during speaking.

4.2.2 Endoscopic Findings

Routinely performed rigid as well as flexible laryngoscopy gives a precise impression of the extent of the immobility of the vocal fold. Due to the lack of an evaluable fundamental frequency, laryngostroboscopy can usually not be performed in cases of complete vocal fold paralysis.

Possible endoscopic and stroboscopic findings in patients with vocal fold immobility are a glottal gap, asymmetric left- and right-sided mucosal wave, impaired mobility of the arytenoid cartilage, forward-tilted arytenoid cartilage, different levels of the vocal folds, vocal fold bowing, signs of reflux, granulomas and signs of swallowing disorders.

4.2.3 CT/MRI

Whether computer tomographic scans (CT) make sense is controversial. CT seems to detect (malignant) diseases of idiopathic paralysis. Other findings suggest that CT has a low yield for occult neck and mediastinal pathology in patients with idiopathic vocal fold paresis [5].

Magnetic resonance imaging (MRI) is the most appropriate imaging technique in patients with vocal fold paralysis. The pathology is likely to be located in the neck or at the skull base or the brain stem. MRI is preferable to CT due to its better soft tissue resolution at the skull base or in the case of intracranial diseases. MRI offers excellent visualization of the morphologic soft tissue structures at and below the skull base [24, 25].

4.2.4 Individual Handicap

The Voice Handicap Index (VHI) [26], the Voice-related Quality of Life (VrQoL) measurement [27], the Voice Outcome Survey (VOS) developed for unilateral laryngeal paralysis [28] and the Voice Activity and Participation Profile (VAPP) [29] are all excellent instruments for measuring the individual handicap in patients with unilateral vocal immobility.

4.2.5 Functional Findings

So far, functional and performance tests of voice quality, such as voice range profile, or the calculation of the dysphonia severity index [30], only have a descriptive function. But they do provide information about the vocal fold losses caused by ULVFI. This is of importance for the recognition of the personal handicap and thus for the therapeutic strategy.

In cases of vocal fold immobility, all voice-related aerodynamic measurements are relevant and meaningful diagnostic parameters, such as maximum phonation time (on the sustained [a:]), vital capacity with the help of a spirometric test system, calculation of phonation quotient (=vital capacity in ml/maximum phonation time on [a:] in s) and calculation of s/z ratio (fortis [s]/lenis [z]) ([31, 32]).

4.2.6 Electromyography of the Larynx (Details in Chap. 1)

Sittel et al. [33, 34] evaluate electromyography of the larynx (LEMG) as an important examination in the case of paralysis of the recurrent laryngeal nerve. LEMG is able to detect 94.4% of possible defect healing. It does not allow prediction of long-term voice quality, e.g. in vocal fold paralysis in paramedian or median position, where, in spite of pathologic LEMG results, a good voice may be present [35]. But unilateral vocal fold paresis (ULVFP) can be defined in terms of results from EMG assessment, and LEMG provides additional information about the functional status of voice-related muscles [5].

4.3 Treatment of ULVFI

The goal of any therapy in unilateral vocal fold immobility is the activation of the paralyzed vocal fold and improvement of the glottic closure. Phonosurgical procedures are used to change the vocal fold position (vertical and horizontal), the vocal fold volume (e.g. by grafting and implant placement), the adduction and abduction (e.g. by arytenoid adduction) as well as the tension of the vocal folds (e.g. by reinnervation). Maintenance or optimization of the vocal fold vibration, especially the mucosal wave of the vocal fold, is an additional purpose of the therapy. The three-dimensionality of the vocal fold movement must be considered when selecting the surgical procedure.

This aims to improve the quality of voice, vocal performance and control of airflow with special consideration of best synchronized oscillation frequencies and phases of the vocal folds. It also focusses on the conservation and restoration of abdominal pressure ability and cough effectiveness.

In analogy to Friedrich's remarks on endolaryngeal phonosurgery [36], conservative voice therapy (vocal exercises/voice techniques) is an important component of the holistic treatment concept. This is due to the inherent multidimensional pathogenesis of immobility of vocal folds. The choice of the optimal treatment method should be based on an interdisciplinary assessment and decision made by otolaryngologists, phoniatricians, voice therapists and other involved professions, such as psychologists.

4.3.1 Conservative Voice Therapy (Vocal Function Exercises)

Conservative voice therapy with voice function exercises for the treatment of ULRP may already be sufficient but may only achieve satisfactory results in cases of minor glottal gap [37]. Sittel et al. noticed a regained satisfactory-to-usable vocal performance in 75–90% of patients with ULVFP, although a complete recovery of vocal fold mobility was observed only in 10–40%. Voice function exercises may facilitate glottal compensation and should be prescribed generously [34]. Conservative voice therapy should begin when wound healing is completed.

Aims of voice function exercises are stimulating the nerve, preventing atrophy, improving glottal closure and supporting the unimpaired vocal fold to cross the middle line for better glottal closure.

As an interim solution, glottal closure can be improved by lateral manual pressure (thumb or index finger and middle finger) on the contralateral outside of the thyroid cartilage or by rotation of the head and neck in the direction of the paralyzed vocal fold [38].

Selection of the optimal voice therapy method depends on the symptoms, etiology and pathogenesis of vocal fold immobility. Voice function exercises should focus on vocal fold physiology as a part of the inspiratory sphincter system, because all muscle groups involved in respiration are determined by body posture and body movement. To improve glottal closure, the inspiration-related sphincter should be activated, for example, through pull-ups [39, 40]. In the case of unilateral vocal fold paralysis, a combination with an electrical stimulation therapy may prove successful [41].

4.3.2 Phonosurgery for Treatment of Vocal Fold Immobility (More Details in Chaps. 10, 11, and 12)

Vocal fold immobility may be treated phonosurgically if the larynx EMG indicates a poor prognosis, or the results of conservative voice therapy are not satisfactory enough, or time limitations make conservative treatment less attractive.

The choice of a particular phonosurgical treatment primarily depends on the pathogenesis of the VFI and the needs of the patient regarding voice function and quality. The best way to treat vocal fold immobility is a "sandwich method", i.e. phonosurgery accompanied by conservative voice therapy.

A proposal for the classification of phonosurgical procedures was published by the Phonosurgery Committee of the ELS (see also Chap. 12). Phonosurgical procedures for treatment of ULVFI are vocal fold surgery (VFS), laryngeal framework surgery (LFS) and neuromuscular surgery (NMS) [42]. The phonosurgical methods for ULFVI include injection, implantation, mobilization, correction of position of arytenoid cartilage and reinnervation.

There are two possible surgical approaches: transoral or transcervical (open surgery or percutaneous). Under functional aspects, special attention must be paid in phonosurgery for resection of tumours to resect only as much as necessary and as little as possible. The superficial layer of the lamina propria, the epithelium and the free edge of the vocal fold should be protected.

4.3.3 Mobilization of the Cricoarytenoid Joint (CAJ)

In cases of luxation or subluxation after intubation, mobilization of the CAJ is an appropriate technique.

This can be performed during full anaesthesia as described by [43]. The authors prefer office-based mobilization [44] of the (sub)luxated arytenoid cartilage in respiration and under phonatory control with specially designed instruments which are regularly used for transoral biopsies during laryngoscopy under local anesthesia.

4.3.4 Vocal Fold Injection (Syn. Injection Laryngoplasty or Injection Augmentation)

The most frequently applied phonosurgical procedure is vocal fold injection. This may be used to treat permanent causes of mild-to-moderate glottal insufficiency [45]. It is easier to perform than an implantation augmentation and other methods of transcervical surgery and can also be carried out office-based under functional endoscopic control during indirect laryngoscopy (more on office-based procedures in Chap. 11).

Thus, this technique can be applied to patients with high anesthetic risk. For injection augmentation under local anesthesia and general anesthesia, comparable results are reported [46]. The aim of vocal fold injection is the medialization of the vocal fold through volume increase (augmentation) and level correction of the paralyzed vocal fold resulting in sufficient glottal closure. The Anglo-American term is "injection laryngoplasty".

Vocal fold injections can be performed transorally as well as transcervically and are primarily used in the treatment of mild-to-moderate glottal gaps. Injection laryngoplasty is useful in partial and total vocal fold paralysis.

The injection material should be placed laterally between the thyroid cartilage and the vocalis muscle [47]. The localization of the material depends on its viscosity. Our clinical experiences are consistent with those of Mallur and Rosen [45], who report poor vibratory properties after superficial injections.

An individual decision should be made after taking further study results according to typical rheological properties of various materials (e.g. [48, 49]) into consideration. Additionally, pathogenetic and prognostic factors as well as personal needs (occupational, aesthetic, ethical, etc.) have to be taken into account when selecting the optimal therapy and injection material.

4.3.5 Injection Material

In 1911, Brünings reported for the first time the possibility of an endolaryngeal injection with paraffin wax in the vocal folds [50]. Since then, various materials have been applied with varying degrees of success, like paraffin, silicone, Teflon® and others. Because of foreign body and inflammatory reaction, paraffin and Teflon® have been abandoned as augmentation materials [51, 52].

The current standard materials differ in their features, e.g. applicability, resorption, compatibility and viscoelasticity, and also in their costs. The various materials are classified according to their absorbability [53] (Fig. 4.10). The advantage of resorbable materials is the possibility of temporary augmentations, e.g. in questionable reversible vocal fold paralysis and in vocal fold reconstruction after unsatisfying thyroplasty type I, e.g. with fat [45], or to verify the usefulness of

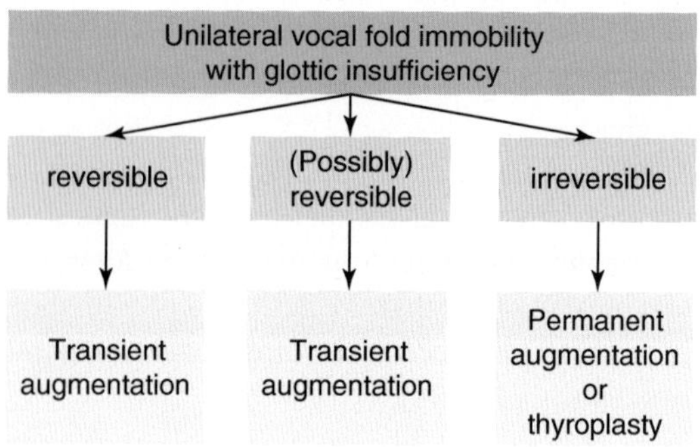

Fig. 4.10 Treatment concept of augmentation in unilateral vocal fold paralysis (ULVFI)

a permanent augmentation (augmentation trial) [54–56].

Indications for permanent injection augmentation are vocal fold atrophy, paralysis (i.e. the LEMG showed a poor prognosis or the paralysis has existed for at least 6 months) and augmentation after previous framework surgery [45].

4.3.6 Resorbable Materials

Hyaluronic acid, which is resorbed within an average of 3–6 months [53], is preferably injected as a hydrogel. Pei et al. [57] have investigated the neurologic and functional effect of early intracordal hyaluronan injections in acute unilateral vocal fold paralysis (UVFP). Early hyaloronic acid injection cannot improve nerve regeneration, but can prevent voice functional compensation, leading to long-lasting improvements of patients' psychosocial well-being. The injection augmentation should be performed after three to four weeks of intensive voice therapy.

Autologous materials include the patient's own fat [58] and fascia lata [59]. Autologous fat has good viscoelastic properties. However, its absorbability is not exactly predictable. In fact, 41% of the patients need additional procedures to attain an acceptable voice [60]. Because of its well-known resorption, fat usually needs to be over-injected.

Autologous fascia is well tolerated, but, on the one hand, it is stiffer compared to fat. On the other hand, the duration of the effect is longer. Fascia can be cut into small pieces and injected or implanted. It can be advantageous for improvement of glottal closure. Reijonen et al. [61] and Cheng et al. [62] recommend that wide glottal gaps should not be treated with fascia injection.

Calcium hydroxylapatite microspheres (CaHA implants) are among the most resorbable materials [63]. They have been tested successfully in patients with unilateral vocal fold paralysis [64] with moderate (38%) to significant results (56%) [63]. It is a material with very good properties in terms of stiffness and viscosity [65]. Chang et al. [66] report that vocal fold medialization with CaHA injection remains a safe and efficacious treatment for UVFP in both irradiated and nonirradiated patients. Mallur et al. [67] confirm the effect of carboxymethyl cellulose injection for the temporary treatment of glottic insufficiency with minimal risk of permanent adverse voice outcomes.

4.3.7 Permanent Materials

The non-absorbable substances include polydimethylsiloxane (VOX Implant®) [45], which is injected far laterally with a water-soluble carrier material in the paraglottic space without overcorrection. After injection, the vocal fold has to be formed with a forceps to avoid bowing of the augmented part in order to create a sufficient counterpart for the intact contralateral vocal fold.

For the treatment of unilateral vocal fold paralysis, this material seems to be most suitable because it is safe and durable. Functional outcome and voice parameters are comparable to those of laryngeal framework surgery [68]. Allergic reactions are unknown [53]. In rare cases, the injected material can change its form secondary to heavy coughing, which may result in bulging of the middle part of the vocal fold. Verma and Dailey [69] report successful office-based injection laryngoplasty for the management of unilateral vocal fold paralysis using a transoral route (85.6%) and rigid angled telescope as well as a curved injection needle. Yung et al. [70] describe that patients with UVFP who underwent vocal fold injection with an agent intended to provide temporary medialization were statistically significantly less likely to undergo permanent medialization laryngoplasty compared to those patients who were treated with conservative management only.

4.3.8 Transoral Implantation

Transoral implantation is a good alternative to injection augmentation. The implantation material (e.g. fascia lata or septal cartilage) is placed laterally between the thyroid cartilage and the vocalis muscle in a prepared pocket (Fig. 4.11a–d).

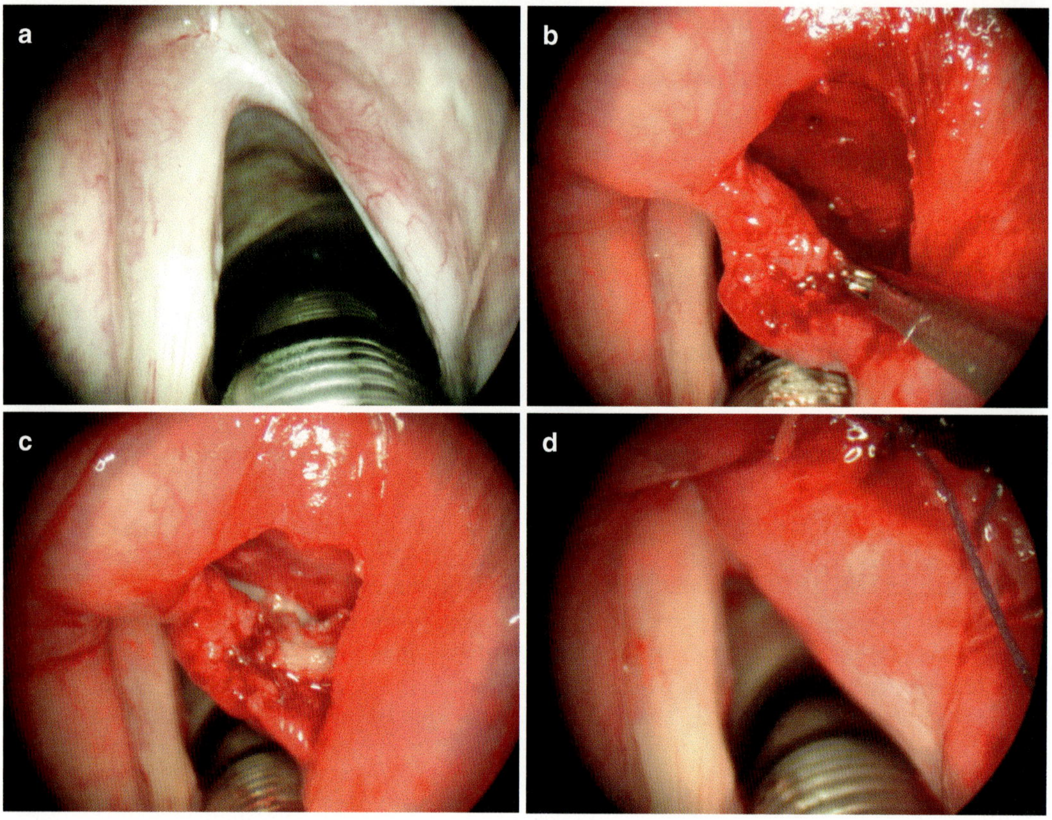

Fig. 4.11 (**a–d**) Implantation augmentation for improving the glottal gap in a case of vocal fold immobility on the right side because of scares after tumour surgery

"Injection augmentation", "implantation augmentation" and "thyroplasty" (open surgery) can be used as complementary methods to improve glottic closure.

4.3.9 Laryngeal Framework Surgery

Four different types of laryngeal framework surgery are suitable for treating vocal fold immobility. These are methods to improve approximation (medialization), relaxation and tension of the vocal folds.

Type I thyroplasty by Isshiki (medialization thyroplasty) is the most commonly used type of laryngeal framework surgery for paralysis of the vocal folds [71]. The advantage of this method is that the complex relevant structures of the vocal fold remain untouched.

During transcervical thyroplasty, a defined thyroid cartilage window is created to medialize the vocal fold by an inwardly pressed tissue or silicon block. Other materials are Gore-Tex® or titanium vocal fold medializing implant (TVFMI) by Friedrich (Fig. 4.12a, b) or autologous cartilage (septum or thyroid cartilage).

Tucker [11] and Friedrich [73] recommend not performing irreversible phonosurgery within 1 year after onset of the paresis, because about 60% of cases of idiopathic unilateral vocal fold paralysis improve in this time period, 80% of those even within the first 6 months—unless the cause is known and the probability of regression of paralysis can thus be anticipated.

Reversible vocal fold medialization using reversible filler material, e.g. hyaluronic acid, can be carried out before the end of the possible reinnervation phase [73]. Paralysis of the vagal nerve

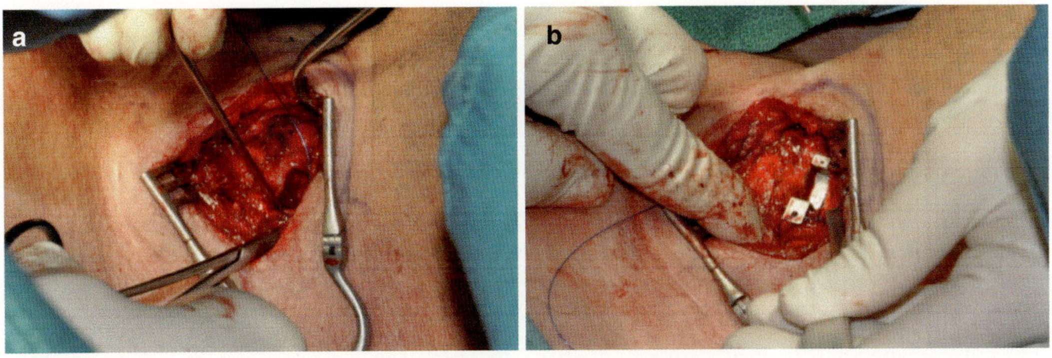

Fig. 4.12 Thyroplasty type I with titanium vocal fold medializing implant (TVFMI): (**a**) Creation of thyroid cartilage window. (**b**) Implantation and fixation of the TVFMI [Reprinted from [72]. With permission from Springer Science + Business Media]

needs a more extensive medialization involving the supraglottic structures as well as the impaired vocal fold.

Benninger et al. [74] report short-term and long-term vocal outcomes after medialization laryngoplasty using a silastic implant in patients with unilateral vocal fold paralysis. Results were comparable with the literature. ML with silastic implant alone can be effective in managing ULVFP.

4.3.10 Arytenoid Adduction for Unilateral Vocal Fold Immobility

Paralyzed arytenoids tend to fall forward and laterally, which shortens the vocal folds and excavates and relocates them from the midline. Surgical methods for adduction of the arytenoid cartilage in unilateral vocal fold paralysis and arthrogenic dysphonia improve the position of the arytenoid cartilage and thus the vocal process. Isshiki [75] reported for the first time a method of medialization of the vocal process by lateral "strain" (pull) by muscle tension through a previously created ipsilateral thyroid cartilage window. Iwamura and Kurita [76] describe a modified technique, the so-called lateral cricoarytenoid muscle pull under local anaesthesia through a thyroid cartilage window.

Maragos [77] and Zeitels et al. [78] describe different methods for fixation. Maragos uses a posterior approach to the thyroid cartilage by creating a semicircular "posterior window technique". In a second step, he fixes the arytenoid cartilage at the upper middle edge of the cricothyroid cartilage. Zeitels et al. [78] fix the manually medially positioned arytenoid cartilage with a special suture to the posterior cricoid cartilage (two-point fixation).

In patients with irreversible unilateral vocal fold paralysis in a lateral position, strong excavation and a large vertical gap, arytenoid adduction is an important method of improving and correcting the vertical difference between the two vocal folds.

Minimally invasive procedures to provide adduction of the arytenoid cartilages are described by Murata et al. [79] and Hess et al. [80]. Under local anaesthesia and endoscopic control, a needle is introduced through the cricothyroid ligament on the affected side with a non-resorbable thread (see also Chap. 11). A second needle with a metal wire loop is placed parallel to the first needle over the arytenoids. The introduced thread is first captured with the loop and then wrapped around the arytenoids. This will allow an adduction of the arytenoid cartilages without resection of the posterior thyroid cartilage.

In the case of a very large glottal gap where a thyroplasty type I is not sufficient and the vocal folds are atrophied, adduction of the arytenoid cartilages and medialization thyroplasty can be combined [77]. Another possible combination is that of adduction of the arytenoid cartilages and reinnervation surgery [81, 82].

4.3.11 Nerve Reconstruction (More Details in Chap. 15)

Injection laryngoplasty, medialization thyroplasty and arytenoid adduction are not able to maintain muscle tension in the paralyzed vocal fold. This can only be attained through nerve reconstruction [83]. Horsley was the first to report the possibility of re-anastomosis of the recurrent laryngeal nerve [84, 85]. The mobility of the paralyzed vocal fold cannot improve, but atrophy can be prevented.

In cases of visible nerve injury during thyroid surgery or after laryngeal trauma, Tucker recommends direct end-to-end anastomosis [11]. Wang et al. [86] describe the following methods of nerve reconstruction: direct end-to-end anastomosis of RLN, free nerve grafting, neuromuscular pedicle, nerve implantation, hypoglossal nerve to RLN anastomosis and ansa cervicalis to RLN anastomosis. A disadvantage of the first two methods is a synkinesis of the abductor and adductor nerve fibres due to misdirected sprouting.

Marie [83], Crumley [87] and Wang et al. [86] describe the possibility of reinnervation by anastomosis between the ansa cervicalis and the recurrent laryngeal nerve in the case of persistent unilateral vocal fold paralysis. This can be combined with arytenoid adduction [88]. The preconditions are an intact ansa cervicalis and a mobile arytenoid. Laryngeal reinnervation by ansa cervicalis is an effective treatment for laryngeal paralysis related to thyroid gland surgery [89].

In the case of a nonviable distal stump of the recurrent laryngeal nerve, which precludes the procedure of nerve transfer, nerve implantation to the thyroarytenoid muscle by the ansa cervicalis is an option [90].

Another technique is the nerve-muscle pedicle technique described by Tucker [91]. This technique uses the ansa cervical omohyoid pedicle muscle for reinnervation of the paralyzed laryngeal adductors.

Because of the different diameters of the neural stumps, the different axon densities and potential impairment of hypoglossal nerve function [92], recurrent laryngeal-hypoglossal nerve anastomosis requires critical discussion.

References

1. Rosenthal LH, Benninger MS, Deeb RH. Vocal fold immobility: a longitudinal analysis of etiology over 20 years. Laryngoscope. 2007;117(10):1864–70.
2. Nawka T, Hosemann W. Chirurgische Verfahren bei gestörter Stimme. Laryngorhinootol. 2005;84:201–12.
3. Brunner E, Friedrich G, Kiesler K, Chibidziura-Priesching J, Gugatschka M. Subjective breathing impairment in unilateral vocal fold paralysis. Folia Phoniatr Logop. 2011;63(3):142–6. doi:10.1159/000316320.
4. Domer AS, Leonard R, Belafsky PC. Pharyngeal weakness and upper esophageal sphincter opening in patients with unilateral vocal fold immobility. Laryngoscope. 2014;124(10):2371–4.
5. Stager SV. Vocal fold paresis: etiology, clinical diagnosis and clinical management. Curr Opin Otolaryngol. Head Neck Surg. 2014;22(6):444–9.
6. Reiter R, Hoffmann TK, Rotter N, Pickhard A, Scheithauer MO, Brosch S. Etiology, diagnosis, differential diagnosis and therapy of vocal fold paralysis. Laryngorhinootol. 2014;93(3):161–73.
7. Rosato L, Avenia N, Bernante P, De Palma M, Gulino G, Nasi PG, Pelizzo MR, Pezzullo L. Complications of thyroid surgery: analysis of a multicentric study on 14,934 patients operated on in Italy over 5 years. World J Surg. 2004;28(3):271–6.
8. Jeannon JP, Orabi AA, Bruch GA, Abdalsalam HA, Simo R. Diagnosis of recurrent laryngeal nerve palsy after thyroidectomy: a systematic review. Int J Clin Pract. 2009;63(4):624–429.
9. Bayar N, Kara SA, Keleş I, Koç C, Altinok D, Orkun S. Cricoarytenoiditis in rheumatoid arthritis: radiologic and clinical study. J Otolaryngol. 2003;32(6):373–8.
10. Eckel HE, Wittekindt C, Klussmann JP, Schroeder U, Sittel C. Management of bilateral arytenoid cartilage fixation versus recurrent laryngeal nerve paralysis. Ann Otol Rhinol Laryngol. 2003;112(2):103–8.
11. Tucker HM. Laryngeal reinnervation. In: Rubin J, Sataloff RT, Korovin G, editors. Diagnosis and treatment of voice disorders. San Diego: Plural Publishing; 2006. p. 727–33.
12. Rieger A, Hass I, Gross M, Gramm HJ, Eyrich K. Intubation trauma of the larynx–a literature review with special reference to arytenoid cartilage

dislocation. Anasthesiol Intensivmed Notfallmed Schmerzther. 1996;31(5):281–7.
13. Wang RC. Three-dimensional analysis of cricoarytenoid joint motion. Laryngoscope. 1998;108(4 Pt 2 Suppl 86):1–17.
14. Sataloff RT, Bough ID Jr, Spiegel JR. Arytenoid dislocation: diagnosis and treatment. Laryngoscope. 1994;104(11 Pt 1):1353–61.
15. Yamanaka H, Hayashi Y, Watanabe Y, Uematu H, Mashimo T. Prolonged hoarseness and arytenoid cartilage dislocation after tracheal intubation. Br J Anaesth. 2009;103(3):452–5.
16. Norris BK, Schweinfurth JM. Arytenoid dislocation: an analysis of the contemporary literature. Laryngoscope. 2011;121(1):142–6.
17. Copeman WS, Elkin AC, Pearce R. A case of rheumatoid arthritis with ankylosis of the crico-arytenoid joints. Br Med J. 1959;1(5137):1575.
18. Arviso LC, Klein AM, Johns MM. The management of postintubation phonatory insufficiency. J Voice. 2012;26(4):530–3.
19. Woo P, Casper J, Colton R, Brewer D. Diagnosis and treatment of persistent dysphonia after laryngeal surgery: a retrospective analysis of 62 patients. Laryngoscope. 1994;104(9):1084–91.
20. Hirano M, Kurita S, Matsuoka H, Tateishi M. Vocal fold fixation in laryngeal carcinomas. Acta Otolaryngol. 1991;111(2):449–54.
21. Brasnu D, Laccourreye H, Dulmet E, Jaubert F. Mobility of the vocal cord and the arytenoid in cancer of the larynx and the hypopharynx. Anatomo-clinical study. Ann Otolaryngol Chir Cervicofac. 1988;105(6):435–41.
22. Dejonckere PH, Bradley P, Clemente P, Cornut G, Crevier-Buchman L, Friedrich G, Van De Heyning P, Remacle M, Woisard V, Committee on Phoniatrics of the European Laryngological Society (ELS). A basic protocol for functional assessment of voice pathology, especially for investigating the efficacy of (phonosurgical) treatments and evaluating new assessment techniques. Guideline elaborated by the committee on Phoniatrics of the European laryngological society (ELS). Eur Arch Otorhinolaryngol. 2001;258(2):77–82.
23. Dejonckere PH, Crevier-Buchman L, Marie JP, Moerman M, Remacle M, Woisard V, European Research Group on the Larynx. Implementation of the European laryngological society (ELS) basic protocol for assessing voice treatment effect. Rev Laryngol Otol Rhinol (Bord). 2003;124(5):279–83.
24. Kwong Y, Boddu S, Shah J. Radiology of vocal cord palsy. Clin Radiol N. 2012;67(11):1108–14.
25. Pretorius PM, Milford CA. Investigating the hoarse voice. BMJ. 2008;337:a1726.
26. Jacobson BH, Johnson A, Grywalsky C, Silbergleit A, Jacobson G, Benninger MS, Newman CW. The voice handicap index (VHI): development and validation. Am J Speech Lang Pathol. 1997;6:66–70.
27. Hogikyan ND, Sethuraman G. Validation of an instrument to measure voice-related quality of life (V-RQOL). J Voice. 1999;13(4):557–69.
28. Gliklich RE, Glovsky RM, Montgomery WW. Validation of a voice outcome survey for unilateral vocal cord paralysis. Otolaryngol Head Neck Surg. 1999;120(2):153–8.
29. Spector BC, Netterville JL, Billante C, Clary J, Reinisch L, Smith TL. Quality-of-life assessment in patients with unilateral vocal cord paralysis. Otolaryngol Head Neck Surg. 2001;125(3):176–82.
30. Wuyts FL, De Bodt MS, Molenberghs G, Remacle M, Heylen L, Millet B, Van Lierde K, Raes J, Van de Heyning PH. The dysphonia severity index: an objective measure of vocal quality based on a multiparameter approach. J Speech Lang Hear Res. 2000;43(3):796–809.
31. Eckel FC, Boone DR. The S/Z ratio as an indicator of laryngeal pathology. J Speech Hear Disord. 1981;46(2):147–9.
32. Iwata S, von Leden H. Phonation quotient in patients with laryngeal diseases. Folia Phoniatr. 1970;22(2):117–28.
33. Sittel C, Stennert E, Thumfart WF, Dapunt U, Eckel HE. Prognostic value of laryngeal electromyography in vocal fold paralysis. Arch Otolaryngol Head Neck Surg. 2001;127(2):155–60.
34. Sittel C, Bosch N, Plinkert PK. Surgical voice rehabilitation in unilateral vocal fold paralysis. Chirurg. 2008;79(1):1055–64.
35. Schuster M, Eysholdt U. Therapy for unilateral vocal fold palsy. HNO. 2005;53(9):756–65.
36. Friedrich G. Endolaryngeal Phonosurgery. In: Remacle M, Eckel HE, editors. Surgery of larynx and trachea. Berlin Heidelberg: Springer; 2010. p. 39–43.
37. Heuer RJ, Sataloff RT, Emerich K, Rulnick R, Baroody M, Spiegel JR, Durson G, Butler J. Unilateral recurrent laryngeal nerve paralysis: the importance of "preoperative" voice therapy. J Voice. 1997;11(1):88–94.
38. Wendler J, Seidner W. Klinik. In: Wendler J, Seidner W, Eysholdt U, editors. Lehrbuch der Phoniatrie und Pädaudiologie. 4th ed. Stuttgart: Thieme; 2005. p. 139–91.
39. Kruse E. Conservative approaches to the management of voice disorders. GMS Curr Top Otorhinolaryngol Head Neck Surg. 2005;4:1–18.
40. Kruse E. Funktionale Stimmtherapie–Therapeutisch konzeptionelle Konsequenz der laryngealen Doppel ventilfunktion. Sprache Stimme Gehör. 1991;15: 127–34.
41. Ptok M, Strack D. Electrical stimulation-supported voice exercises are superior to voice exercise therapy alone in patients with unilateral recurrent laryngeal nerve paresis: results from a prospective, randomized clinical trial. Muscle Nerve. 2008;38(2):1005–11.
42. Friedrich G, Remacle M, Birchall M, Marie JP, Arens C. Defining phonosurgery: a proposal for classification and nomenclature by the Phonosurgery Committee of the European Laryngological Society (ELS). Eur Arch Otorhinolaryngol. 2007;264(10):1191–200.
43. Rudert H. Uncommon injuries of the larynx following intubation. Recurrent paralysis, torsion and luxation of the cricoarytenoid joints. HNO. 1984;32(9):393–8.

44. Pascher W, Dzirsk B. The treatment of dislocation of the arytenoid cartilage by mobilization in indirect microlaryngoscopy. Vestn Otorinolaringol. 1996;6:27–9.
45. Mallur PS, Rosen CA. Vocal fold injection: review of indications, techniques, and materials for augmentation. Clin Exp Otorhinolaryngol. 2010;3(4):177–82.
46. Sulica L, Rosen C, Postma G, Simpson B, Amin M, Courey M, Merati A. Current practice in injection augmentation of the vocal folds: indications, treatment principles, techniques, and complications. Laryngoscope. 2010;120(2):319–25.
47. Hirano M. Surgical and medical management of voice disorders. In: Colton RH, Casper JK, editors. Understanding voice problems. Baltimore: Williams and Wilkins; 1996. p. 241–69.
48. Caton T, Thibeault SL, Klemuk S, Smith ME. Viscoelasticity of hyaluronan and nonhyaluronan based vocal fold injectables: implications for mucosal versus muscle use. Laryngoscope. 2007;117(3):516–21.
49. Klemuk SA, Titze IR. Viscoelastic properties of three vocal-fold injectable biomaterials at low audio frequencies. Laryngoscope. 2004;114(9):1597–603.
50. Brünings W. Über eine neue Behandlungsmethode der Rekurrenslähmung. Ver Deutsch Laryng. 1911;18:93–151.
51. Anderson TD, Sataloff RT. Complications of collagen injection of the vocal fold: report of several unusual cases and review of the literature. J Voice. 2004;18(3):392–7.
52. Varvares MA, Montgomery WW, Hillman RE. Teflon granuloma of the larynx: etiology, pathophysiology, and management. Ann Otol Rhinol Laryngol. 1995;104(7):511–5.
53. Sittel C, Plinkert PK. Vocal fold augmentation. HNO. 2005;53(1):6–10.
54. Kwon TK, Rosen CA, Gartner-Schmidt J. Preliminary results of a new temporary vocal fold injection material. J Voice. 2005;19(4):668–73.
55. Kwon TK, Buckmire R. Injection laryngoplasty for management of unilateral vocal fold paralysis. Curr Opin Otolaryngol Head Neck Surg. 2004;12(6):538–42.
56. Carroll TL, Rosen CA. Trial vocal fold injection. J Voice. 2010;24(4):494–8.
57. Pei YC, Fang TJ, Hsin LJ, Li HY, Wong AM. Early hyaluronate injection improves quality of life but not neural recovery in unilateral vocal fold paralysis: an open-label randomized controlled study. Restor Neurol Neurosci. 2015;33(2):121–30.
58. Laccourreye O, Papon JF, Kania R, Crevier-Buchman L, Brasnu D, Hans S. Intracordal injection of autologous fat in patients with unilateral laryngeal nerve paralysis: long-term results from the patient's perspective. Laryngoscope. 2003;113(3):541–5.
59. Rihkanen H. Vocal fold augmentation by injection of autologous fascia. The Laryngoscope. 1998;108(1Pt.1):51–54.
60. McCulloch TM, Andrews BT, Hoffman HT, Graham SM, Karnell MP, Minnick C. Long-term follow-up of fat injection laryngoplasty for unilateral vocal cord paralysis. Laryngoscope. 2002;112(7 Pt1):1235–8.
61. Reijonen P, Tervonen H, Harinen K, Rihkanen H, Aaltonen LM. Long-term results of autologous fascia in unilateral vocal fold paralysis. Eur Arch Otorhinolaryngol. 2009;66(8):1273–8.
62. Cheng Y, Li ZQ, Huang JZ, Xue F, Jiang MJ, Wu KM, Wang QP. Combination of autologous fascia lata and fat injection into the vocal fold via the cricothyroid gap for unilateral vocal fold paralysis. Arch Otolaryngol Head Neck Surg. 2009;135(8):759–63.
63. Rosen CA. Phonosurgical vocal fold injection: procedures and materials. Otolaryngol Clin N Am. 2000;33(5):1087–95.
64. Storck C, Brockmann M, Schnellmann E, Stoeckli SJ, Schmid S. Functional outcome of vocal fold medialization thyroplasty with a hydroxyapatite implant. Laryngoscope. 2007;117(6):1118–22.
65. Kimura M, Mau T, Chan RW. Viscoelastic properties of phonosurgical biomaterials at phonatory frequencies. Laryngoscope. 2010;120(4):764–8.
66. Chang J, Courey MS, Al-Jurf SA, Schneider SL, Yung K. Injection laryngoplasty outcomes in irradiated and nonirradiated unilateral vocal fold paralysis. Laryngoscope. 2014;124(8):1895–9.
67. Mallur PS, Morrison MP, Postma GN, Amin MR, Rosen CA. Safety and efficacy of carboxymethylcellulose in the treatment of glottic insufficiency. Laryngoscope. 2012;122(2):322–6.
68. Bergamini G, Alicandri-Ciufelli M, Molteni G, Villari D, Luppi MP, Genovese E, Presutti L. Therapy of unilateral vocal fold paralysis with polydimethylsiloxane injection laryngoplasty: our experience. J Voice. 2010;24(1):119–25.
69. Verma SP, Dailey SH. Office-based injection laryngoplasty for the management of unilateral vocal fold paralysis. J Voice. 2014;28(3):382–6.
70. Yung KC, Likhterov I, Courey MS. Effect of temporary vocal fold injection medialization on the rate of permanent medialization laryngoplasty in unilateral vocal fold paralysis patients. Laryngoscope. 2011;121(10):2191–4.
71. Isshiki N. Progress in laryngeal framework surgery. Acta Otolaryngol. 2000;120(2):120–7.
72. Voigt-Zimmermann S, Arens C. Treatment of glottal gap. HNO. 2013;61(2):117–34.
73. Friedrich G. External vocal cord medialization: functional outcome. Laryngorhinootologie. 1998;77(1):18–26.
74. Benninger MS, Manzoor N, Ruda JM. Short- and long-term outcomes after silastic medicalization laryngoplasty: are arytenoid procedures needed? J Voice. 2015;29(2):236–40.
75. Isshiki G. Arytenoid adduction for unilateral vocal fold paralysis. Arch Otolaryngol. 1978;104(19):555–8.
76. Iwamura S, Kurita N. A newer arytenoids adduction technique for one vocal fold paralysis. Head Neck Surg Jpn. 1996;6:1–10.
77. Maragos NE. Arytenoid fixation surgery for the treatment of arytenoid fractures and dislocations. Laryngoscope. 1999;109(5):834–7.

78. Zeitels SM, Hochman I, Hillman RE. Adduction arytenopexy: a new procedure for paralytic dysphonia with implications for implant medialization. Ann Otol Rhinol Laryngol. 1998;107:2–24.
79. Murata T, Yasuoka Y, Shimada T, Shino M, Iida H, Takahashi K, Furuya N. A new and less invasive procedure for arytenoid adduction surgery: endoscopic-assisted arytenoid adduction surgery. Laryngoscope. 2011;121(6):1274–80.
80. Hess M, Schroeder P, Pueschel K. Sling arytenoid adduction. Eur Arch Otorhinolaryngol. 2011;268(7):1023–8.
81. Hassan MM, Yumoto E, Kumai Y, Sanuki T, Kodama N. Vocal outcome after arytenoid adduction and ansa cervicalis transfer. Arch Otolaryngol Head Neck Surg. 2012;138(1):60–5.
82. Yumoto E. Nerve-muscle pedicle flap implantation combined with arytenoid adduction. Arch Otolaryngol Head Neck Surg. 2010;136(10):965–9.
83. Marie JP. Nerve reconstruction. In: Remacle M, Eckel HE, editors. Surgery of larynx and trachea. Berlin: Springer; 2010. p. 279–94.
84. Horsley JS. Suture of the recurrent laryngeal nerve with report of a case. Trans South Surg Gynecol Assoc. 1909;22:161–7.
85. Horsley JS. Suture of the recurrent laryngeal nerve: with report of a case. Ann Surg. 1910;51(4):524–48.
86. Wang W, Chen D, Chen S, Li D, Li M, Xia S, Zheng H. Laryngeal reinnervation using ansa cervicalis for thyroid surgery-related unilateral vocal fold paralysis: a long-term outcome analysis of 237 cases. PLoS One. 2011;6(4):e19128.
87. Crumley RL. Update: ansa cervicalis to recurrent laryngeal nerve anastomosis for unilateral laryngeal paralysis. Laryngoscope. 1991;101(4 Pt 1):384–8.
88. Chhetri DK, Gerratt BR, Kreiman J, Berke GS. Combined arytenoid adduction and laryngeal reinnervation in the treatment of vocal fold paralysis. Laryngoscope. 1999;109(12):1928–36.
89. Palamarchuk VA. Larynx reinnervation by the main branch of ansa cervicalis use in the thyroid surgery in cases of unilateral vocal fold paralysis. Klin Khir. 2013;8:75–9.
90. Su WF, Hsu YD, Chen HC, Sheng H. Laryngeal reinnervation by ansa cervicalis nerve implantation for unilateral vocal cord paralysis in humans. J Am Coll Surg. 2007;204:64–72.
91. Tucker HM. Reinnervation of the paralyzed larynx: a review. Head Neck Surg. 1979;1(3):235–42.
92. Paniello RC. Laryngeal reinnervation with the hypoglossal nerve: II. Clinical evaluation and early patient experience. Laryngoscope. 2000;110(5 Pt 1):739–48.

Vocal Fold Immobility: Bilateral

5

Gerd Fabian Volk and Orlando Guntinas-Lichius

Abstract

Bilateral vocal fold immobility occurs mainly as unilateral or less frequently as bilateral immobility. Numerous metabolic, neurologic, and mechanical conditions can cause bilateral loss of vocal fold abduction. The most important reason is a bilateral vocal fold paralysis related to a lesion of the recurrent laryngeal nerve. Etiologies and key epidemiological numbers are summarized in this chapter. Severity of symptoms of bilateral vocal fold immobility is highly variable depending on the duration of the disease. To decide on the optimal treatment for the individual patient, a sequence of otolaryngological, phoniatric, respiratory, and other functional tests is performed. This will help to find the optimal surgical treatment. The same diagnostic procedures are needed to follow up the patient after surgery to evaluate the efficacy of the applied therapy.

5.1 Introduction

Bilateral vocal fold immobility (BVFI; old incorrect term: bilateral vocal cord immobility) is a rare condition. BVFI can be a neural disease due to paralysis of either recurrent or vagal nerves (bilateral vocal fold paralysis [BVFP]) or due to fixation of the vocal folds, for instance, due to a bilateral tumor infiltration. Other reasons are extremely rare. BVFI results in a narrowed glottic area and airway. BVFI is in most cases associated with significant morbidity and functional disability leading to the presentation for surgery. In case of BVFP and most cases of BVFI, both vocal folds become unable to open during inspiration because of the bilateral loss of the abductor function due to impaired innervation of the posterior cricoarytenoid muscles (PCA). Thus during inspiration both vocal folds remain in the paramedian position causing the narrowing or even the blockage of the airway, depending on the size of the free space left between the immobile vocal

Electronic Supplementary Material The online version of this chapter (doi:10.1007/978-3-319-61724-4_5) contains supplementary material, which is available to authorized users.

G.F. Volk
Department of Otorhinolaryngology,
Jena University Hospital, Jena, Germany

O. Guntinas-Lichius (✉)
Department of Otorhinolaryngology,
Institute of Phoniatry/Pedaudiology,
Jena University Hospital, Jena, Germany
e-mail: orlando.guntinas@med.uni-jena.de

C. Sittel, O. Guntinas-Lichius (eds.), *Neurolaryngology*,
https://doi.org/10.1007/978-3-319-61724-4_5

folds. Vocal fold position and compensatory behavior and the degrees of dyspnea, dysphonia, and dysphagia are highly variable depending on the underlying etiology and comorbidity of the patient. BVFI can be treated by surgery. Tracheotomy still is frequently required in an emergency situation with severe dyspnea that became acute at the moment of occurrence of BVFI or if additional factors like an acute laryngitis worsened the situation. In elective case, the aim of surgery is to widen the glottic area. At best, this widening results in a symptomatic relief but preserves swallowing and voice function.

5.2 Etiology and Epidemiology

A distinction should be made between bilateral paralysis and immobility of the vocal folds. In the narrow sense, BVFI is a more general term covering all causes. A bilaterally paralyzed fold in BVFP implies disruption of neuromuscular innervation, whereas an immobile vocal fold can be the result of multiple causes, including both paralysis and mechanical fixation. BVFI can occur as a result of a primary disorder or as an iatrogenic complication of surgery or intubation. There are numerous metabolic, neurologic, and mechanical conditions that can cause bilateral loss of vocal fold abduction [1]. The etiologies of congenital BVFP may be traumatic (delivery, surgery), neurologic, and idiopathic, with an estimated incidence of 40%, 40%, and 30%, respectively [2]. The most important causes of BVFI are listed in Table 5.1.

Table 5.1 Etiology of bilateral vocal fold immobility

Etiology	Comment
Paralytic etiology	
Traumatic	Lesion of the recurrent laryngeal nerve or of the vagal nerve on both sides
Iatrogenic	Mainly during thyroid surgery
Neurologic	Myasthenia gravis, stroke, and amyotrophic lateral sclerosis are typical examples
Idiopathic	Reason remains unclear after complete diagnostic work-up
Non-paralytic etiology	
Neoplastic	Tumorous infiltration of the vocal folds on both sides
Traumatic	Actually, posttraumatic, when an endolaryngeal lesion or endolaryngeal surgery has led to scar tissue formation hindering the vocal fold movements on both sides
Inflammatory	Seldom, for instance, by inflammatory reaction of the arytenoid cartilages due to rheumatoid arthritis

Overall, thyroidectomy still is the most frequent cause of BVFI, mostly by bilateral lesion of the recurrent laryngeal nerve. A steady decline in the proportion of BVFI attributed to thyroidectomy is seen in the last decades with a concurrent rise in trauma and malignancy. The proportion for BVFI due to thyroidectomy, malignancy, traumatic reason, neurologic disease, idiopathic reason, and nonclassified reasons is about 60%, 8%, 13%, 10%, 5%, and 6% [1]. BVFI due to a malignancy is more frequent in recurrent and metastatic than in primary disease. Most important malignancies beyond thyroid cancer are laryngeal cancer, esophageal cancer, and mediastinal lymph node metastasis. Traumatic lesions include blunt and open neck trauma but also other iatrogenic lesions than post-thyroidectomy (carotid endarterectomy, anterior cervical fusion, esophageal surgery). Bilateral trauma due to prolonged endotracheal tube intubation is very rare. When a BVFI occurs due to intubation, then it is mainly delayed due to subglottic or interarytenoid fibrosis and cricoarytenoid ankylosis. If BVFI occurs immediately after extubation, three reasons are discussed: cricoarytenoid joint inflammation, cricoarytenoid joint dislocation, and recurrent laryngeal nerve neurapraxia. It may occur when the endotracheal tube cuff lies immediately inferior to the true vocal folds. It is meant that the cuff can compress recurrent nerve fibers as they enter through the thyroid cartilage lamina [1].

BVFP is less frequent than unilateral paralysis. The ratio is about 1:5 [3]. The annual incidence of post-thyroidectomy BVFP for benign disease is estimated with <0.1–2.3% calculated on hospital-based data [4, 5]. The annual incidence of BVFP after total thyroidectomy for thyroid cancer is about 1.3% [4]. The true incidence of BVFI or BVFP based on population-based data is unknown. The annual surgical rate for BVFI calculated from population-based data is given with about 2.8/100,000 population [3].

Congenital BVFP in the neonate is very rare. Never the less, vocal fold paralysis is the second most common congenital laryngeal anomaly in newborns (30–60% of all laryngeal anomalies) [2]. The estimated incidence of congenital BVFP is 0.75 cases per million births per year [6].

5.3 Symptoms and Diagnostics

5.3.1 Symptoms

The classical presentation of patients with peripheral BVFI is the inability to abduct the vocal folds resulting in a narrow glottic chink. The presentation of a patient with BVFI varies. Initially a patient may have a breathy voice without respiratory complaints. Over time the voice can improve as airway symptoms worsen. Such patients may be in a precarious position with respect to the airway. Depending on the width of the remaining glottic chink, their body mass, the presence of comorbidity, and their usual physical activity, the patients may develop severe dyspnea. About 4–14% of these patients tolerates this condition and does not require any surgical treatment, though some of them may decompensate after years and surgery becomes inevitable [7]. In the worst case, BVFI, especially in cases of BVFP, after acute damage of the recurrent laryngeal nerve on both side or if on side was damaged already chronically and the other side is damaged during revision surgery, the free space left between the immobile vocal folds can be very small. Then, BVFP can even become life-threatening.

If no reinnervation occurs, BVFP results in progressive atrophization of the denervated laryngeal muscles, a process starting after nerve injury and causing the consequent gradual reduction of the muscle mass. Usually it is assumed that some spontaneous reinnervation due to axonal regeneration takes place within a year since the occurrence of BVFP. Hence, permanent surgical solutions are often applied only after six upon the occurrence of recurrent laryngeal nerve injury. Reinnervation after severe nerve lesion with muscle fiber degeneration is expected to require between 6 and 12 months to be completed but leads to misdirected reinnervation due to nerve sprouting. This results clinically in increase of muscle mass, i.e., less atrophy of the vocal folds and better resting tone, but still and permanently no movement is regained. Hence, permanent surgical solutions are often applied only after 6–12 months upon the occurrence of recurrent nerve injury.

Most patients with BVFI presenting for surgery are patients with BVFP. When these patients with BVFI present for surgical management, they often have dyspnea or stridor with an apparently normal voice. Voice quality is often better in patients with BVFI than in patients with unilateral immobility. Congenital BVFP causes stridor and respiratory distress in the neonate and infant.

5.3.2 Diagnostics

Diagnostics for BVFI have several important aims: clarifying the reason and type of BVFI, determining the need for surgery, as well as assessing the outcome. Investigations comprise review of patient's history, physical examination with endoscopy, phoniatric examinations including stroboscopy, voice and speech tests, and electrophysiological tests. Testing the airway function includes imaging, pulmonary function testing, sleep studies, and validated quality of life questionnaires. Imaging is not described in more detail in this chapter as imaging is related to the underlying etiology or assumed cause. A sleep study might be indicated if sleep disturbances occur in a patient with BVFI as the disease might be compensated in the daytime but decompensated during the night. Table 5.2 gives an overview about the most important diagnostic investigations.

Table 5.2 Overview about the most important diagnostic investigations for patients with bilateral vocal fold immobility (BVFI)

Diagnostic investigation	Comment
History	Comorbidity and for instance smoking habits can have influence on the functional severity of BVFI
Physical examination	Physical resilience is important in the early postoperative phase, because due to laryngeal swelling, the symptoms can be transiently even more severe after surgery
Laryngoscopy	Important to detect residual movement, tension of the vocal folds, and position of the arytenoid cartilages
Stroboscopy	To confirm the immobility
Voice and speech tests	Voice pathology has to be quantified at best before treatment and during follow-up after treatment
Pulmonary function tests	At least a peak flow meter should be used, or, at best, spirometry should be performed together with a pulmonologist
Sleep studies	Indicated in patients with breathing problems especially during the night
Swallowing tests	Important when the patients has also swallowing complaints as some type of surgery might impair swallowing function
Electrophysiological tests	Means mainly laryngeal electromyography, important to differentiate between paralytic and non-paralytic etiologies of BVFI. Import prognostic tool in patients with paralytic etiology
Patient-related outcome measures (PROM) and quality of life assessments	Important instruments to evaluate the outcome of treatment
Miscellaneous	Six-minute walk test gives a good impression about the functional impairment of the patient
	Imaging studies: necessary to clarify the etiology of BVFI

5.3.3 Medical History and Demographic Data

The following symptoms, if present, should be addressed: breathing problems, snoring problems, voice quality, swallowing problems, problems while performing indoor activities, problems while performing outdoor activities, issues at workplace, and issues during leisure time. All comorbidities and long-term medication should be recorded. Severe illnesses and surgeries related to or which may be related to the BVFI should be reported. Not only standard demographic data can be relevant for treatment decision-making, but also data on smoking and drinking habits, body weight, and body mass index are relevant.

5.3.4 Physical Examination and Standard Otolaryngology Examination

Physical examination to assess the subject's physical status is very important to estimate the physical resilience of the patients. Especially after transoral surgery, there might be a transient critical phase due to local postoperative swelling with even poorer respiratory function than before surgery. The most important step of the otolaryngological examination is the transnasal or transoral (rigid and/or flexible) endoscopic evaluation of the larynx. Endoscopy is needed to document the bilateral vocal fold immobility, the tension, flaccidity or atrophy of the vocal fold, and, where appropriate, endolaryngeal lesions or scar tissue. The position of both arytenoid cartilages is described (normal position, signs of fixation, medial tilting). At best, laryngoscopy is performed as videolaryngoscopy. Videolaryngocopy allows recording the natural status of the vocal folds and the configuration of the glottic gap during phonation and sniffing.

5.3.5 Phoniatric Examinations

Videostroboscopy should be part of the videolaryngoscopy. The videostrip should include,

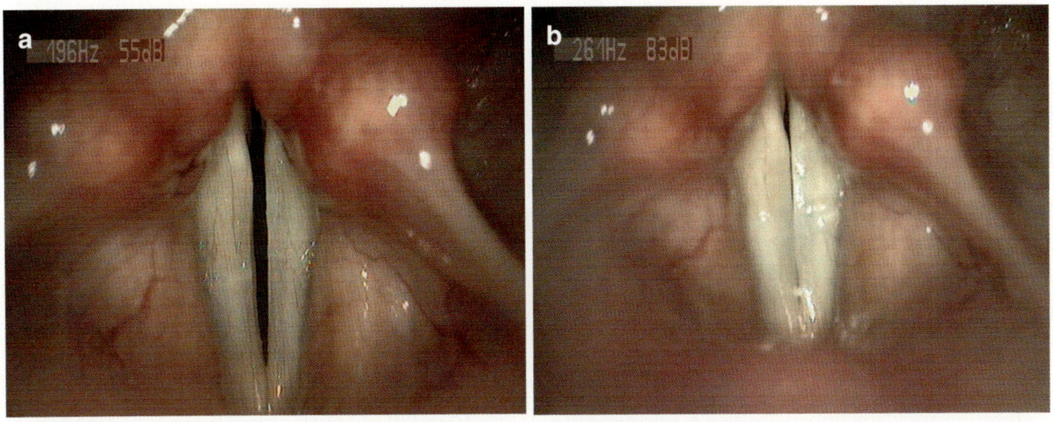

Fig. 5.1 The videolaryngoscopy should include a short stroboscopy sequence during phonation vocal [ee:] at the normal speech frequency level with and without pitch. (**a**) The larynx at rest; (**b**) during phonation. Evaluation of the videostroboscopy is descriptive (impression of the examiner concerning, e.g., laryngeal tissue abnormalities, tissue appearance, vocal fold edge, ample laryngeal movement, arytenoid movement, supraglottic compression, vibratory characteristics, glottic closure, vibratory amplitude, vibratory symmetry, mucosal wave, appearance of laryngeal anatomy, and physiology description of vocal use)

if possible, a short stroboscopy sequence during phonation vocal [ee:] at the normal speech frequency level with and without pitch (Fig. 5.1). Evaluation of the videostroboscopy is descriptive (impression of the examiner concerning, e.g., laryngeal tissue abnormalities, tissue appearance, vocal fold edge, ample laryngeal movement, arytenoid movement, supraglottic compression, vibratory characteristics, glottic closure, vibratory amplitude, vibratory symmetry, mucosal wave, appearance of laryngeal anatomy, and physiology description of vocal use).

There are manifold test procedures but no international standard for the evaluation of voice pathologies. Some of the procedures presented here are described in more detail in the guideline of the European Laryngological Society [8]. The following diagnostic procedure allows a comprehensive and detailed picture of the functional deficits of a patient with BVFI.

The text passage and roughness-breathiness-hoarseness (RBH) test help to semiquantify the quality of the patient's voice [9]. This perceptive voice analysis is based on the examiner's ear response. The RBH is used to evaluate the severity of roughness (R), breathiness (B), and hoarseness (H). Briefly, roughness is the impression of the irregularity of the vibration of the vocal folds, and breathiness (B) is the audible impression of turbulent air leakage through insufficient glottic closure, while hoarseness (H) describes the overall voice quality. All three parameters have to be scored on a scale from 0 to 3 (0 = not existing, 0 = normal, 1 = mild, 2 = moderate, 3 = severe). The auditive rating is made based on 1 min audio recording of a standardized text.

Jitter is a popular quantifiable parameter for voice pathology. The perturbation parameter jitter in percentage is recorded in room bearing an ambient noise level below 40 dB and showing the characteristics of a "living room." The patient is asked to vocalize using a head-mounted microphone with 30 cm microphone-mouth distance. The recording is stored typically with a sampling rate of 22 kHz. Acoustic analysis is conducted offline using the most stable part of the phonation. Subjects are asked to "sustain /a/ for one to three seconds at normal pitch and habitual loudness". Other parameters are the maximum phonation time (MPT) and the voice range profile (VRP). MPT is measured on a sustained /a/ after full inspiration in a comfortable loudness and pitch. VRP identifies the minimal I (low) and maximal amplitude and the lowest and highest frequency F0 (high) of the voice range.

5.3.6 Airway Function Tests

Airway function tests are not routinely performed during the diagnostic work-up of patients with BFVI. Nevertheless, in order to select patients for surgery or to evaluate the effect of different therapy strategies, these tests are very important (see also Chap. 2).

The easiest instrument to test the patient's airway function is the peak flow meter. It enables the subject to estimate the peak expiratory flow (PEF) as an important surrogate marker of the respiratory function herself/himself. Furthermore, it can be used, if appropriate, also at home. PEF is the maximum flow generated during expiration performed with maximal force and started after a full inspiration. The subject is instructed to inhale as deeply as possible and to exhale as much as possible through the mouthpiece. The measurement is repeated three times. The best result is recorded.

Spirometry is another relatively simple test for the evaluation of the patient's airway function [10]. The spirometer consists of a mouthpiece and tubing connected to a recording device. The subject's lips should form a tight seal around the mouthpiece, and nose clips should be worn to ensure that all the air inhaled or exhaled goes through the mouth. Spirometry analysis will primarily also be performed to evaluate the PEF as most important parameter. Like using the peak flow meter, the subject is instructed to inhale as deeply as possible and to exhale as much as possible through the mouthpiece. The measurement is repeated three times. PEF has to be reached within 120 ms after commencement of exhalation. Exhalation is finished if the continuous air flow falls below 0.1 l/sec. The best result is recorded. There are other three important spirometry parameters: To measure the forced vital capacity (FVC), the subject is instructed to exhale as much as possible and thereafter to inhale as deeply as possible through the mouthpiece. The measurement is repeated three times. Another important parameter is the forced expiratory volume (FEV1). The FEV1 is the volume exhaled during the first second of a forced expiratory flow started from the level of total lung capacity. The start point of the FEV1 is obtained by linear extrapolation of the steepest part of the volume-time diagram. The extrapolated volume should not be >5% of the FVC. Finally, peak inspiratory flow (PIF): it is the maximum flow generated during inspiration performed with maximal force and started after a full expiration. The subject is instructed to exhale as much as possible and to inhale as deeply as possible through the mouthpiece. The measurement is repeated three times. Other helpful parameters might be:

(a) FEV1/FVC ratio: this ratio is calculated from the FEV1 and FVC best results. It indicates what percentage of the total FVC was expelled from the lungs during the first second of forced exhalation.
(b) Two forced expiratory flow at 50% of vital capacity (FEF50): this measurement describes the amount of air expelled from the lungs during the first half (50%) of the forced vital capacity test.
(c) Forced inspiratory flow at 50% of vital capacity (FIF50): is obtained from the flow volume diagram by measuring the inspiratory flow at 50% of vital capacity (VC).
(d) Finally, the FEF50/FIF50 ratio is calculated from the FEF50 and FIF50 best results.

The most complex investigation, normally performed by pneumologists but the golden standard, is whole-body plethysmography [11]. Briefly, the body plethysmograph consists of an airtight box with constant volume and electronic compensation for body temperature and water vapor saturated pressure, as well as a mouthpiece and tubing connected to a recording device. The subject's lips should form a tight seal around the mouthpiece, and nose clips should be worn to ensure that all the air inhaled or exhaled goes through the mouth. Briefly, body plethysmography allows the measurement of the inspiratory resistance (Rin), expiratory resistance (Rex), total resistance (Rtot), and specific Resistance (sR) at different breathing frequencies. Additionally, the intrathoracic gas volume (ITGV) is measured while the patient is breathing against the occluded tubing (shutter).

5.3.7 Swallowing Test

A standard procedure to evaluate the swallowing function is the fiber-optic endoscopic evaluation of swallowing (FEES) [12]. In the FEES procedure, a flexible fiber-optic endoscope is introduced transnasally to the patient's hypopharynx where the clinician can clearly view laryngeal and pharyngeal structures. Briefly, the subject swallows two test boluses: 5 mL liquid (methylene blue or vital blue diluted in water), from a cup, and 15 mL yogurt (methylene blue or vital blue diluted in smooth yogurt), from a standard dessert spoon. Subjects also swallow an undyed 5 mL water bolus immediately after swallowing the liquid test bolus. The water bolus is given to rinse the pharynx and is not recorded. The yogurt bolus is swallowed immediately after the water bolus. All participants swallowed the three boluses in the same sequence: (a) liquid test bolus, (b) water, and (c) yogurt test bolus. The subject is asked to take a gulp into her/his mouth and swallows upon the sign of the investigator. The depth of dye entry into the larynx and/or trachea is graded according to the penetration-aspiration scale (PAS) [13]. Accordingly, the most critical finding is aspiration, and the literature demonstrates that FEES is able to detect this finding with good sensitivity. PAS is an 8-point clinical scale for rating penetration and aspiration. The severity of the rating depends on the perceived depth of entry of food or fluid material into the airway and clearance of material from the airway.

5.3.8 Other Functional Tests

The 6-min walk test (6MWT) is the most frequently used exercise test in pulmonary rehabilitation and is considered to provide a reliable and valid measure of functional exercise capacity [14]. This test will be carried out according to the guidelines of the American Thoracic Society [15]. Patients are instructed to try to cover as long a distance as possible within 6 min without running. They are instructed to wear comfortable shoes and clothing and told that they may rest or stop when necessary. At the end of the 6 min, the subject will be told to stop and the distance walked will be recorded.

5.3.9 Electrophysiological Testing

In a strict sense, a neurogenic origin of BVFI can only be proven by laryngeal electrophysiological testing (see Chap. 1). Electrophysiological testing in the larynx is basically restricted in clinical routine to laryngeal electromyography (LEMG). LEMG is a procedure that records the electrical activity produced by voice box muscles in action. LEMG gives specific information as to whether the nerve input into a particular muscle is normal or abnormal. During LEMG, electrical activity is recorded, amplified, and displayed on a screen and played on a loudspeaker to allow visual and sound analysis. Most frequently, LEMG is recorded by transcutaneous placement of the recording needles. Only this approach is described in detail here. The patient is asked to assume a comfortable position with slightly reclined head, and if necessary, her/his larynx is locally anesthetized with lidocaine or tetracaine either applied transorally to the mucosal surface or with a transcutaneous intraluminal injection. Afterward the investigator inserts the electrodes into the laryngeal muscles. Both transdermal insertion with a concentric bipolar needle and transoral with hooked wire electrodes are possible, according to the patient's needs and the experience of examiner. Alternatively, during suspension laryngoscopy, hooked wire electrodes can be inserted into the vocalis/thyroarytenoid muscles (TA) and the m. cricoarytenoideus posterior/posterior cricoarytenoid muscle (PCA). When the sedation fades, respiration activity should become stronger, so that EMG activity from both muscles can be recorded simultaneously (Fig. 5.2). Examination usually starts with both TA, followed by examination of both cricothyroid muscles (CT), and may be extended to the PCA. Phonation is the agonistic maneuver for the TA and the antagonistic maneuver for the PCA. Forced sniffing inspiration is the antagonistic maneuver for the TA and the agonistic maneuver for the PCA. In case of BVFP and an acute flaccid palsy or in case of no regeneration, no activity can be recorded at least from the TA during phonation. In case of a synkinetic reinnervation, regeneration potential will be seen during agonistic and antagonistic maneuvers but not movement of the vocal folds. If the BVFI is not related to a nerve palsy but, for instance, to a fixation of the vocal fold by tumor or scar tissue, LEMG will show normal activity during agonistic maneuvers only and no or only little EMG activity during antagonistic maneuvers but no movements of the vocal fold.

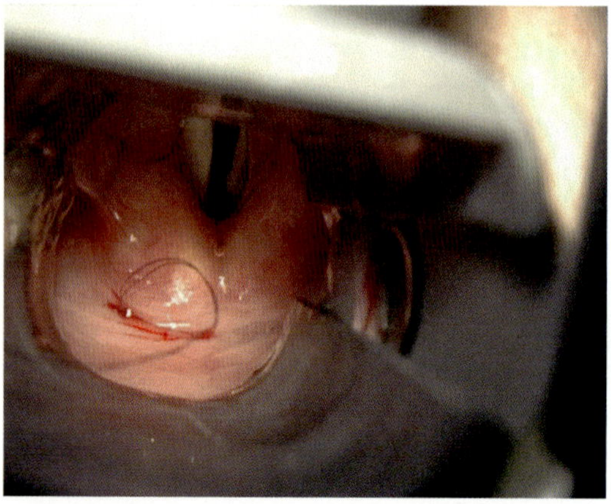

Fig. 5.2 During suspension laryngoscopy, hooked wire electrodes have been inserted into the left vocalis/thyroarytenoid muscles (TA) and the left m. cricoarytenoideus posterior/posterior cricoarytenoid muscle (PCA). Only the thin *black* wires remain in the larynx after retraction of the insertion tool. When the sedation fades, respiration activity should become stronger, so that EMG activity from both muscles can be recorded simultaneously

A new procedure is the electrical laryngeal stimulation as part of the diagnostic work-up in patients selected for laryngeal pacemaking (see Chap. 14). The electrical laryngeal stimulation can be applied on both PCAs to determine and to confirm the results of the LEMG performed and help to localize the optimal side (hot spot) for the surgery. During electrical laryngeal stimulation of the PCA, the stimulated vocal fold should show a movement. The stimulator used can be either a needle electrode inserted into the PCA or a surface electrode inserted postcricoidally during microlaryngoscopy in general anesthesia. For the application of the surface electrode, the investigator shall gain an optimal overview over the arytenoid cartilage as well as the entrance to the piriform recess by using either a flexible or rigid endoscope (Fig. 5.3). The hot spot for electrically evoked vocal fold abduction is located by inserting the surface electrode postcricoidally and applying continuous biphasic pulses of variable duration and amplitude. During this process, the Investigator may try different insertion angles and depths, as well as current rates (Video 5.1). A

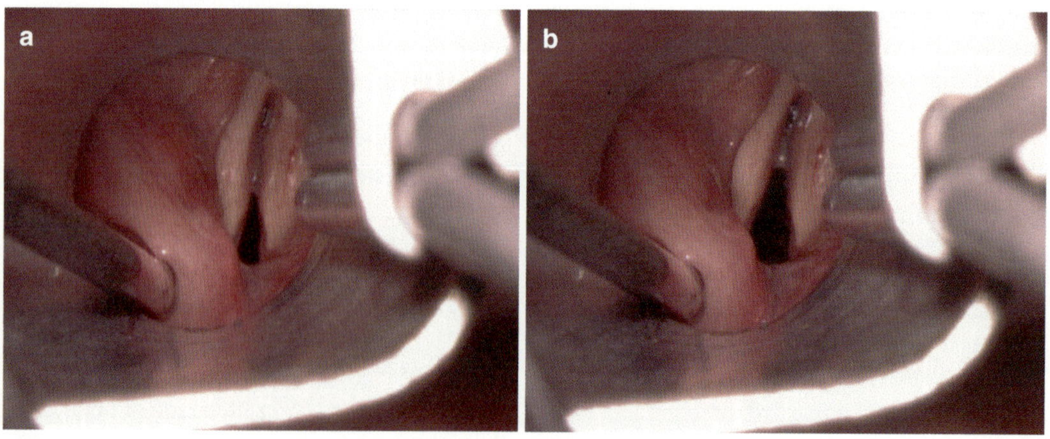

Fig. 5.3 For the application of the surface electrode, the investigator has directed the rigid laryngoscope toward the left arytenoid cartilage as well as the entrance to the piriform recess. The hot spot for electrically evoked vocal fold abduction is located by inserting the surface electrode postcricoidally and applying continuous biphasic pulses of variable duration and amplitude. (**a**) Setting without electrostimulation; (**b**) during electrostimulation causing an abduction of the left vocal fold

stimulation frequency below 30 Hz is recommended in order to detect movements of the arytenoid cartilage. In general, 2–3 mA should suffice to evoke visible vocal fold abduction. In order to affirm the hot spot and distinguish between evoked abduction and adduction, a stimulation frequency of 30 Hz should be applied.

5.3.10 Patient-Related Outcome Measures (PROM) and Quality of Life Assessments

The SF-36 is a well-known and validated instrument for the self-assessment of general health status, principally used to gather a generic measure of the burden of a disease [16]. Therefore, the SF-36 can also be applied in patients with BVFI. The SF-36 is a self-administered instrument. It can also be used to evaluate the efficacy of a specific treatment of patients with BVFI. Another general measurement tool of subject benefit, which can be used for surgically treated patients, is the Glasgow Benefit Inventory (GBI) [17]. Any improvement in her/his health status resulting from healthcare intervention is considered to be a subject's benefit. The GBI was developed to be subject-oriented and specifically accurate and sensitive in the evaluation of all kind of otolaryngological interventions. The GBI is also a self-administered instrument. In contrast to SF-36 and GBI, the Voice Handicap Index (VHI) is a specific voice and voice-related handicap assessment. The VHI is a test developed on the basis of subject survey studies for subjective evaluation of impairments of voice quality [18]. Subjects are asked to respond to questions about their voice problems, including loss of self-confidence because of impaired communication power and/or social rejection, and/or psychological problems, such as depression and self-isolation.

5.4 Therapy and Outcome

Standard therapy and outcome is described in an own chapter (see Chap. 13). A prospective clinical trial on standard surgical procedures for treatment of BVFI was published recently [19, 20]. New strategies as laryngeal pacing and reinnervation surgery are described in Chaps. 14 and 15, respectively.

5.4.1 Postoperative Care

Especially after transoral surgery, there is an increased risk for transient laryngeal swelling with dyspnea and swallowing problems. Typically, prednisolone (1.5 mg/kg body weight per day) is recommended directly at the end of surgery and the following days as long as needed against laryngeal swelling. Transoral laser surgery can lead, whether intended or not, to exposure or lesion of laryngeal cartilage and increased risk of cartilage infection. Therefore, a prophylactic antibiotic treatment (for instance, 1 g metamizole per day) can be recommended in such a situation.

References

1. Feehery JM, Pribitkin EA, Heffelfinger RN, Lacombe VG, Lee D, Lowry LD, et al. The evolving etiology of bilateral vocal fold immobility. J Voice. 2003;17(1):76–81.
2. Lesnik M, Thierry B, Blanchard M, Glynn F, Denoyelle F, Couloigner V, et al. Idiopathic bilateral vocal cord paralysis in infants: case series and literature review. Laryngoscope. 2015;125(7):1724–8.
3. Djugai S, Boeger D, Buentzel J, Esser D, Hoffmann K, Jecker P, et al. Chronic vocal cord palsy in Thuringia, Germany: a population-based study on epidemiology and outcome. Eur Arch Otorhinolaryngol. 2014;271(2):329–35.
4. Francis DO, Pearce EC, Ni S, Garrett CG, Penson DF. Epidemiology of vocal fold paralyses after total thyroidectomy for well-differentiated thyroid cancer in a Medicare population. Otolaryngol Head Neck Surg. 2014;150(4):548–57.
5. Enomoto K, Uchino S, Watanabe S, Enomoto Y, Noguchi S. Recurrent laryngeal nerve palsy during surgery for benign thyroid diseases: risk factors and outcome analysis. Surgery. 2014;155(3):522–8.
6. Murty GE, Shinkwin C, Gibbin KP. Bilateral vocal fold paralysis in infants: tracheostomy or not? J Laryngol Otol. 1994;108(4):329–31.
7. Sapundzhiev N, Lichtenberger G, Eckel HE, Friedrich G, Zenev I, Toohill RJ, et al. Surgery of adult bilateral vocal fold paralysis in adduction: history and trends. Eur Arch Otorhinolaryngol. 2008;265(12):1501–14.

8. Dejonckere PH, Bradley P, Clemente P, Cornut G, Crevier-Buchman L, Friedrich G, et al. A basic protocol for functional assessment of voice pathology, especially for investigating the efficacy of (phonosurgical) treatments and evaluating new assessment techniques. Guideline elaborated by the committee on phoniatrics of the European laryngological society (ELS). Eur Arch Otorhinolaryngol. 2001;258(2):77–82.
9. Ptok M, Schwemmle C, Iven C, Jessen M, Nawka T. On the auditory evaluation of voice quality. HNO. 2006;54(10):793–802.
10. Giner J, Plaza V, Rigau J, Sola J, Bolibar I, Sanchis J. Spirometric standards and patient characteristics: an exploratory study of factors affecting fulfillment in routine clinical practice. Respir Care. 2014;59(12):1832–7.
11. Criee CP, Baur X, Berdel D, Bosch D, Gappa M, Haidl P, et al. Standardization of spirometry: 2015 update. Published by German Atemwegsliga, German respiratory society and German Society of Occupational and Environmental Medicine. Pneumologie. 2015;69(3):147–64.
12. Lim SH, Lieu PK, Phua SY, Seshadri R, Venketasubramanian N, Lee SH, et al. Accuracy of bedside clinical methods compared with fiberoptic endoscopic examination of swallowing (FEES) in determining the risk of aspiration in acute stroke patients. Dysphagia. 2001;16(1):1–6.
13. Rosenbek JC, Robbins JA, Roecker EB, Coyle JL, Wood JL. A penetration-aspiration scale. Dysphagia. 1996;11(2):93–8.
14. Guyatt GH, Sullivan MJ, Thompson PJ, Fallen EL, Pugsley SO, Taylor DW, et al. The 6-minute walk: a new measure of exercise capacity in patients with chronic heart failure. Can Med Assoc J. 1985;132(8):919–23.
15. Laboratories ATSCoPSfCPF. ATS statement: guidelines for the six-minute walk test. Am J Respir Crit Care Med. 2002;166(1):111–7.
16. Ware JE Jr, Gandek B. Overview of the SF-36 health survey and the international quality of life assessment (IQOLA) project. J Clin Epidemiol. 1998;51(11):903–12.
17. Robinson K, Gatehouse S, Browning GG. Measuring patient benefit from otorhinolaryngological surgery and therapy. Ann Otol Rhinol Laryngol. 1996;105(6):415–22.
18. Jacobson BH, Johnson A, Grywalski C, Silbergleit A, Jacobson G, Benninger MS. The voice handicap index (VHI): development and validation. J Speech Lang Path. 1997;6:66–70.
19. Nawka T, Sittel C, Gugatschka M, Arens C, Lang-Roth R, Wittekindt C, et al. Permanent transoral surgery of bilateral vocal fold paralysis: a prospective multicenter trial. Laryngoscope. 2015;125(6):1401–8.
20. Nawka T, Sittel C, Arens C, Lang-Roth R, Wittekindt C, Hagen R, et al. Voice and respiratory outcomes after permanent transoral surgery of bilateral vocal fold paralysis. Laryngoscope. 2015;125(12):2749–55.

Vocal Cord Immobility: Central Origin

6

Gerd Fabian Volk and Orlando Guntinas-Lichius

Abstract

Vocal cord immobility of central origin, mainly as unilateral or less frequently as bilateral vocal cord palsy, is a rare symptom considering the incidence of central nervous system diseases. Theoretically, any cerebral or cerebellar disease affecting motor neurons or motor neuron pathways that are involved in laryngeal muscle movement may lead to vocal cord palsy. The most important causes are stroke, Parkinson's disease, and multiple system atrophy. These diseases and characteristic laryngeal findings are presented in detail in this chapter. The differentiation of vocal cord immobility of central origin and diseases like essential voice tremor and laryngeal dystonia is explained. Finally, a subchapter deals with the special situation of congenital vocal cord immobility of central origin. Treatment is dominated by the treatment of the underlying neurological disease. Nevertheless, as in vocal cord immobility of peripheral origin, modern phonosurgery plays an important role in the curative or palliative care of these patients.

6.1 Introduction

Movement of the vocal cords depends on complex neuromotor coordination (Fig. 6.1). The most important relay stations are the motor cortex, brainstem centers for the breathing pattern, reflex control, the vagal nerve with its branches to the larynx, and the neuromuscular terminals on the laryngeal muscles. In most cases a paralysis of the vocal fold is caused by a lesion of the vagal nerve or more precise mainly by a lesion of

Electronic Supplementary Material The online version of this chapter (doi:10.1007/978-3-319-61724-4_6) contains supplementary material, which is available to authorized users.

G.F. Volk
Department of Otorhinolaryngology,
Jena University Hospital, Jena, Germany

O. Guntinas-Lichius (✉)
Department of Otorhinolaryngology,
Institute of Phoniatry/Pedaudiology, Jena University Hospital, Jena, Germany
e-mail: orlando.guntinas@med.uni-jena.de

C. Sittel, O. Guntinas-Lichius (eds.), *Neurolaryngology*,
https://doi.org/10.1007/978-3-319-61724-4_6

the recurrent nerve (cf. Chaps. 3, 4, and 5). Such a vocal fold paralysis of the lower motor neuron type is typically characterized by a flaccid paralysis, muscle atrophy in the further course of disease, or defective healing in the case of spontaneous regeneration. In contrast, symptoms of vocal fold dysfunction of the upper motor neuron type, as an expression of a central nervous system disease, are much more variable. Typically, several components of voice production are affected because multiple cranial nerves might be affected (Table 6.1). The type of voice dysfunction can help to diagnose the underlying neurological disease (Table 6.2). Furthermore, in cases of laryngeal upper motor neuron-type disease, the symptoms are not restricted to the larynx and can be found in other parts of the body (Table 6.3). Spastic paralysis is a symptom of cerebral disorders. Resting tremor, dystonia, or rigidity of the laryngeal muscles is usually found in disorders affecting the basal ganglia. Cerebellar disorders can lead to intention tremor of the vocal folds and dysdiadochokinesis. Myoclonus and choreatic movements of the vocal folds are found irregularly and cannot be related to a specific central nervous system disease. When a vocal cord palsy is classified as idiopathic, it is worth investigating for a neurological disease, because approximately a quarter of these patients has or will develop a neurological disease in the next months [1].

In a wider sense, laryngeal dystonia also belongs to laryngeal upper motor neuron-type diseases (see Chap. 8). Beyond vocal fold paralysis, upper motor neuron disorders can also lead to dysphagia and other phonatory diseases. The most important types of vocal cord immobility due to central origin are presented in this chapter.

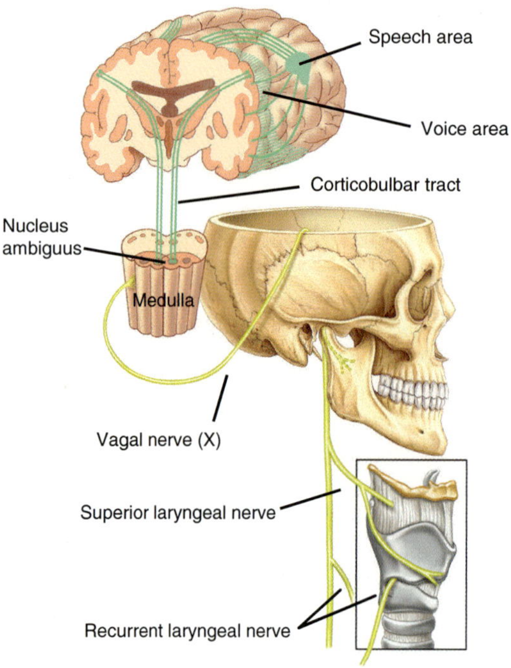

Fig. 6.1 Pathway of volitional phonation. The most important relay stations are the motor cortex, brainstem centers for the breathing pattern, reflex control, and the vagal nerve with its branches to the larynx

Table 6.1 Possible affected nerves in case of a central nervous system disease and related dysfunction of the larynx and the voice

Affected nerve	Affected organs/muscles	Related dysfunction
Phrenic nerve	Diaphragm, lungs	Impaired respiration
Vagal nerve (X)	Vocal folds	Impaired phonation, respiration, pitch changes
Facial nerve (VII) and vagal nerve (X)	Supraglottis, pharynx, oral cavity, nasal cavities	Impaired resonance, rhinophonia, disturbed articulation
Trigeminal nerve (V), facial nerve (VII), and hypoglossal nerve (XII)	Lips, cheeks, mandible, tongue	Disturbed articulation
Facial nerve (VII), glossopharyngeal nerve (IX), vagal nerve (X), and hypoglossal nerve (XII)	Oral cavity, pharynx, larynx	Dysphagia

Based on data from Ref. [7]

Table 6.2 Typical voice dysfunction and related neurological disease

Voice type	Characteristics	Disease localization	Possible etiologies	Comment
Flaccid	Slurred speech with weak voice	Lower motor neuron disease or laryngeal muscles	Stroke, bulbar palsy, myasthenia gravis	Vocal fatigue and combination with flaccid dysarthria are important hint for the differential diagnosis of myasthenia gravis
Spastic	Strained and strangled voice	Bilateral upper motor neuron disease	Pseudobulbar palsy, stroke, any kind of motor neuron disease	Differential diagnosis: Laryngeal dystonia
Ataxic	Slow speech rate, monopitch voice	Cerebellum	Cerebellar ataxia, multiple sclerosis	Symptoms must not be present constantly
Hypokinetic	Progressive deterioration of articulation, drop-off phases	Extrapyramidal neural paths	Parkinson's disease	Vocal fold bowing is typical
Hyperkinetic	Involuntary spastic-like movements, dysprosody	Extrapyramidal neural paths	Huntington's disease, myoclonus	Look for choreiform movements, dystonia, and dyskinesia
Mixed spastic-flaccid	Weak articulation, spastic voice with low volume	Combined upper and lower motor neuron disease	Amyotrophic lateral sclerosis	Can be combined with weakened respiratory support

Based on data from Ref. [7]

Table 6.3 Affected central nervous system region of upper motor neuron disease and related symptoms

Affected region	Symptom
Cerebrum	Spastic paresis, decreased agility
Basal ganglia	Resting tremor, dystonia, rigidity
Cerebellum	Intention tremor, dysdiadokinesis
Cortical and subcortical motor and sensory pathways	Vocal fold discoordination
Dento-olivary pathway	Myoclonus
Lateral medulla	Paresis, pharyngeal dysphasia, palatal incompetence, vertigo, facial pain, and Horner syndrome (Wallenberg syndrome)

Principally, the diagnostic work-up in children is not different to adults (see Chaps. 3 and 4). Therefore, diagnostics including electrophysiology (Chap. 1) are not presented in detail. In younger patients some investigations are only feasible with anesthesia. This might limit the significance of the investigation.

6.2 Stroke

Laryngeal manifestations of stroke via both direct and indirect mechanisms play a significant role in the morbidity and mortality of stroke (Videos 6.1 and 6.2). Airway protection, respiration, and phonation can be affected. Poststroke dysphagia and aspiration are topics of Chap. 11. Primary dysfunction of the larynx following stroke is often the result of an insult to the nucleus ambiguus and the nucleus solitarius. Insults to the cortical and subcortical pathways can result in loss of the laryngeal cough reflex [2]. Patients with hemispheric stroke show delayed laryngeal elevation and delayed laryngeal closure affecting the airway protection [3]. Stroke is an uncommon cause of vocal fold paralysis. In cases of stroke, an isolated vocal paralysis is uncommon [4]. In this setting, vocal fold paralysis is usually associated with a brainstem stroke, or lateral medullary syndrome (Wallenberg syndrome), which is characterized by severe pharyngeal dysphasia, palatal incompetence, vertigo, facial pain, and Horner syndrome [5]. Infarction of the nucleus ambiguus is usually related to occlusion of the posterior inferior cerebellar artery (PICA), which also results in lateral medullary infarction (Wallenberg syndrome). Infarction of the cortical and subcortical motor and sensory pathways may result in vocal fold incoordination rather than paresis or paralysis [6].

Laryngoscopy should be performed while the patient is at rest and during phonation. Dysphagia assessment is not presented here. The resting tone and position of the vocal folds should be noted. Involuntary motion of the vocal folds, including tremor, myoclonus, and spasm, should be identified. Laryngeal tremor is characterized by involuntary rhythmic movements of the vocal folds during rest and during phonation. In contrast to tremor, myoclonus is characterized by an abrupt, nonrhythmic nature of the movement, although slow (4–6 Hz) rhythmic movements may also be observed. Unilateral weakness of laryngeal mobility suggests a lower motor neuron lesion, whereas global weakness suggests upper motor neuron dysfunction. Motion-induced movement disorders (laryngeal dystonia) may also be observed. A supranuclear lesion may result in dysphonia without obvious vocal fold paralysis. In such a case, additional diagnostics are necessary for proper diagnosis. Although dysphonia must be differentiated from pure dysarthria, aphasia, or dyspraxia, phonatory dysfunction (frequently resulting from presbylarynx as many stroke patients are older than 60 years of age) is very common as a comorbid condition in patients with dysarthria [7].

Concerning prognosis, recovery from vascular insult to the motor innervation of the larynx is similar to that of other central nervous system motor deficits. The clinical consequences of vocal fold paralysis may range from none (asymptomatic) to airway obstruction that requires urgent tracheostomy [7].

6.3 Parkinson's Disease

Parkinson's disease is the most common movement disorder in patients older than 55 years of age. The disease is characterized by progressive degeneration of the brainstem nuclei, particularly the substantia nigra. Dysphonia can be the first presenting sign. Characteristic tremors (arm, leg, pill-rolling), rigidity, festinating gate, and slow initiation of movement are common. About 70–90% of the patients have voice difficulties. In about a third of these patients, the voice disorder is the most disabling part of the disease. Patients present with a typically soft, breathy, monotone voice. The voice is perceived by the patient to be of normal loudness. Additional components of Parkinson's dysphonia include voice tremor, poor articulation, variable rate, stuttering-like quality, difficulty initiating speech, and a "flat" effect [8].

Laryngoscopy and stroboscopy show that vocal fold bowing, midfold opening of the glottis on phonation, and slowed vibration are common characteristics. Glottal incompetence has been one of the most consistent findings described. Nowadays, if vocal fold immobility is present (in <5–10% of patients [9]), it is often considered a sign of a Parkinson's plus syndrome. Parkinson's plus syndromes include multisystem atrophy (see next Sect. 4), basal ganglia degeneration, and progressive supranuclear palsy. These disorders show rapidly progressive deterioration of motor function, with significantly worse speech deficits. Laryngeal electromyography findings demonstrate a decreased firing rate and increased variability of the interspike interval of single laryngeal motor units in older males only. This is a possible contributing factor to the pathophysiology of Parkinson's dysphonia.

Standard Parkinson's treatment with L-dopa has had mixed results in dysphonia. Sanabria et al. showed decreased jitter and increased fundamental frequency in a mildly affected population, but other investigators have shown no statistical improvement [10]. Deep brain stimulation has shown limited improvement in voice and speech function despite significant changes in limb movements [11]. Despite the many therapies tried, only behavioral therapy has shown a sustained beneficial effect on the voice and speech function of patients with Parkinson's disease [9].

6.4 Multiple System Atrophy

Multiple system atrophy (MSA) is a degenerative neurological disorder with a typical age of onset in the late 50s to early 60s [12]. The cause is unknown. The main symptoms of MSA are movement and balance disturbances. Often autonomic functions such as bladder control or blood pressure regulation are affected. MSA often presents with some of the same symptoms as Parkinson's disease (see above Sect. 3), but MSA does not show a significant response to dopamine medication. MSA is characterized by a slowness of the initiation of movements (like in Parkinson's disease), i.e., in the larynx by slowness of vocal cord movement (mimicking a vocal cord palsy). Like in Parkinson's disease, the patients can also show signs of muscle rigidity, tremor, and/or ataxia. Additionally, MSA patients present with symptoms of autonomic dysfunction (p.e. dysregulation of body temperature due to sweating deficiency, dry mouth and skin). In the past, the term Shy–Drager syndrome was sometimes used when autonomic dysfunction predominated. This term should not be used anymore, given terminology changes. In rare cases, the patients have a vocal cord paralysis. Even bilateral vocal ford paralysis has been recognized in patients with MSA [13]. Other typical otorhinolaryngological symptoms are loud snoring, sleep apnea, abnormal breathing, or inspiratory stridor during sleep. Therefore, work-up should also include polysomnography [13].

Laryngoscopy shows vocal cord bowing and glottic incompetence, and open-phase configuration is shown on stroboscopy. Frequently, the vocal folds cannot abduct past the paramedian position, but adduction may be normal [13].

Primary medical treatment of MSA is similar to Parkinson's disease although the efficacy is much lower. Patients with sleep-related disorders may respond to continuous positive or bi-level airway pressure therapy. In case of bilateral vocal ford paralysis, especially when combined with a severe sleep-related disorder, a tracheotomy might be necessary.

6.5 Other Central Nervous System Diseases

Amyotrophic lateral sclerosis (ALS) is an idiopathic and progressive degeneration of upper and lower motor neurons, with muscle wasting, fasciculations, and weakness [14]. Vocal cord dysfunction, including hoarseness and stridor, may be part of the clinical picture of ALS. Unilateral or bilateral vocal cord palsy in ALS patients is described in the literature but is rare in onset [15]. Multiple sclerosis (MS) is a diffuse autoimmune inflammatory disease of the central nervous system resulting in demyelination. The specific symptoms depend on the portions of the brain or spinal cord that are affected. Therefore, MS can present as an upper and/or lower motor neuron disease, but vocal fold immobility is a rare event [16]. Guillain–Barré syndrome (GBS), also known as acute idiopathic polyneuritis, is the most common acquired demyelinating neuropathy. It is characterized by muscular weakness and mild distal sensory loss [17]. However, unilateral or bilateral vocal fold immobility is a rare occurrence. In contrast to the fatal course in ALS or MS, GBS patients show a full recovery in two thirds of all cases within several weeks or up to 2 years. Therefore, if surgery is planned for treatment, transient or reversible methods should be favored for GBS patients.

6.6 Important Differential Diagnoses: Essential Voice Tremor and Laryngeal Dystonia

Essential voice tremor and laryngeal dystonia (details in Chap. 8) are not characterized by vocal cord immobility. However, both diseases can be confused with vocal cord immobility.

The type of essential voice tremor is important in the differential diagnosis of movement disorders of the larynx caused by a central nervous disease. Essential voice tremor is the phonatory manifestation of essential tremor; an age-related disease of involuntary movement [18]. Essential tremor is among the most common adult-onset movement disorders [8]. The pathophysiology is not well understood. The tremor may be mild enough to go unnoticed in many of the persons affected [18]. In many cases, the disease is an inherited and autosomal dominant disorder. The other cases are of sporadic origin [19]. The tremor occurs during voluntary movement (so-called kinetic tremor), and often to some degree with posture holding (so-called postural tremor), without task-specific characteristics. Tremor at rest, which occurs when the affected body part is in repose and completely supported against gravity, is far less common but can occur in up to 20% of clinic-derived cases and in particular in cases of long-standing or severe disease. Essential tremor begins insidiously and progresses at a variable rate but generally slowly [20]. Most commonly, the tremor begins in the upper extremities, i.e., the tremor does not begin in the larynx. A tremor frequency of 4–10 Hz is considered characteristic, but there is some overlap with enhanced physiologic tremor (8–12 Hz) and intention tremor (2–5 Hz). Symptoms of laryngeal dystonia may also include a tremor component. This might be the reason why some cases of essential voice tremor are misdiagnosed as laryngeal dystonia. Laryngeal dystonia is characterized by irregular, nonperiodic vocal fold movements.

Laryngoscopy shows that essential tremor affects the whole phonatory apparatus, albeit variably from patient to patient. The extension of involuntary motion beyond the muscles of the vocal folds is typical. This is also the reason why it is better to use the term "essential voice tremor" instead of "laryngeal tremor" or "vocal cord tremor."

The first line of treatment of essential tremor is pharmacologic. Propranolol and primidone are first-line treatments [18]. Botulinum toxin treatment is not as effective as in laryngeal dystonia.

6.7 Congenital Vocal Cord Immobility of Central Origin

Vocal fold immobility in children can result from birth trauma, central nervous system abnormalities, or surgical trauma, which is often related to the repair of congenital heart anomalies [21]. Therefore, the left side is affected more frequently than the right side. Vocal fold immobility in children accounts for approximately 10% of all congenital laryngeal abnormalities. This is second to laryngomalacia [22]. The Arnold–Chiari malformation is the most classic central nervous system disease associated with bilateral vocal fold palsy. The key symptom of congenital vocal cord immobility in children is stridor. The children also typically show increased work of breathing, hoarseness, and/or an impaired cough reflex leading to aspiration (depending on laterality of the paralyzed vocal folds and laryngeal muscles affected) [23]. It is usually secondary to an impairment of the nerve supply to the larynx. This impairment can be congenital or acquired (e.g., iatrogenic, neurologic insults, or systemic muscular diseases). Oftentimes, laryngeal paralysis is labeled as idiopathic because an etiology cannot be elicited [24]. The immobility can be unilateral or bilateral, with the presentation varying accordingly. Moreover, the disease can affect the laryngeal abductors and/or adductors.

In very young children, the diagnosis is made with bedside flexible laryngoscopy. Direct suspension laryngoscopy might be needed to rule out vocal fold fixation and comorbid conditions, for instance, a laryngotracheomalacia. If laryngeal EMG is not possible in the alert patient, surgery can be combined with intraoperative EMG. Cerebral MRI is mandatory in all cases of bilateral paralysis to diagnose underlying neurologic diseases.

Spontaneous recovery of vocal cord immobility in children is more common than in adults. Nevertheless, the etiology and the results of electrophysiological testing give the most reliable prognosis (see Chap. 1).

6.8 Treatment

Principally, the underlying central nervous system disease should be treated. Normally, this will also have an impact on the voice disorder. Further symptomatic medical and surgical treatment shall be considered in the two following sections.

6.8.1 Medical Treatment

Medical treatment is performed, if possible, according to the underlying neurological disease. Unfortunately, a medical treatment of the underlying disease is rarely possible. An exception is in Parkinson's disease. In Parkinson's disease the first line of treatment to improve the laryngeal functions is the standard Parkinson's treatment to improve the general condition of the patient. However, the effect on vocal fold function is not as good as for other Parkinson's symptoms. In most cases, for instance, in stroke patients or degenerative disorders like ALS, a specific medical treatment for the laryngeal symptoms is not available.

6.8.2 Surgical Treatment

As in vocal fold immobility of other origin, the selection of the optimal surgical procedure depends on several factors. The most important factors are emergency or elective surgery, unilateral or bilateral disease, prognosis, and the wishes of the patient. Age itself is not a predominant factor, as the principles of surgery are valid for adults as for children [21]. Surgery might be indicated for curative or palliative purposes [25].

In the rare cases of bilateral vocal fold paralysis due to central origin, the surgical therapy is the same as for bilateral cases of other origin; in urgent cases, a tracheostomy may be necessary. Posterior laser cordotomy, arytenoidectomy, and suture lateralization of the arytenoid cartilage are three standard surgical options that are available to attempt decannulation or to prevent tracheostomy (see also Chaps. 5 and 13 for surgical details). Each of these procedures is used in an attempt to provide an adequate posterior glottic airway, with continued anterior glottic closure for phonation. The results in cases of central origin are principally no different to cases of peripheral origin. Limiting factors might be the comorbidity and other neurological symptoms.

Patients who have dysphonia due to unilateral vocal fold paralysis for less than 6 months are candidates for vocal fold injection thyroplasty [26]. The techniques are the same as those used for unilateral palsy due to peripheral origin (details of the surgical technique in Chap. 4). If it is clear that the lesion will be permanent, medialization thyroplasty may be performed at any time as a first-choice surgery. Otherwise, for patients whose paralysis lasts 12 months or more or for patients with no evidence of electrical recovery on electromyography after 6 months, medialization thyroplasty and arytenoid repositioning procedures are indicated. Again, the technique is the same as for unilateral palsy due to peripheral origin (details of the surgical technique in Chaps. 4 and 12).

Literature on results of phonosurgery for unilateral or bilateral vocal fold immobility due to central origin is very limited. Due to the underlying neurological diseases, it seems that the effectiveness in general is not as high as after surgery in patients with palsies of peripheral origin [27].

References

1. Urquhart AC, St Louis EK. Idiopathic vocal cord palsies and associated neurological conditions. Arch Otolaryngol Head Neck Surg. 2005;131(12):1086–9.
2. Addington WR, Stephens RE, Widdicombe JG, Rekab K. Effect of stroke location on the laryngeal cough reflex and pneumonia risk. Cough. 2005;1:4.
3. Power ML, Hamdy S, Singh S, Tyrrell PJ, Turnbull I, Thompson DG. Deglutitive laryngeal closure in stroke patients. J Neurol Neurosurg Psychiatry. 2007;78(2):141–6.

4. Senatorov VV, Satpute S, Perry K, Kaylie DM, Cole JW. Aphonia induced by simultaneous bilateral ischemic infarctions of the putamen nuclei: a case report and review of the literature. J Med Case Rep. 2013;7:83.
5. Venketasubramanian N, Seshadri R, Chee N. Vocal cord paresis in acute ischemic stroke. Cerebrovasc Dis. 1999;9(3):157–62.
6. Ishibashi A, Fujishima I. Lesion of the nucleus solitarius leads to impaired laryngeal sensation in bulbar palsy patients. J Stroke Cerebrovasc Dis. 2012;21(3):174–80.
7. Altman KW, Schaefer SD, Yu GP, Hertegard S, Lundy DS, Blumin JH, et al. The voice and laryngeal dysfunction in stroke: a report from the neurolaryngology subcommittee of the American academy of otolaryngology-head and neck surgery. Otolaryngol Head Neck Surg. 2007;136(6):873–81.
8. Merati AL, Heman-Ackah YD, Abaza M, Altman KW, Sulica L, Belamowicz S. Common movement disorders affecting the larynx: a report from the neurolaryngology committee of the AAO-HNS. Otolaryngol Head Neck Surg. 2005;133(5):654–65.
9. Blumin JH, Pcolinsky DE, Atkins JP. Laryngeal findings in advanced Parkinson's disease. Ann Otol Rhinol Laryngol. 2004;113(4):253–8.
10. Sanabria J, Ruiz PG, Gutierrez R, Marquez F, Escobar P, Gentil M, et al. The effect of levodopa on vocal function in Parkinson's disease. Clin Neuropharmacol. 2001;24(2):99–102.
11. Kompoliti K, Wang QE, Goetz CG, Leurgans S, Raman R. Effects of central dopaminergic stimulation by apomorphine on speech in Parkinson's disease. Neurology. 2000;54(2):458–62.
12. Ozawa T, Paviour D, Quinn NP, Josephs KA, Sangha H, Kilford L, et al. The spectrum of pathological involvement of the striatonigral and olivopontocerebellar systems in multiple system atrophy: clinicopathological correlations. Brain. 2004;127(Pt 12):2657–71.
13. Blumin JH, Berke GS. Bilateral vocal fold paresis and multiple system atrophy. Arch Otolaryngol Head Neck Surg. 2002;128(12):1404–7.
14. Woodson G. Management of neurologic disorders of the larynx. Ann Otol Rhinol Laryngol. 2008;117(5):317–26.
15. Bigliardi G, Malaguti MC, Sola P, Georgoulopoulou E, Tondelli M, Barbi F, et al. Bilateral vocal cord paralysis: a rare onset of amyotrophic lateral sclerosis. Arch Neurol. 2010;67(7):897–8. author reply 8-9
16. Rontal E, Rontal M, Wald J, Rontal D. Botulinum toxin injection in the treatment of vocal fold paralysis associated with multiple sclerosis: a case report. J Voice. 1999;13(2):274–9.
17. Yoskovitch A, Enepekides DJ, Hier MP, Black MJ. Guillain-Barre syndrome presenting as bilateral vocal cord paralysis. Otolaryngol Head Neck Surg. 2000;122(2):269–70.
18. Sulica L, Louis ED. Clinical characteristics of essential voice tremor: a study of 34 cases. Laryngoscope. 2010;120(3):516–28.
19. Elble RJ. Diagnostic criteria for essential tremor and differential diagnosis. Neurology. 2000;54(11 Suppl 4):S2–6.
20. Cohen O, Pullman S, Jurewicz E, Watner D, Louis ED. Rest tremor in patients with essential tremor: prevalence, clinical correlates, and electrophysiologic characteristics. Arch Neurol. 2003;60(3):405–10.
21. Gardner GM, Altman JS, Balakrishnan G. Pediatric vocal fold medialization with silastic implant: intraoperative airway management. Int J Pediatr Otorhinolaryngol. 2000;52(1):37–44.
22. Dedo DD. Pediatric vocal cord paralysis. Laryngoscope. 1979;89(9 Pt 1):1378–84.
23. Bathini L, Jomah M, Krajacic A, Jeffery C, Campbell S, El-Hakim H. Acquired bilateral adductor laryngeal paralysis in neonates and children: a case series and a systematic review. Int J Pediatr Otorhinolaryngol. 2014;78(11):1866–9.
24. King EF, Blumin JH. Vocal cord paralysis in children. Curr Opin Otolaryngo Head Neck Surg. 2009;17(6):483–7.
25. Cohen SM, Elackattu A, Noordzij JP, Walsh MJ, Langmore SE. Palliative treatment of dysphonia and dysarthria. Otolaryngol Clin N Am. 2009;42(1):107–21.
26. Hill AN, Jankovic J, Vuong KD, Donovan D. Treatment of hypophonia with collagen vocal cord augmentation in patients with parkinsonism. Mov Disord. 2003;18(10):1190–2.
27. Sinclair CF, Gurey LE, Brin MF, Stewart C, Blitzer A. Surgical management of airway dysfunction in Parkinson's disease compared with Parkinson-plus syndromes. Ann Otol Rhinol Laryngol. 2013;122(5):294–8.

Thyroid and Parathyroid Surgery Intraoperative Nerve Monitoring and Management of Iatrogenic Vocal Cord Paralysis

7

Ricard Simo, Iain J. Nixon, and Enyinnaya Ofo

Abstract

Thyroid and parathyroid surgeries are common procedures undertaken worldwide by a variety of surgeons ranging from highly specialised endocrine and head-and-neck surgeons in high-volume centres to surgeons in district general hospitals.

Recurrent laryngeal nerve (RLN) injury is a well-known and serious complication of thyroid and parathyroid surgery and can lead to serious consequences in addition to important medicolegal implications.

The general basic principles of thyroid and parathyroid surgery include the removal of the involved pathological tissue, with preservation of the functioning vital structures including the external branch of the superior laryngeal nerve (EBSLN) and the recurrent laryngeal nerve (RLN).

Over the years surgeons have developed strategies to avoid damage of above-mentioned anatomical structures culminating in the development of intraoperative neuromonitoring (IONM). Despite of the use of IONM, the rate of recurrent laryngeal nerve palsy (RLNP) is clearly underestimated. The true rate varies widely according to the method of laryngeal examination. The average incidence of temporary RLNP following thyroid surgery is 9.8% with a 2.3% rate of permanent RLNP.

The risk factors for RLNP include malignant histology, neck dissection and revision surgery. Additionally it appears that high-volume departments doing more than 150 thyroid procedures per year seem to perform significantly better.

R. Simo (✉)
Otorhinolaryngology Head and Neck Surgery, Guy's and St Thomas' Hospital NHS Foundation Trust, Guy's Hospital, St. Thomas' Street, London SE1 9RT, UK
e-mail: ricardsimo1@icloud.com; ricard.simo@gstt.nhs.uk

I.J. Nixon
Otorhinolaryngology/Head and Neck Surgery, NHS Lothian/Edinburgh University, Lauriston Building, Lauriston Place, Edinburgh, UK

E. Ofo
Department of Otorhinolaryngology Head and Neck Surgery, St George's University Hospital, Blackshaw Road, London, London, SW17 0QT, UK

C. Sittel, O. Guntinas-Lichius (eds.), *Neurolaryngology*, https://doi.org/10.1007/978-3-319-61724-4_7

This chapter addresses the principles of thyroid and parathyroid surgery as applied to the intraoperative management of the RLN, the pre- and postoperative laryngeal evaluation in thyroid and parathyroid surgery, the surgical anatomy of the EBSLN and RLN nerves, identification and preservation of these nerves during thyroid and parathyroid surgery, intraoperative neuromonitoring of both nerves and the intraoperative management of the injured nerve during thyroid and parathyroid surgery. It also addresses the general principles of managing recurrent laryngeal nerve paralysis.

7.1 Introduction and Principles of Thyroid and Parathyroid Surgery

Thyroid and parathyroid pathology is very common. Thyroid and parathyroid surgeries are common procedures undertaken worldwide by a variety of surgeons ranging from highly specialised endocrine and head-and-neck surgeons in high-volume centres to either ear, nose and throat or general surgeons in district general hospitals.

Recurrent laryngeal nerve (RLN) injury is a well-known and serious complication of thyroid and parathyroid surgery and can lead to significant morbidity and even mortality as well as have important medicolegal implications [1].

The general basic principles of thyroid surgery include the removal of thyroid tissue either in the form of lobectomy or total thyroidectomy, with preservation of the functioning vital structures including the external branch of the superior laryngeal nerve (EBSLN), the recurrent laryngeal nerve (RLN) and the parathyroid glands.

In the case of parathyroid surgery, the main principle of the surgery is to remove the affected parathyroid gland or glands with the preservation of the RLN.

Over the years surgeons have developed various strategies to avoid damage of the abovementioned anatomical structures including leaving a cuff of thyroid tissue next to the RLN and the parathyroid glands. However this surgical technique is no longer advisable as this may cause significant problems in the event that revision thyroid surgery is required.

The rate of recurrent laryngeal nerve palsy (RLNP) is clearly underestimated. The true rate varied widely according to the method used for laryngeal examination. In a recent review of 27 articles and 25,000 patients, the average incidence of temporary RLNP after thyroid surgery was 9.8%, and the incidence of permanent RLNP was 2.3%. The rate of RLNP varied according to the method of examining the larynx and ranged from 26% to 2.3%. The best method of laryngeal examination is currently through the use of flexible nasal fibre-optic laryngoscopy [2].

The risk factors for RLP include malignant histology, neck dissection and previous performed surgery. Additionally it appears that high-volume departments doing more than 150 thyroid procedures per year have significantly lower complication rates [1].

This chapter addresses the management of the RLN in the preoperative, intraoperative and postoperative setting, intraoperative neuromonitoring (IONM) and its iatrogenic injury.

7.2 Pre and Postoperative Laryngeal Evaluation in Thyroid and Parathyroid Surgery

Pre and postoperative laryngeal examination is imperative when performing thyroid or parathyroid surgery. There are several clinical reasons in favour of a laryngeal examination.

7.2.1 Preoperative Evaluation

Preoperative voice symptoms or a normal voice is not a reliable indicator of RLN function with a sensitivity ranging from 33% to 68%. This is especially true in patients with long-standing pathology or those that have had previous thyroid or neck surgery many years prior, given that compensatory mechanisms may have stabilised the voice.

Preoperative recognition of RLNP is an essential element for the planning of the surgical procedure especially in those cases with malignant extra-thyroidal invasion. In addition evidence of intact preoperative laryngeal function is essential from the medicolegal perspective.

For the same reasons, to offer patients an adequate standard of care, evidence of pre- and postoperative function is essential. Knowing that there has been nerve injury, clinicians should then adopt a more proactive approach to the management of these injuries that may produce better outcomes [2].

7.2.2 Postoperative Evaluation

Voice changes are common following thyroid and parathyroid surgery. These are often caused by oedema of the larynx due to the placement of the endotracheal tube during surgery, postsurgical venous congestion of the larynx and not necessarily by injury to the RLN. The main reason for postoperative evaluation as already stated is accurate visualisation of the vocal cords and their function and therefore provides the measurement of one of the main outcomes of surgery.

The postoperative evaluation also provides functional information that allows accurate correlation with the interpretation of the EMG during neuromonitoring of the RLN. Finally, RLP has implications for safety of swallowing and of future contralateral surgery.

Guidance across the world has been varied. However recent reliable guidance has suggested a more proactive approach recommending pre- and postoperative evaluation in all thyroid and parathyroid surgery procedures.

7.3 Surgical Anatomy of the Superior and Recurrent Laryngeal Nerves

7.3.1 Superior Laryngeal Nerve (SLN)

The SLN is one of the first branches of the vagus nerve. It has branches from the vagus at the nodose ganglion (inferior ganglion), approximately 4 cm above the carotid bifurcation. The SLN divides 1.5 cm caudally into two branches, the internal and the external branch (EBSLN). The EBSLN continues in a caudal course, then crosses the carotid sheath medially and then goes into the larynx. Its length is variable ranging from 8.0 to 8.9 cm, and the entry into the larynx varies depending on its relationship with the superior thyroid vessels and the upper border of the superior thyroid pole [3] (Fig. 7.1).

In 1992 Cernea [4] classified the EBSLN into three types:

Type 1: Nerve crossing the superior thyroid vessels 1 cm or more above a horizontal plane passing through the upper border of the superior thyroid pole

Type 2a: Nerve crossing the vessels less than 1 cm above the aforementioned horizontal plane

Type 2b: Nerve below the plane

It is obvious that type 2b nerves are most at risk of iatrogenic injury; however, in most cadaveric studies, up to 68% of nerves appear to be

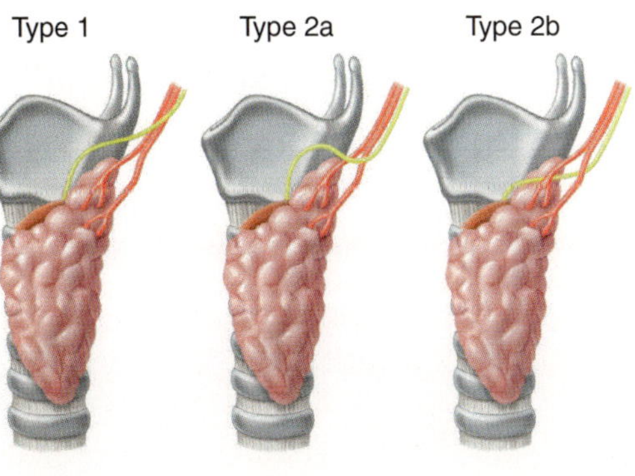

Fig. 7.1 Cernea's classification of the external branch of the superior laryngeal nerve (EBSLN)

type 1 nerves. Over the past two decades, several authors have published other EBSLN classifications; however Cernea's one has been the most commonly accepted by most surgeons [5, 6].

However Morton et al., in a recent review article, have criticised all these EBSLN classifications indicating that they have failed to provide an adequate anatomic landmark to safely identify and protect the EBRL from injury [7].

7.3.2 Recurrent Laryngeal Nerve (RLN)

The RLN is a branch of the vagus nerve. As the heart descents during embryological development, the RLN on the left is dragged down by the aortic arch; however, on the right, it remains high around the subclavian artery (Fig. 7.2).

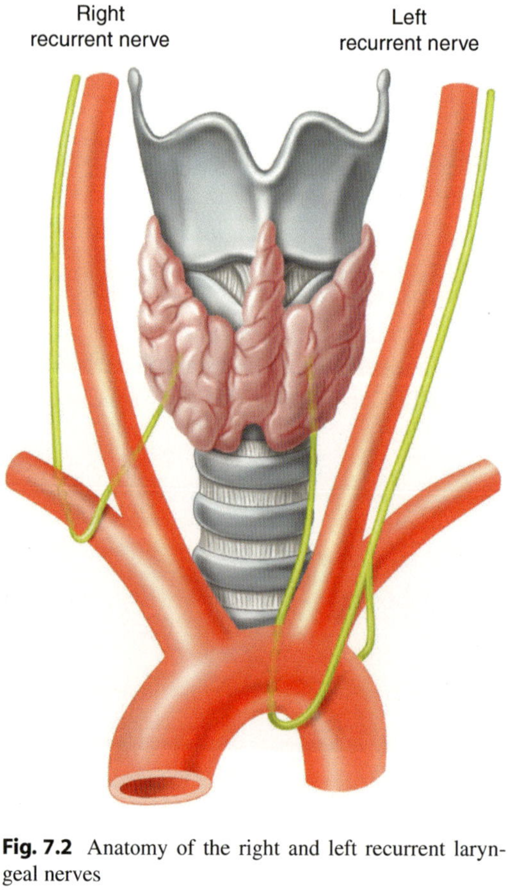

Fig. 7.2 Anatomy of the right and left recurrent laryngeal nerves

7.3.3 Right Recurrent Laryngeal Nerve

As indicated the right RLN loops round the subclavian artery and enters the base of the neck at the thoracic inlet in a more lateral oblique direction.

7.3.4 Left Recurrent Laryngeal Nerve

The left RLN loops around the aortic arch just lateral to the obliterated ductus arteriosus and ascends along the tracheo-oesophageal groove before its entry in the larynx at the level of the cricothyroid joint. It has been noted that typically the left RLN forms an angle of between 15 and 30° relative to the trachea, but the right RLN appears to cross the neck in a more oblique angle [8].

Hisham et al. found that in 60% of cases, the nerve on both sides is located in the tracheo-oesophageal groove, 5% more lateral to the trachea and 28% directly posterior to the thyroid lobe [9].

7.3.5 Recurrent Laryngeal Nerve Extra-Laryngeal Branching

Although most RLNs are single, up to 30% of nerves can branch before entering the larynx, and this may lead to higher risk of injury [10, 11] (Fig. 7.3).

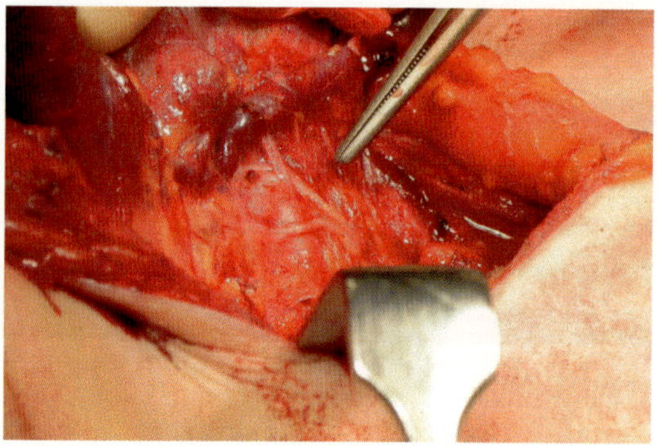

Fig. 7.3 Extra-laryngeal branching of the right RLN

7.4 Identification and Preservation of the Superior and Recurrent Laryngeal Nerves During Thyroid and Parathyroid Surgery

As stated the identification and preservation of the external branch of the superior laryngeal nerve (EBSLN) and the recurrent laryngeal nerves (RLN) during thyroid and parathyroid surgery are essential. In every thyroidectomy, an attempt should be made to identify the RLN. Without this attention to detail, injury rates may be unacceptably high.

7.4.1 Management of the EBSLN

This is done during the dissection of the superior pole. The external branch of the superior laryngeal nerve should be identified whenever possible [4, 12, 13]. This is done at the sternothyrolaryngeal or Joll's triangle which is delimited by the superior thyroid pedicle and upper lobe of the gland, the cricothyroid muscle and the lower edge of the thyroid cartilage (Fig. 7.4).

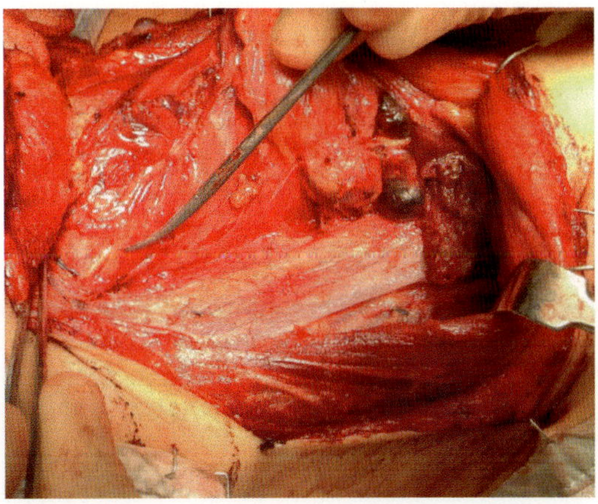

Fig. 7.4 External branch of right superior laryngeal nerve

7.4.2 Management of the RLN

The position of the recurrent laryngeal nerve varies depending on the side as previously described in the anatomy section.

7.4.2.1 Lateral Approach

The nerve is usually identified in the Beahrs' triangle, which is located in the lateral lower part of the neck. This triangle is defined by the inferior thyroid artery superiorly, the trachea medially and the common carotid artery laterally. Once the nerve is identified, this is dissected in a cranial direction tunnelling the tissue surrounding the nerve and gradually dissecting the thyroid tissue from its medial side. This is the most common and safest way of identifying the RLN (Fig. 7.9) [14] (Fig. 7.5).

7.4.2.2 Superior Approach

The nerve can be identified at the level of the cricothyroid junction at its entry in the larynx. This approach can be very useful in cancer patients with extensive nodal disease, re-operative surgery, when other approaches have failed and when considering a nonrecurrent laryngeal nerve. Once the nerve is identified, this should be dissected in a caudal direction tunnelling the tissue surrounding the nerve with a mosquito fine-tip dissector. The tissue above the tunnel is then diathermised with bipolar diathermy and divided (Fig. 7.6) [14].

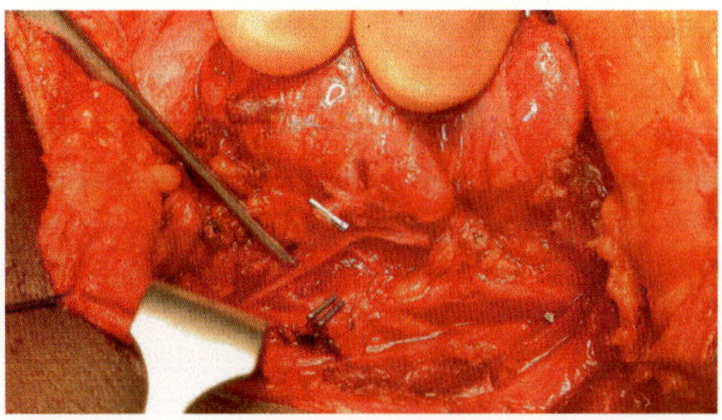

Fig. 7.5 Identification of the left RLN via a lateral approach once the inferior thyroid artery has been divided

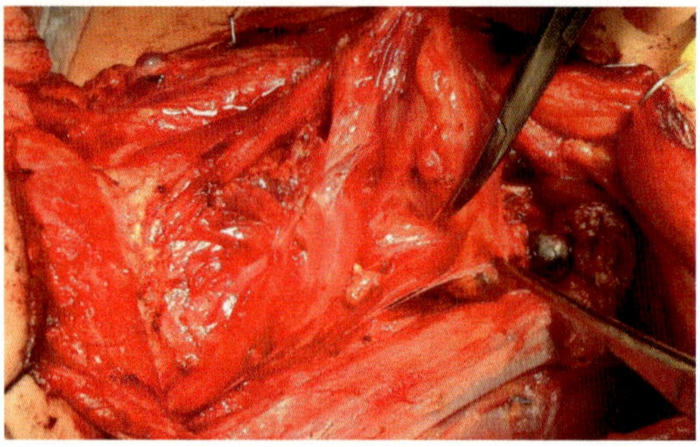

Fig. 7.6 Identification of the right RLN using a superior approach. The mosquito forceps indicates the position of the nerve at its entry in the cricothyroid joint

7.4.2.3 Inferior Approach

In large goitres or revision surgery, an inferior approach can be used. This allows for identification of the nerve in a virgin site (Fig. 7.7) [14].

Having identified the nerve, there is usually no need for it to be traced for any great distance. With experience, the surgeon will come to recognise the importance of the relationship between the level of Berry's ligament and the nerve. In patients with a low Berry's ligament, which sits posterior on the trachea, the nerve will be in close proximity to the gland at this crucial point. In these cases the nerve must be carefully traced and the gland mobilized off the nerve. When the Berry's ligament is high, the nerve is often quite laterally placed in comparison, and minimal dissection will be required. This minimises the chance of inadvertent injury.

Nonrecurrent RLN occurs in 2–3% of patients and is invariably present on the right side. Preoperative imaging, which identifies situs inversus, or more commonly a retro-oesophageal subclavian artery, may raise the index of suspicion. If the RLN cannot be identified in the traditional position, the surgeon must consider the possibility of a nonrecurrent nerve. This structure will be running inferomedially from the vagus nerve and will be wide in comparison with a normal RLN (Fig. 7.8).

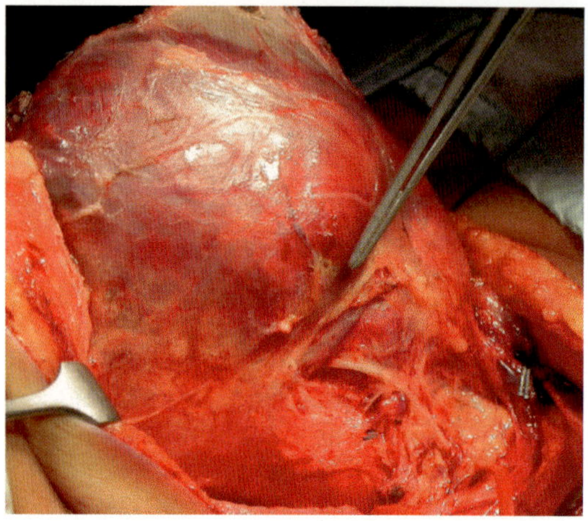

Fig. 7.7 Identification of the right RLN using an inferior approach

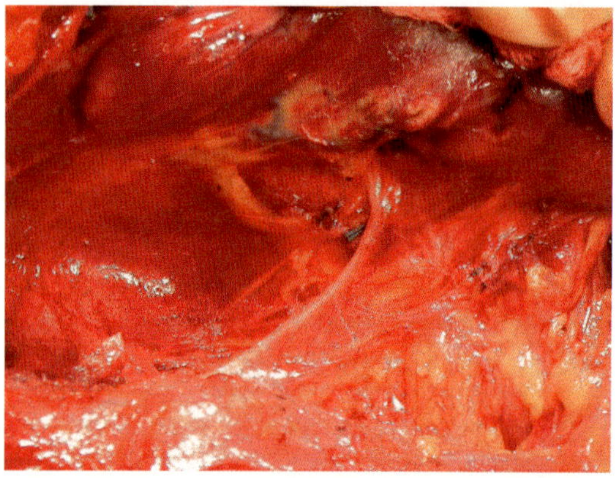

Fig. 7.8 Right nonrecurrent RLN

7.5 Intraoperative Monitoring of the Superior and Recurrent Laryngeal Nerves

The RLN and ESBLN are at risk of iatrogenic injury during thyroidectomy given their close anatomical relationship to the thyroid and parathyroid glands. Despite appropriate surgical training and experience, these nerves may be difficult to identify and protect intraoperatively, especially in cases of invasive thyroid cancer, large goitres or revision surgery. Intraoperative neuromonitoring (IONM) is a useful aid for localising and monitoring the electrophysiological status of the RLN and EBSLN during surgery; however routine use of IONM remains controversial, as will be discussed later.

Current guidelines recommend definitive visual identification of the RLN and EBSLN during thyroid surgery being this the most reliable method of reducing the rate of injury [15, 16]. Historical surgical training promoted complete avoidance of the RLN as a means of preventing nerve injury. However, following descriptions of newer surgical techniques over 70 years ago [17, 18], during which an attempt was made to systematically recognise the RLN, visual nerve identification became an acceptable practice. Further supporting evidence for routine RLN visualisation to prevent iatrogenic injury comes from Hermann et al. [19] who compared two historical cohorts (of over 26,000 patients) undergoing thyroidectomy for benign disease, from a period when RLN identification was not performed (1979–1990), to more recent times (1991–1998), when RLN visualisation was routine practice, and the authors demonstrated that the rate of permanent RLN palsy was significantly lower with RLN identification (0.4%) versus non-identification (1.1%).

In spite of relatively low rates of permanent vocal fold paralysis with RLN visualisation alone during thyroidectomy (i.e. <2%) [20], the negative impact on laryngeal function [21–24] and the medicolegal implications [25, 26] of vocal fold paralysis have prompted thyroid surgeons to seek further reductions in the incidence of RLN injury, through the use of surgical adjuncts such as IONM. Notwithstanding the purported benefits, several studies over the past 20 years have failed to demonstrate an obvious statistically significant difference in the rates of permanent vocal fold paralysis when comparing routine use of IONM versus visual RLN identification alone [20, 27–29], a result that was confirmed in a recent systematic review of 42 studies and over 64,000 nerves at risk [30]. With the lack of strong evidence for a clinical advantage of IONM in thyroid surgery, the additional costs associated with specialised equipment and consumables [31], surgeon learning curve and theatre staff training time are cited as further reasons why its routine use may not be justified. However, whilst the benefits of IONM for routine thyroid surgery are debated, IONM has been shown to reduce the rate of RLN injury during revision surgery [32] or when neck anatomy is complex, e.g. large goitres [33]. Therefore, in the context of high-risk thyroidectomies, IONM is widely accepted to be beneficial. Conversely, for surgeons to gain experience with IONM for difficult cases, it is important that they are familiar with its use during routine procedures, so that they can precisely interpret electrophysiological information acquired during complex surgeries.

There are several additional benefits of routine IONM during thyroid surgery which include earlier identification of the RLN and EBSLN and a consequent reduction in operative time [33, 34], more accurate prediction of postoperative vocal fold palsy, given that an anatomically intact RLN may not be functional (especially if neuropraxia has occurred secondary to blunt or stretch injury) and clearer identification of the site of neuronal injury. Surgeon recognition of RLN injury from visual inspection only is very poor, at around 15% of cases [35], and this is particularly relevant in the context of bilateral RLN injury which is also poorly recognised from inspection alone [36]. The use of IONM can prevent bilateral RLN paralysis and its life-threatening complication of airway obstruction. Failed IONM stimulation of the RLN after hemithyroidectomy has resulted in some surgeons changing the operative strategy and delaying contralateral thyroid lobectomy, with a significant reduction in bilateral RLN palsy rates, compared to a reliance on visual neural integrity alone [37]. Overall, the benefits of IONM appear to outweigh any potential disadvantage from increased equipment or training costs; hence current guidelines recommend the use of laryngeal electromyography (EMG) monitoring during thyroid surgery [16].

The principles of IONM are twofold:

1. Stimulation of the RLN or EBSLN
2. Evaluation of vocal fold musculature response to RLN or EBSLN stimulation

Stimulation of the RLN or EBSLN may be achieved using low current (1–2 mA) applied directly to the nerves or indirectly by stimulation of the ipsilateral vagus nerve. Stimulator probes may be monopolar or bipolar, with the latter producing less stimulation artefact and consequently has a greater sensitivity. Bipolar stimulating electrodes must be used in the correct orientation of the anode and cathode for effective nerve stimulation [38].

Monitoring of vocal fold response to RLN or vagal stimulation can be accomplished in a number of ways:

a. Finger palpation of the posterior cricoarytenoid muscle during stimulation [14, 39–42]
b. Direct observation of vocal fold mobility via flexible laryngoscopy [43]
c. Interpretation of EMG data acquired from intramuscular vocal fold electrodes [44, 45]
d. Interpretation of EMG data acquired from endotracheal tube (ET) surface electrodes [32, 46]

Of all the monitoring techniques mentioned above, endotracheal tube surface electrodes are most commonly used worldwide [38], because it is a simple, non-invasive, commercially available technique that does not require additional skill or expertise from the operating surgeon for correct electrode placement. There are several manufacturers of neuromonitoring equipment, and a popular commercially available system is the Medtronic Nerve Integrity Monitoring (NIM®) 3.0 unit (Fig. 7.9) which consists of surface electrodes integrated into endotracheal tubes and a monitor that provides a visual EMG waveform and auditory signal of vocal fold activity following appropriate stimulation using a probe attached to the NIM system. An advantage of the NIM unit is that it is also widely used to facial nerve monitoring during parotid or otological surgery, making it readily available in most hospitals. However the use of ET tubes with integrated electrodes restricts the anaesthetist to using Medtronic supplied tubes, which reduces flexibility given the limited range of Medtronic endotracheal tube sizes. Other manufacturers, such as Inomed (Inomed Medizintechnik GmbH), produce adhesive laryngeal electrodes for use with their nerve-monitoring units that can be applied to standard endotracheal tubes.

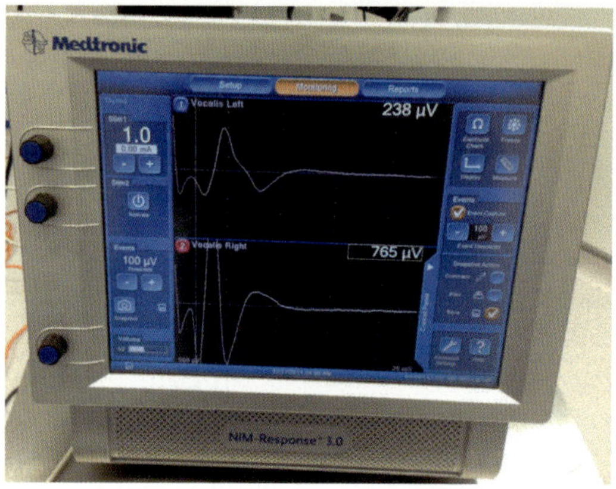

Fig. 7.9 Medtronic Nerve Integrity Monitoring (NIM®) demonstrating active waveforms in standard settings

Regardless of the ET surface electrode or EMG monitoring system employed, a number of essential aspects require consideration prior to IONM use. The surgeon must be familiar with the neuromonitoring equipment and may have to attend additional training sessions with the manufacturer to achieve this. Unambiguous communication between the operating surgeon and anaesthetist on the preoperative laryngoscopy findings, especially if abnormal, is also important. The anaesthetist should be made aware of the need for accurate placement of the ET tube so that surface electrodes are between the vocal folds, a process that should be relatively straightforward, especially if the vocal folds are clearly visualised during intubation. Long-acting neuromuscular-blocking agents must be avoided during ET intubation, so as not to interfere with neural stimulation.

During thyroid and parathyroid surgery, surgeons may use IONM to aid identification of the RLN or EBSLN. This usually involves intermittent stimulation of the area being dissected with interpretation of the auditory signal and EMG waveform from the nerve monitor to confirm whether or not the RLN has been stimulated. The International Neural Monitoring Study Group (INMSG) has produced thorough guidelines on IONM equipment set-up for thyroid/parathyroid surgery, anaesthetic considerations and interpretation of electrophysiological data and have also standardised loss of signal troubleshooting algorithms [38]. As experience with IONM increases, it has become more evident that reliance on auditory signals of RLN stimulation is unreliable with a reported positive predictive value ranging from 9.2% to 94% [38]. A four-step procedure for IONM during thyroid surgery has been advocated [38, 47]:

1. Initial ipsilateral vagal stimulation prior to RLN identification, i.e. *V1 signal* (Fig. 7.10). An EMG waveform with amplitude >100 μV should be achieved at stimulation currents between 0.5 mA and 1 mA. This initial process confirms integrity of the neuromonitoring circuit and may alert the surgeon of the presence of a nonrecurrent RLN (on the right side) which can occur in up to 3% of patients [48].
2. EMG waveform obtained upon stimulation of the RLN on its first identification, i.e. *R1 signal* (Fig. 7.11).
3. EMG trace derived from stimulation of the most proximal portion of the RLN at the end of thyroidectomy, i.e. *R2 signal* (Fig. 7.12).
4. EMG waveform derived following stimulation of the ipsilateral vagus nerve prior to closure, once haemostasis has been achieved, i.e. *V2 signal* (Fig. 7.13). This final EMG trace again confirms that the whole neuromonitoring circuit remains intact at the end of surgery provided the desired event threshold (i.e., EMG amplitude > 100 μV) is achieved at appropriate stimulation currents.

Quantification of the laryngeal EMG for prognostication of postoperative vocal fold function is a key advantage of neuromonitoring systems which provide a visual EMG waveform; however this requires a basic understanding of waveform amplitude, threshold and latency, for the surgeon to interpret and act on the information provided. The INMSG has attempted to standardise these EMG waveform characteristics [38]. Repeated stimulation of the RLN and vagus nerve has so far not been shown to cause permanent neurological deficits [38].

The EBSLN is closely related to the superior thyroid pole vessels and is at risk of injury during ligation of the superior thyroid pole. This may result in difficulty with voice projection and pitch [49], especially in females. Through the human communicating nerve, the EBSLN innervates the anterior half of the ipsilateral vocal fold in up to 85% of patients [50], and this forms a basis that current IONM systems use can monitor the electrophysiological status of the EBSLN [3].

As with IONM for the RLN, the INMSG has proposed an algorithm with a sequence of neural stimulation steps to minimise the risk of EBSLN injury [3]. Standards for equipment set-up, endotracheal tube placement, anaesthetic considerations etc. are the same as for RLN IONM, with a number of additional steps required for the EBSLN. Similar to the RLN, identification of the EBSLN prior to ligation of superior thyroid pole vasculature is recommended in all patients. The anatomy of the EBSLN has been described earlier. It is worth remembering that the EBSLN may not be visually identifiable in up to 20% of patients because the nerve runs in a subfascial or intramuscular plane. IONM is particularly useful in this case, because neural mapping with a stimulation current of 1–2 mA can be used to detect these otherwise "hidden" nerves.

IONM of the EBSLN is a two-step process. Firstly, upon visualisation of the nerve in the sternothyroid-laryngeal triangle, it is stimulated at a current of 1 mA whilst observing for contraction of the cricothyroid muscle (CTM). The presence of an unambiguous CTM contraction or

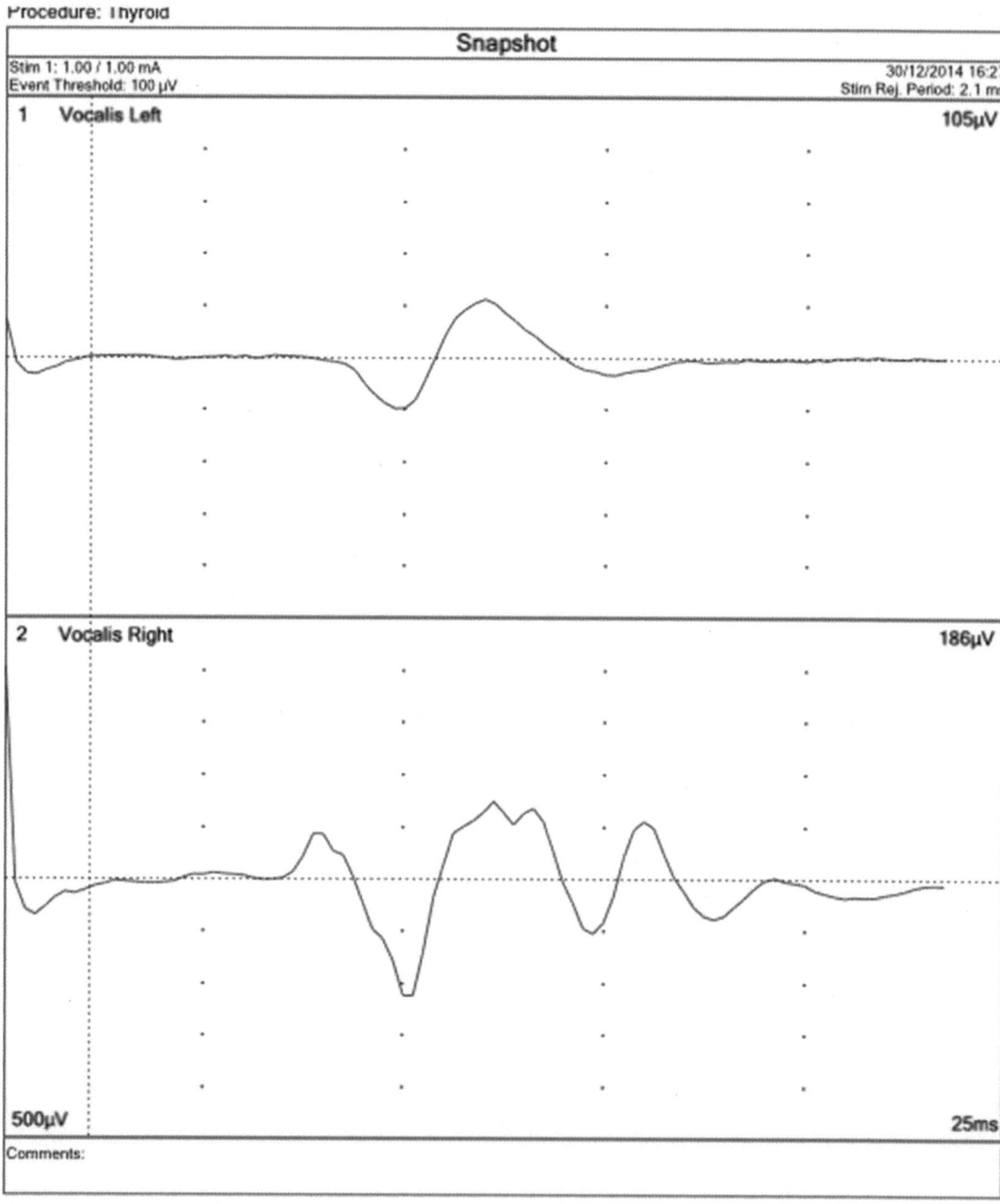

Fig. 7.10 Ipsilateral vagal stimulation V1

"twitch" confirms positive identification of the EBSLN. Additionally, prior to ligation of the superior thyroid pole, stimulation of the tissue to be divided should be performed, with concurrent inspection for a negative CTM twitch to confirm the absence of neural tissue. Secondly, upon EBSLN stimulation, the nerve monitor is observed for a laryngeal EMG waveform, with an amplitude that is usually one-third that of the ipsilateral RLN in comparison. Currently,

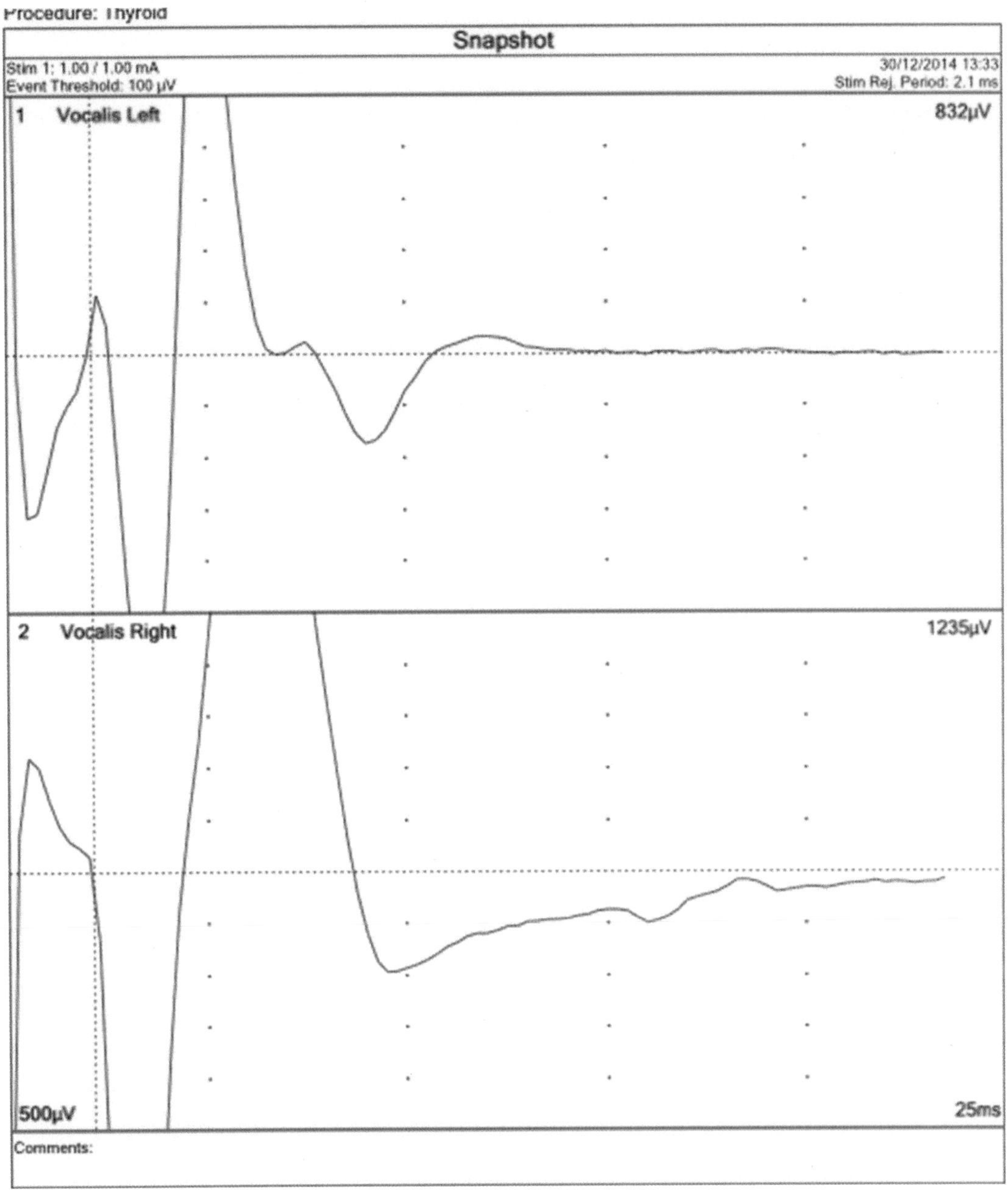

Fig. 7.11 EMG waveform obtained upon stimulation of the RLN on its first identification

EBSLN stimulation will result in an identifiable laryngeal EMG waveform in only 70–80% of patients [3]. The reasons for this are not clearly understood, but the INMSG has proposed that it is more likely related to equipment issues, such as suppression of early evoked potential responses or the influence of endotracheal tube positioning, given that terminal branches of the EBSLN innervate only the anterior 50% of the ipsilateral vocal fold [3]. Using the two techniques described above, the thyroid surgeon should be able to identify the EBSLN in 100% of cases.

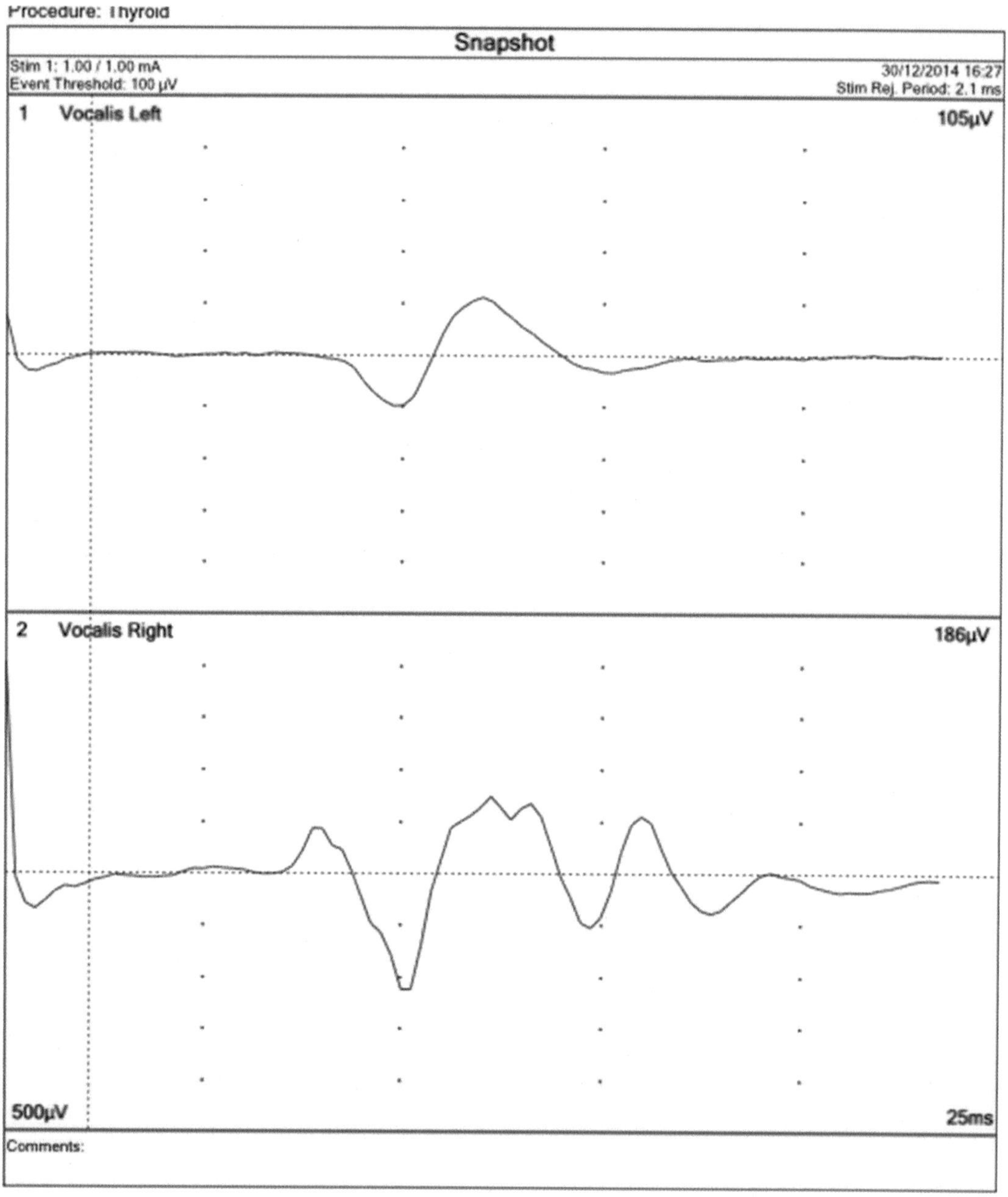

Fig. 7.12 EMG trace derived from stimulation of the most proximal portion of the RLN at the end of thyroidectomy

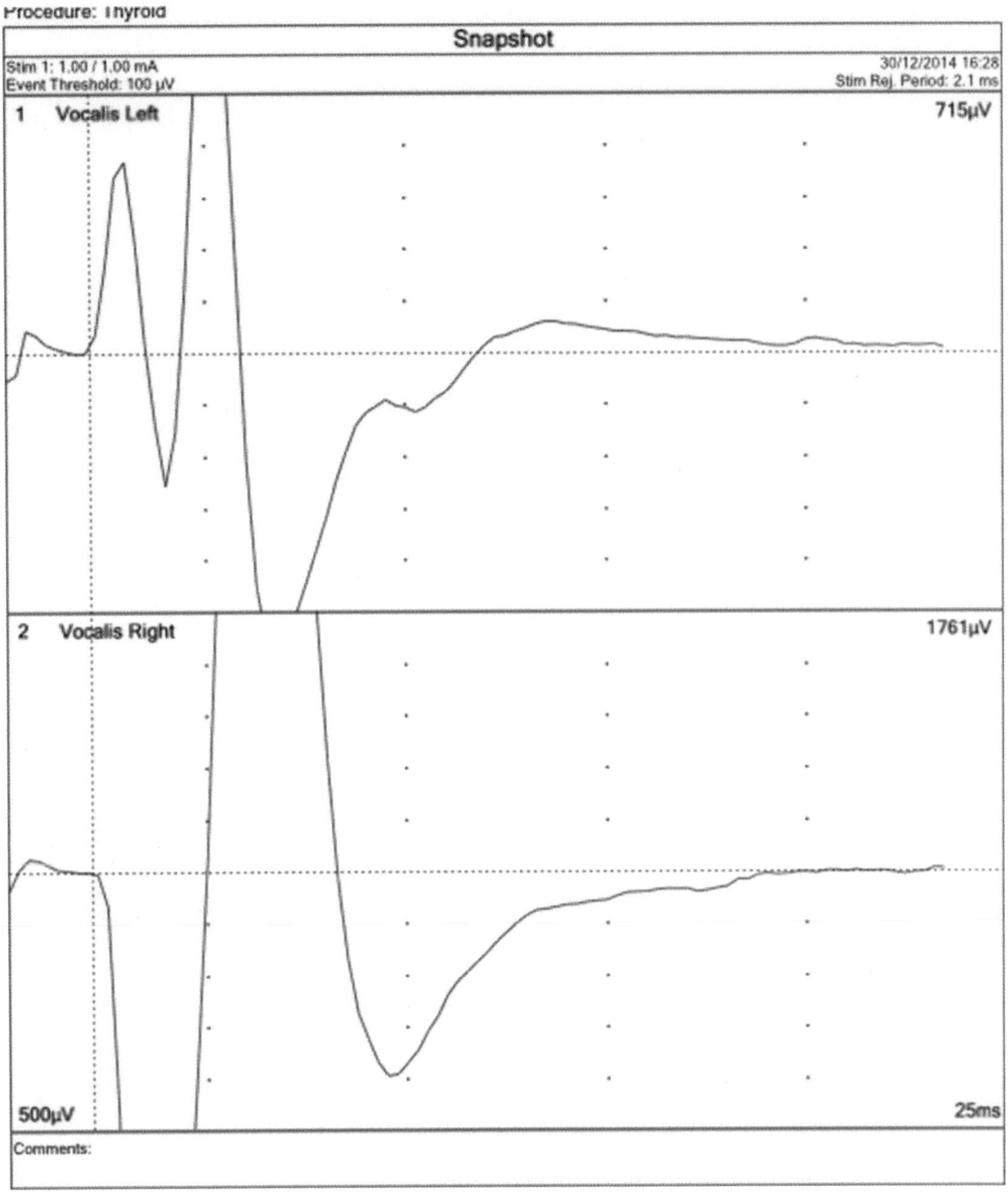

Fig. 7.13 EMG trace derived from stimulation of the most proximal portion of the RLN at the end of thyroidectomy

7.6 Intraoperative Management of the Injured Nerve During Thyroid and Parathyroid Surgery

Injury to the recurrent laryngeal nerve may be identified in the peri or postoperative period. It may also be expected or unexpected, depending on intraoperative findings. If an inadvertent nerve injury is recognised during the initial lobectomy of a total thyroidectomy, careful consideration should be given as to whether to proceed with the contralateral procedure. In the vast majority of cases, the risk will outweigh the benefit. When gross invasion of the nerve is seen and nerve sacrifice is required, many authors would recommend exploration of the contralateral lobe to ensure the integrity of the contralateral nerve prior to sacrifice as a bilateral cord palsy is a devastating complication.

In the event that a unilateral RLN is intentionally sacrificed (e.g. to achieve complete tumour resection) or divided unintentionally and the injury is recognised during the procedure, attempts should be made to perform a primary re-anastomosis of the nerve endings [51]. In patients with a long segment of missing nerve, primary re-anastomosis may be impossible, and consideration should be given to mobilisation of the ansa cervicalis with anastomosis to the laryngeal remnant of the RLN (Fig. 7.14) [52–55] or cable grafting with the greater auricular nerve [56]. Few surgeons have significant experience in this field, and so generalisation of results from expert centres may not be easily reproduced by general thyroid surgeons. If performed, such manoeuvres will not result in a return-to-normal vocal cord function but will optimise the chance of achieving tone within the cord and maximise the potential for rehabilitation.

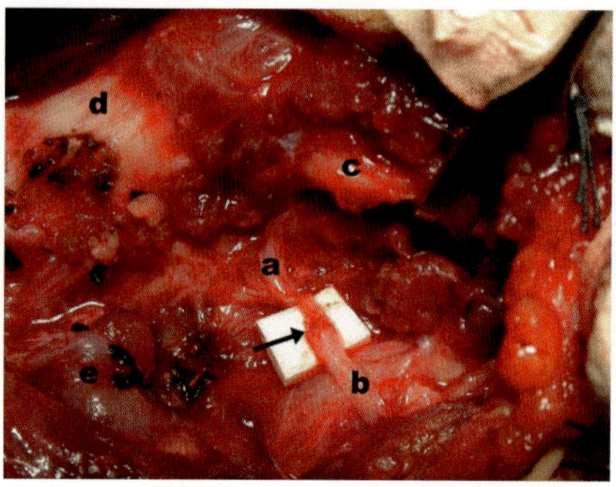

Fig. 7.14 Intraoperative picture of the left RLN remnant anastomosis with left ansa cervicalis

In contrast, if there is suspicion of a nerve injury due to a change in feedback from the nerve monitor but the nerve remains anatomically intact, the structural integrity should be double checked, and the nerve should not be further disturbed.

7.7 Postoperative Management of the Injured Nerve During Thyroid and Parathyroid Surgery

Assuming the procedure went as planned and the RLN was visualised and felt to be intact (whether nerve monitoring is used or not), most authors would not advocate immediate re-exploration. The vast majority of nerve injuries will be temporary [57], and therefore conservative management seems most appropriate. In the event that there was concern over a nerve injury at the time of surgery, re-exploration should be considered, with evidence suggesting that results of early exploration exceed those of late procedures [51, 56, 57]. In this uncommon event, the surgeon should proceed as for an intraoperatively recognised injury.

Those patients in who re-exploration is not performed are candidates for medical therapy. A randomised controlled trial of dexamethasone use in the immediate preoperative period suggested lower rates of temporary palsy in the treatment group [58]. For this reason, consideration should be given to the routine use of steroids in patients undergoing thyroid surgery. In addition, it seems reasonable to continue steroid use in those patients in whom nerve palsy is identified, although duration and dose are unclear. The use of vasodilators such as nimodipine has also been suggested [59, 60]. Experimental work in animal models suggests that improvements in regeneration of neuromuscular function may be possible, although this is yet to be confirmed in work on human subjects.

An essential aspect of the management of postoperative RLN or EBSLN injury is voice therapy. The basic principles of voice therapy include ensuring understanding and knowledge of laryngeal function and rationale of therapeutic input, maximising voice care, reducing glottal insufficiency and increasing range of vocal fold adduction, reducing transglottal airflow and improving subglottal air pressure, preventing supraglottic activity/hyperfunction, optimising resonance and pitch and reducing aspiration and improving airway clearance. This is best done as early as possible to ensure best outcomes and should be done by a dedicated speech and language therapist or pathologist [61, 62].

In patients with bilateral vocal cord palsy, airway compromise should be expected. In this setting the intraoperative condition of the nerves should be considered. Assuming the nerves were considered intact, the patient should be re-intubated and managed in a critical care setting with intravenous steroid administration and a trial of extubation after 48 h.

Patients with an intraoperatively recognised bilateral nerve injury should be extremely uncommon. Some patients still will require immediate tracheostomy to secure a safe airway. Further management will depend on patient and tumour factors. For those patients with advanced disease or significant co-morbidities, no further therapy may be suitable. For fit motivated patients with reasonable pulmonary reserve, arytenoidectomy with or without posterior cordotomy may be possible with the aim of avoiding or achieving early decannulation [63].

7.8 Summary

Recurrent laryngeal nerve (RLN) injury is a well-known and serious complication of thyroid and parathyroid surgery and can lead to serious consequences as well as have important medicolegal implications [1].

IONM is no substitute for detailed knowledge of RLN, EBSLN anatomy and their variations, as well as meticulous and careful surgical technique in dissecting and visualising these nerves during thyroid or parathyroid surgery. IONM is however a useful tool in reducing the rate of iatrogenic neural injury especially during complex thyroid/parathyroid cases.

Visual assessment on the integrity of the RLN or EBSLN is poorly correlated with postoperative vocal fold function, and IONM not only aids earlier identification of the RLN and EBSLN but also helps determine the nature of neural injury if present (i.e. segmental vs. global); it also has a very high positive predictive value for normal post-surgery vocal fold function if vagal, RLN and EBSLN stimulation result in appropriate laryngeal muscle responses and EMG waveforms. Important considerations need to be given to equipment and set-up, endotracheal tube placement and confirmation of appropriate positioning, avoidance of long-acting neuromuscular-blocking agents, interpretation of graphic laryngeal EMG data and loss of signal evaluation standards, amongst other things, for the surgeon and patient to derive maximum benefits from IONM. Other complimentary neuromonitoring techniques during thyroidectomy, such as continuous vagal IONM, which aims to provide an early warning system of impending RLN injury, are currently being evaluated [64] and may offer another useful adjunct in reducing the incidence of permanent vocal fold paralysis, especially with complex cases.

Early recognition of injury either intraoperatively or postoperatively should instigate appropriate prompt management, which will lead to best results. The importance of early voice therapy should be not underestimated.

References

1. Godballe C, Madsen AR, Sorensen CH, Schytte S, Trolle W, Helweg-Larsen J, Pedersen HB. Risk factors for recurrent nerve palsy after thyroid surgery: a national study of patients treated at Danish departments of ENT head and neck surgery. Eur

Arch Otorhinolaryngol. 2014;271(8):2267–76. doi:10.1007/s00405-013-2767-7.
2. Jeannon JP, Orabi AA, Bruch GA, Abdalsalam HA, Simo R. Diagnosis of recurrent laryngeal nerve palsy after thyroidectomy: a systematic review. Int J Clin Pract. 2009;63(4):624–9. doi:10.1111/j.1742-1241.2008.01875.x.
3. Barczynski M, Randolph GW, Cernea CR, Dralle H, Dionigi G, Alesina PF, International Neural Monitoring Study, Group. External branch of the superior laryngeal nerve monitoring during thyroid and parathyroid surgery: international neural monitoring study group standards guideline statement. Laryngoscope. 2013;123(Suppl 4):S1–14. doi:10.1002/lary.24301.
4. Cernea CR, Ferraz AR, Furlani J, Monteiro S, Nishio S, Hojaij FC, Bevilacqua RG. Identification of the external branch of the superior laryngeal nerve during thyroidectomy. Am J Surg. 1992;164(6):634–9.
5. Friedman M, LoSavio P, Ibrahim H. Superior laryngeal nerve identification and preservation in thyroidectomy. Arch Otolaryngol Head Neck Surg. 2002;128(3):296–303.
6. Kierner AC, Aigner M, Burian M. The external branch of the superior laryngeal nerve: its topographical anatomy as related to surgery of the neck. Arch Otolaryngol Head Neck Surg. 1998;124(3):301–3.
7. Morton RP, Whitfield P, Al-Ali S. Anatomical and surgical considerations of the external branch of the superior laryngeal nerve: a systematic review. Clin Otolaryngol. 2006;31(5):368–74. doi:10.1111/j.1749-4486.2006.01266.x.
8. Shindo ML, Wu JC, Park EE. Surgical anatomy of the recurrent laryngeal nerve revisited. Otolaryngol Head Neck Surg. 2005;133(4):514–9. doi:10.1016/j.otohns.2005.07.010.
9. Hisham AN, Lukman MR. Recurrent laryngeal nerve in thyroid surgery: a critical appraisal. ANZ J Surg. 2002;72(12):887–9.
10. Barczynski M, Nowak W, Sancho JJ, Sitges-Serra A. The motor fibers of the recurrent laryngeal nerves are located in the anterior extralaryngeal branch. Ann Surg. 2010;251(4):773–774.; author reply 774–775. doi:10.1097/SLA.0b013e3181d57a59.
11. Sancho JJ, Pascual-Damieta M, Pereira JA, Carrera MJ, Fontane J, Sitges-Serra A. Risk factors for transient vocal cord palsy after thyroidectomy. Br J Surg. 2008;95(8):961–7. doi:10.1002/bjs.6173.
12. Aina EN, Hisham AN. External laryngeal nerve in thyroid surgery: recognition and surgical implications. ANZ J Surg. 2001;71(4):212–4.
13. Pagedar NA, Freeman JL. Identification of the external branch of the superior laryngeal nerve during thyroidectomy. Arch Otolaryngol Head Neck Surg. 2009;135(4):360–2. doi:10.1001/archoto.2009.9.
14. Randolph GW, Kobler JB, Wilkins J. Recurrent laryngeal nerve identification and assessment during thyroid surgery: laryngeal palpation. World J Surg. 2004;28(8):755–60. doi:10.1007/s00268-004-7348-x.
15. Barczynski M, Konturek A, Pragacz K, Papier A, Stopa M, Nowak W. Intraoperative nerve monitoring can reduce prevalence of recurrent laryngeal nerve injury in thyroid reoperations: results of a retrospective cohort study. World J Surg. 2014;38(3):599–606. doi:10.1007/s00268-013-2260-x.
16. Chandrasekhar SS, Randolph GW, Seidman MD, Rosenfeld RM, Angelos P, Barkmeier-Kraemer J, Robertson PJ. Clinical practice guideline: improving voice outcomes after thyroid surgery. Otolaryngol Head Neck Surg. 2013;148(6 Suppl):S1–37. doi:10.1177/0194599813487301.
17. Lahey F. Routine dissection and demonstration of the recurrent laryngeal nerve in subtotal thyroidectomy. Surg Gynecol Obstet. 1938;66:775–7.
18. Riddell VH. Injury to recurrent laryngeal nerves during thyroidectomy; a comparison between the results of identification and non-identification in 1022 nerves exposed to risk. Lancet. 1956;271(6944):638–41.
19. Hermann M, Alk G, Roka R, Glaser K, Freissmuth M. Laryngeal recurrent nerve injury in surgery for benign thyroid diseases: effect of nerve dissection and impact of individual surgeon in more than 27,000 nerves at risk. Ann Surg. 2002;235(2):261–8.
20. Shindo M, Chheda NN. Incidence of vocal cord paralysis with and without recurrent laryngeal nerve monitoring during thyroidectomy. Arch Otolaryngol Head Neck Surg. 2007;133(5):481–5. doi:10.1001/archotol.133.5.481.
21. Brunner E, Friedrich G, Kiesler K, Chibidziura-Priesching J, Gugatschka M. Subjective breathing impairment in unilateral vocal fold paralysis. Folia Phoniatr Logop. 2011;63(3):142–6. doi:10.1159/000316320.
22. Leder SB, Ross DA. Incidence of vocal fold immobility in patients with dysphagia. Dysphagia. 2005;20(2):163–167.; discussion 168–169. doi:10.1007/s10350-005-0002-4.
23. Ollivere B, Duce K, Rowlands G, Harrison P, O'Reilly BJ. Swallowing dysfunction in patients with unilateral vocal fold paralysis: aetiology and outcomes. J Laryngol Otol. 2006;120(1):38–41. doi:10.1017/S0022215105003567.
24. Stojadinovic A, Shaha AR, Orlikoff RF, Nissan A, Kornak MF, Singh B, Kraus DH. Prospective functional voice assessment in patients undergoing thyroid surgery. Ann Surg. 2002;236(6):823–32.
25. Kern KA. Medicolegal analysis of errors in diagnosis and treatment of surgical endocrine disease. Surgery. 1993;114(6):1167–73. discussion 1173-1164
26. Singer MC, Iverson KC, Terris DJ. Thyroidectomy-related malpractice claims. Otolaryngol Head Neck Surg. 2012;146(3):358–61. doi:10.1177/0194599811430898.
27. Barczynski M, Konturek A, Cichon S. Randomized clinical trial of visualization versus neuromonitoring of recurrent laryngeal nerves during thyroidectomy. Br J Surg. 2009;96(3):240–6. doi:10.1002/bjs.6417.

28. Dralle H, Sekulla C, Haerting J, Timmermann W, Neumann HJ, Kruse E, Gimm O. Risk factors of paralysis and functional outcome after recurrent laryngeal nerve monitoring in thyroid surgery. Surgery. 2004;136(6):1310–22. doi:10.1016/j.surg.2004.07.018.
29. Dralle H, Sekulla C, Lorenz K, Brauckhoff M, Machens A, German, Ionm Study Group. Intraoperative monitoring of the recurrent laryngeal nerve in thyroid surgery. World J Surg. 2008;32(7):1358–66. doi:10.1007/s00268-008-9483-2.
30. Higgins TS, Gupta R, Ketcham AS, Sataloff RT, Wadsworth JT, Sinacori JT. Recurrent laryngeal nerve monitoring versus identification alone on post-thyroidectomy true vocal fold palsy: a meta-analysis. Laryngoscope. 2011;121(5):1009–17. doi:10.1002/lary.21578.
31. Dionigi G, Bacuzzi A, Boni L, Rausei S, Rovera F, Dionigi R. Visualization versus neuromonitoring of recurrent laryngeal nerves during thyroidectomy: what about the costs? World J Surg. 2012;36(4):748–54. doi:10.1007/s00268-012-1452-0.
32. Chan WF, Lang BH, Lo CY. The role of intraoperative neuromonitoring of recurrent laryngeal nerve during thyroidectomy: a comparative study on 1000 nerves at risk. Surgery. 2006;140(6):866–872.; discussion 872-863. doi:10.1016/j.surg.2006.07.017.
33. Chiang FY, Lu IC, Chen HC, Chen HY, Tsai CJ, Lee KW, Wu CW. Intraoperative neuromonitoring for early localization and identification of recurrent laryngeal nerve during thyroid surgery. Kaohsiung J Med Sci. 2010;26(12):633–9. doi:10.1016/S1607-551X(10)70097-8.
34. Sari S, Erbil Y, Sumer A, Agcaoglu O, Bayraktar A, Issever H, Ozarmagan S. Evaluation of recurrent laryngeal nerve monitoring in thyroid surgery. Int J Surg. 2010;8(6):474–8. doi:10.1016/j.ijsu.2010.06.009.
35. Lo CY, Kwok KF, Yuen PW. A prospective evaluation of recurrent laryngeal nerve paralysis during thyroidectomy. Arch Surg. 2000;135(2):204–7.
36. Bergenfelz A, Jansson S, Kristoffersson A, Martensson H, Reihner E, Wallin G, Lausen I. Complications to thyroid surgery: results as reported in a database from a multicenter audit comprising 3,660 patients. Langenbeck's Arch Surg. 2008;393(5):667–73. doi:10.1007/s00423-008-0366-7.
37. Goretzki PE, Schwarz K, Brinkmann J, Wirowski D, Lammers BJ. The impact of intraoperative neuromonitoring (IONM) on surgical strategy in bilateral thyroid diseases: is it worth the effort? World J Surg. 2010;34(6):1274–84. doi:10.1007/s00268-009-0353-3.
38. Randolph GW, Dralle H, Abdullah H, Barczynski M, Bellantone R, Brauckhoff M, Woodson G. Electrophysiologic recurrent laryngeal nerve monitoring during thyroid and parathyroid surgery: international standards guideline statement. Laryngoscope. 2011;121(Suppl 1):S1–16. doi:10.1002/lary.21119.
39. Cavicchi O, Caliceti U, Fernandez IJ, Ceroni AR, Marcantoni A, Sciascia S, Piccin O. Laryngeal neuromonitoring and neurostimulation versus neurostimulation alone in thyroid surgery: a randomized clinical trial. Head Neck. 2012;34(2):141–5. doi:10.1002/hed.21681.
40. James AG, Crocker S, Woltering E, Ferrara J, Farrar W. A simple method for identifying and testing the recurrent laryngeal nerve. Surg Gynecol Obstet. 1985;161(2):185–6.
41. Loch-Wilkinson TJ, Stalberg PL, Sidhu SB, Sywak MS, Wilkinson JF, Delbridge LW. Nerve stimulation in thyroid surgery: is it really useful? ANZ J Surg. 2007;77(5):377–80. doi:10.1111/j.1445-2197.2007.04065.x.
42. Tomoda C, Hirokawa Y, Uruno T, Takamura Y, Ito Y, Miya A, Miyauchi A. Sensitivity and specificity of intraoperative recurrent laryngeal nerve stimulation test for predicting vocal cord palsy after thyroid surgery. World J Surg. 2006;30(7):1230–3. doi:10.1007/s00268-005-0351-z.
43. Eltzschig HK, Posner M, Moore FD Jr. The use of readily available equipment in a simple method for intraoperative monitoring of recurrent laryngeal nerve function during thyroid surgery: initial experience with more than 300 cases. Arch Surg. 2002;137(4):452–6. discussion 456-457.
44. Rice DH, Cone-Wesson B. Intraoperative recurrent laryngeal nerve monitoring. Otolaryngol Head Neck Surg. 1991;105(3):372–5.
45. Tschopp KP, Gottardo C. Comparison of various methods of electromyographic monitoring of the recurrent laryngeal nerve in thyroid surgery. Ann Otol Rhinol Laryngol. 2002;111(9):811–6.
46. Eisele DW. Intraoperative electrophysiologic monitoring of the recurrent laryngeal nerve. Laryngoscope. 1996;106(4):443–9.
47. Chiang FY, Lu IC, Kuo WR, Lee KW, Chang NC, Wu CW. The mechanism of recurrent laryngeal nerve injury during thyroid surgery--the application of intraoperative neuromonitoring. Surgery. 2008;143(6):743–9. doi:10.1016/j.surg.2008.02.006.
48. Donatini G, Carnaille B, Dionigi G. Increased detection of non-recurrent inferior laryngeal nerve (NRLN) during thyroid surgery using systematic intraoperative neuromonitoring (IONM). World J Surg. 2013;37(1):91–3. doi:10.1007/s00268-012-1782-y.
49. Sulica L. The superior laryngeal nerve: function and dysfunction. Otolaryngol Clin N Am. 2004;37(1):183–201. doi:10.1016/S0030-6665(03)00175-0.
50. Maranillo E, Leon X, Quer M, Orus C, Sanudo JR. Is the external laryngeal nerve an exclusively motor nerve? The cricothyroid connection branch. Laryngoscope. 2003;113(3):525–9. doi:10.1097/00005537-200303000-00024.
51. Hong JW, Roh TS, Yoo HS, Hong HJ, Choi HS, Chang HS, Kim YS. Outcome with immediate direct anastomosis of recurrent laryngeal nerves injured during thyroidectomy. Laryngoscope. 2013;124(6):1402–8. doi:10.1002/lary.24450.

52. Li M, Chen S, Wang W, Chen D, Zhu M, Liu F, Zheng H. Effect of duration of denervation on outcomes of ansa-recurrent laryngeal nerve reinnervation. Laryngoscope. 2014;124(8):1900–5. doi:10.1002/lary.24623.
53. Lorenz RR, Esclamado RM, Teker AM, Strome M, Scharpf J, Hicks D, Lee WT. Ansa cervicalis-to-recurrent laryngeal nerve anastomosis for unilateral vocal fold paralysis: experience of a single institution. Ann Otol Rhinol Laryngol. 2008;117(1):40–5.
54. Wang W, Chen D, Chen S, Li D, Li M, Xia S, Zheng H. Laryngeal reinnervation using ansa cervicalis for thyroid surgery-related unilateral vocal fold paralysis: a long-term outcome analysis of 237 cases. PLoS One. 2011;6(4):e19128. doi:10.1371/journal.pone.0019128.
55. Wang W, Chen S, Chen D, Xia S, Qiu X, Liu Y, Zheng H. Contralateral ansa cervicalis-to-recurrent laryngeal nerve anastomosis for unilateral vocal fold paralysis: a long-term outcome analysis of 56 cases. Laryngoscope. 2011;121(5):1027–34. doi:10.1002/lary.21725.
56. Yumoto E, Sanuki T, Kumai Y. Immediate recurrent laryngeal nerve reconstruction and vocal outcome. Laryngoscope. 2006;116(9):1657–61. doi:10.1097/01.mlg.0000233245.27582.fc.
57. Jiang Y, Gao B, Zhang X, Zhao J, Chen J, Zhang S, Luo D. Prevention and treatment of recurrent laryngeal nerve injury in thyroid surgery. Int J Clin Exp Med. 2014;7(1):101–7.
58. Schietroma M, Cecilia EM, Carlei F, Sista F, De Santis G, Lancione L, Amicucci G. Dexamethasone for the prevention of recurrent laryngeal nerve palsy and other complications after thyroid surgery: a randomized double-blind placebo-controlled trial. JAMA Otolaryngol Head Neck Surg. 2013;139(5):471–8. doi:10.1001/jamaoto.2013.2821.
59. Hydman J, Remahl S, Bjorck G, Svensson M, Mattsson P. Nimodipine improves reinnervation and neuromuscular function after injury to the recurrent laryngeal nerve in the rat. Ann Otol Rhinol Laryngol. 2007;116(8):623–30.
60. Nishimoto K, Kumai Y, Sanuki T, Minoda R, Yumoto E. The impact of nimodipine administration combined with nerve-muscle pedicle implantation on long-term denervated rat thyroarytenoid muscle. Laryngoscope. 2013;123(4):952–9. doi:10.1002/lary.23698.
61. Chen X, Wan P, Yu Y, Li M, Xu Y, Huang P, Huang Z. Types and timing of therapy for vocal fold paresis/paralysis after thyroidectomy: a systematic review and meta-analysis. J Voice. 2014;28(6):799–808. doi:10.1016/j.jvoice.2014.02.003.
62. Kasterovic B, Veselinovic M, Mitrovic SM. Voice therapy and assistive techniques in voice disorders caused by unilateral vocal cord pareses. Med Pregl. 2014;67(3-4):91–6.
63. Dispenza F, Dispenza C, Marchese D, Kulamarva G, Saraniti C. Treatment of bilateral vocal cord paralysis following permanent recurrent laryngeal nerve injury. Am J Otolaryngol. 2012;33(3):285–8. doi:10.1016/j.amjoto.2011.07.009.
64. Phelan E, Schneider R, Lorenz K, Dralle H, Kamani D, Potenza A, Randolph W. Continuous vagal IONM prevents recurrent laryngeal nerve paralysis by revealing initial EMG changes of impending neuropraxic injury: a prospective, multicenter study. Laryngoscope. 2014;124(6):1498–505. doi:10.1002/lary.24550.

Spasmodic Dysphonia (Laryngeal Dystonia)

8

Claus Wittekindt

Abstract

Spasmodic dysphonia (SD) or laryngeal dystonia is a focal voice disorder that produces involuntary spasms of the vocal folds, resulting in a strained-strangled voice production. Symptoms of SD come in several varieties. The disorder can be broadly divided into three forms: adductor-type SD, abductor-type SD, and mixed-type SD. The most common adductor-type causes a tight, "strangled-sounding" voice quality, often with abrupt starting and stopping of the voice. The abductor-type causes a breathy, whispering voice. Most cases of SD are primary and develop in adults (adult-onset). There is no cure for SD, and little is known on risk factors that contribute to its development. The diagnosis is mainly based on speech analysis. Injecting botulinum toxin has become the treatment of choice for 30 years. However, the disorder typically remains chronic after onset, and repeated injections therefore are needed.

8.1 Introduction

Spasmodic dysphonia (SD) is a primary focal dystonia that affects the larynx. The respective cause of this focal dystonia typically remains enigmatic, i.e., it is a focal dystonia of idiopathic origin. The management continues to be directed at relief of vocal cord spasms rather than cure. SD can be subdivided into adductor-type SD that is mainly characterized by uncontrollable approximation of the vocal folds with intermittent closing of the glottis and staccato phonation. The second subtype, abductor-type SD, is reported to be present in less than 20% of the affected patients with irregular opening of the glottis followed by voiceless consonants [1]. The third type, mixed SD, describes patient with symptoms of adductor-type and abductor-type SD. The most common treatment is the injection of botulinum toxin (BT) directly into the affected muscles in the larynx (more details on BT treatment in Chap. 9).

C. Wittekindt
Department of Otorhinolaryngology, University of Gissen, Klinikstrasse 33, Giessen 35390, Germany
e-mail: Claus.Wittekindt@hno.med.uni-giessen.de

C. Sittel, O. Guntinas-Lichius (eds.), *Neurolaryngology*,
https://doi.org/10.1007/978-3-319-61724-4_8

8.2 Definition

SD is a rare chronic voice disorder of idiopathic origin that is characterized by overly contracting laryngeal muscles during speech. It may manifest as excessive glottic closure (adductor-type SD) or unnatural lateralization of the vocal folds (adductor-type SD). Patterned, repeated "breaks" in speech and strangled phonation characterize adductor-type SD. Abductor-type SD presents with breathy voice or brief vocal loss. Symptoms may overlap—the disease also might take a back-seat in multifocal dystonia as secondary SD. Mixed SD describes the rare involvement of muscles that open and close the glottis and therefore has features of both classical types of SD. Whispering dystonia is a very rare inherited form of SD caused by mutations of the TUBB4 gene that has been described in an Australian family (also called DYT-4 dystonia; see below).

8.3 History

Ludwig Traube first described the symptoms of spasmodic dysphonia in a German pathophysiology book in 1871. He described a nervous hoarseness and invented the term "spastic dysphonia," but the term spasmodic dysphonia (SD) today is more widely accepted. During the next 100 years, SD was predominantly regarded as being a psychogenic disorder, typically observed in anxious individuals. SD today is classified as a focal dystonia that affects the larynx during speech. Therefore, the name laryngeal dystonia might be more exact. Historical treatments include recurrent laryngeal nerve section or laryngeal nerve crush [2].

8.4 Epidemiology and Risk Factors

Limited data are available on prevalence and risk factors for SD. Generally, SD is a rare and idiopathic disorder; however, it might be considerably underdiagnosed. The disease affects females more commonly with a reported male-to-female ratio as high as 1:1–1:7 [3, 4]. SD is the third most common form of focal dystonia; incidence estimates range from 1.2 to 4.26/100.000 annual incidence rate, and it seems to be more frequent in European compared to Asian people [5]. SD typically appears early in the fifth decade of life and remains chronic thereafter; however, the condition may rarely occur in the second decade of life and as late as the ninth decade of life [3]. About 10% of the patients have a positive family history of dystonia [6].

Although the genetic origin of dystonia is not established, genetic etiologies have long been suspected for many types of dystonia. To date 18 different so-called DYT genetic loci have been mapped, e.g., DYT-1 is associated with juvenile-onset dystonia of the limbs. Laryngeal dystonia has been described in DYT-6 families, and DYT-4 has been found in a family with whispering dystonia. The DYT gene loci, however, have variable penetrance and expressivity; none of the described loci are specifically linked to SD. The system of DYT loci is unsatisfactory; the designation of some loci has never been replicated and is of questionable significance [7]. Described environmental risk factors include a personal history of mumps, intense voice use, and family history of tremor [3, 8].

8.5 Pathophysiology

Vocalization is a result of preprogrammed systems for the expression of emotional states such as alarm, aggression, laughter, or cry. In contrast to this innate vocal system, the capacity to produce learned vocal utterances is limited to humans. Only speech is affected in SD, whereas innate vocalizations are spared. Dopaminergic abnormalities in cortical-basal ganglia circuits are believed to impair inhibition of involuntary muscle activity in dystonia [9]. The combination of genetic factors and environmental modifiers, e.g., history of mumps, may lead to SD. These physiological mechanisms have been described in dystonia: abnormal sensory input, increased plasticity, and loss of inhibition. Sensory abnormalities and loss of inhibition with abnormal spinal and brain stem reflexes have been described in detail in patients with writer's cramp but also for SD patients [10]. Onset of SD might follow disordered inhibition in response to sensory feedback. Sensory input includes flow receptors, pressure on the laryngeal mucosa, and muscle activity. Songbirds might act as promising animal models in the future, since they have both innate and learned vocalization. Hormonal contributions might also be explored, because women have higher incidence rates. Recent functional brain imaging studies confirmed abnormalities in the primary somatosensory cortex and abnormal auditory cortical responses [11].

8.6 Clinical Features

Patients tend to report inciting events (upper respiratory tract infections, major life stressor, etc.) that caused their onset of SD; however, taking the idiopathic origin of the disease into consideration, this is doubtful [12]. In the majority of cases, there is sudden-onset of idiopathic origin. Symptoms come in several varieties; one of the most characteristic features is patterned and repeated breaks during speech. In the more common adductor-type SD, a tight, strangled-sounding voice quality, with abrupt starting and stopping is characteristic. Intermitting voice offsets on voicing of vowels and worsening of symptoms under emotional stress are also typical. Symptoms are often reduced in the morning or after drinking alcohol. Hoarseness is not a leading symptom. The essential symptom is voice breaks. During laryngoscopy there is intermittent squeezing of the vocal folds with rapid glottic closures, which results in quick glottic closures.

Abductor-type SD typically leads to prolonged voiceless consonants because of difficulties with voice onset. Further symptoms include pitch change and phonatory breaks during vowels. Laryngoscopy reveals wide-ranging abduction movements for voiceless consonants (p, t, k, f, s, th, sh, ch, h) that are prolonged and interfere with following vowels. An important diagnostic feature is that symptoms may improve when whispering, laughing, or singing. Many of the symptoms vary during the day and particularly become aggravated in certain situations like speaking on the phone or to the public. The combination of adductor-type and abductor-type SD has been described with overlapping symptoms. Patients with SD can be misdiagnosed having voice tremor and vice versa. Voice tremor normally is seen alongside systemic manifestations of the underlying disorder.

8.7 Diagnostic Workup

Thorough neurological examinations are mandatory in every person with suspicion for SD since other neurologic disorders (tremors, myoclonus, progressive supranuclear pathology) may be misdiagnosed as SD. Brain imaging with MRI may be necessary in patients with focal findings beyond the typical clinical presentation of SD. Speech perception and acoustic analysis (jitter, shimmer, signal-to-noise ratio) should be performed. Aerodynamic analysis may range from normal to extremely low in patients with SD. The mainstay of diagnosis is documentation of adductor and abductor breaks during conversational speech. Standard sentences in the respective language might be helpful (e.g., "How high is Harry's hat?"—to trigger abductor breaks). Fiberoptic nasolaryngoscopy without anesthesia is necessary to exclude other reasons for abnormal voice. In SD, normal movement is observed during cough, whistling, and respiration. Vocal fold spasms (adductor-type SD) and prolonged vowels (abductor-type SD) can be observed and monitored during speech.

Electromyography (EMG) is supplementary to the abovementioned tests to confirm SD [13]. Usually it is used to guide botulinum toxin injections into the thyroarytenoid muscles (more details on electrodiagnostics in Chap. 1). Surface or needle electrodes may be used to record muscle activity during phonation and breathing; however, the use of surface electrodes is questionable [14]. EMG also can be performed by transoral direct insertion technique. In adductor-type SD, needle EMG reveals significantly increased amplitudes when monitoring the thyroarytenoid muscle motor unit potentials. In abductor-type SD, the posterior cricoarytenoid muscle is monitored through direct or indirect approach. Recruitment potentials reveal characteristic high-frequency (150–400 Hz) bursts of motor unit potentials that correlate with clinically observed voice interruptions. Significantly increased TA muscle amplitudes in SD patients with reduction after BT treatment have recently been reported [15]. EMG is particularly helpful in differentiating SD from other hyperfunctional voice disorders, e.g., muscle tension dysphonia or tremor with dysphonia.

8.8 Treatment

Botulinum toxin (BT) injection is widely accepted as being an effective treatment for controlling the symptoms of adductor spasmodic dysphonia [16]. In addition to BT, medical treatment, surgery, and other adjuvants such as voice therapy have been reported; the latter mentioned can be regarded as being potentially recommended for selected cases. Appropriate treatment is always dependent upon proper diagnosis, particularly in SD patients since the two different types of SD may overlap and multisegmental dystonia as well as tremor as comorbidity are frequent.

8.8.1 Botulinum Toxin

The treatment of choice for most cases of SD is regular injections of botulinum toxin into the TA muscles (more on BT treatment in Chap. 9). There are a variety of injection techniques, including EMG guidance and percutaneous or transoral/transnasal approaches. Evidence-based reviews have been published in recent years on the effectivity of BT injections. Effectivity has been described in adductor-type SD, but there is insufficient evidence for abductor-type SD [17, 18]. For example, endoscopic versus EMG-guided BT injections in abductor-type SD have been compared in a randomized trial with no effect in both groups [19].

8.8.1.1 Injection Technique

There are several different techniques used to deliver BTX into the intrinsic laryngeal adductor compartment. No particular technique has been shown to be superior to another. The technique first described is a percutaneous injection, guided by EMG signals with a monopolar Teflon-coated hollow needle. The patient is sitting or in nearly supine position (Fig. 8.1). The neck is palpated, and the cricothyroid membrane is identified. Infiltration of lidocaine into the skin and the ligament is recommended.

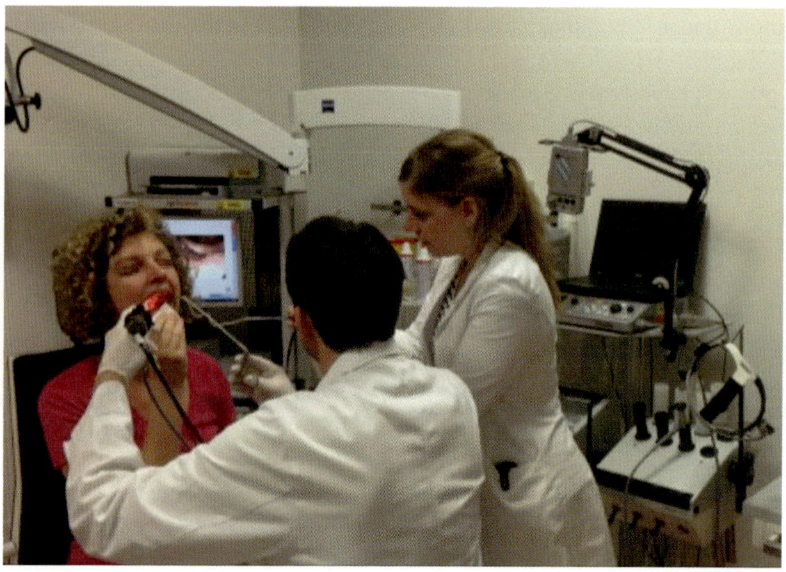

Fig. 8.1 Injection with laryngoscopy guidance. This approach is a direct visualization of the injection point, but is not often tolerated in dystonia patients

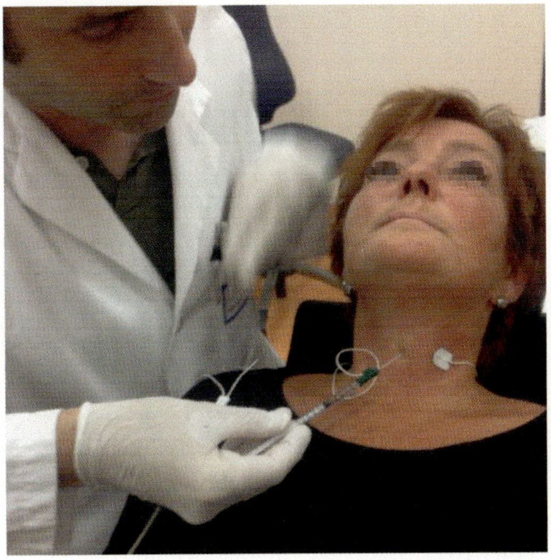

Fig. 8.2 Percutaneous BT injection in spasmodic dysphonia. The patient is in nearly supine position, and the BT is injected via a Teflon-coated monopolar hollow needle with EMG guidance

Additionally, the larynx is anesthetized with lidocaine spray. The needle is then directed 30–45° upward the TA muscle. Alternative approaches have been published to be as effective. These include transoral and transnasal guidance by means of laryngoscopy and transcartilagenous injections. The transoral approach involves direct visualization of the vocal folds by laryngoscopy (Fig. 8.2). The transnasal injection technique needs a flexible nasopharyngoscope with a working channel. In a review on injection techniques, the transnasal and transoral approach led to similar functional benefit with lower failure rates in comparison to EMG-guided methods. However, the application under visualization is less often tolerated by patients [20]. Later, no significant differences between EMG and fiberoptic guidance toward the outcome were shown in a randomized trial [21].

The injection technique for abductor-type SD is technically demanding. The thyroid cartilage is rotated away from the injection site, and the posterior cricoarytenoid muscle (PCA) is identified by EMG signal during sniff after advancement of the needle through the inferior constrictor muscle. Alternatively, the EMG needle can be passed through the cricothyroid ligament and the cricoid plate. Transnasal approach to the PCA muscle has also been published with similar results to transcutaneous approach [19].

8.8.1.2 Dosage

BT is reconstituted with saline before injection. A limited dilution volume is helpful since large amounts of injected volume harbor a higher risk of adverse effects as dysphagia. Typical amounts of saline are 2 ml/100 U of onabotulinum toxin (Botox©, Allergan). The amount of BT needed is unique in each patient; accordingly a standard injection amount does not exist. Typical amounts range between 1 and 5 U of Botox to each side for effect in adductor-type SD. The amount should be titrated at each visit and be well documented. In a large series, the dose range varied between 0.008 and 30 U, with an average of 3 U [6]. A feasible starting dose could be 1 or 1.25 U of Botox per TA muscle. For patients with abductor-type SD, the dose is higher, e.g., 5 U as starting dose. In a retrospective case review of 100 injections, 2.5–7.5 U (mean 4.7 U total dose per patient) was found to be safe with a complication rate below 5% [22]. The long-term BT dose in 150 treatments has been reported to be very consistent with a trend downward over time [23]. The optimal dose normally is found after 2–3 treatments.

8.8.1.3 Complications

Immediately after the injection, a mild edema or hematoma can be expected. BT is effective after a latency time between 2 and 5 days. The major adverse reaction is breathiness together with onset of BT effect; a duration of 4–6 weeks can be expected in case of overdosage. Transient difficulty in swallowing liquids also is a common treatment side effect, reported to be present in 15–50% of the patients [24, 25]. To summarize, technically, there are no side effects, BT might be ineffective in case of underdosing, or benefit will only last for a shorter time. In case of overdosage, the injection will result in longer-lasting relief, but the side effects appear in a dose-dependent proportion. Breathiness after the BT injection goes in line with a longer-lasting relief of symptoms. Improper localization or deposition of the toxin too far behind into the larynx will enhance the risk of swallowing disorders after the procedure. Severe adverse events include bilateral abductor paralysis; the risk of stridor after bilateral injection has been numbered 8/352 (2.3%) with one patient needing a tracheotomy in a retrospective review [26]. The rule of thumb is 4–6 weeks after the injection, adverse effects always will disappear.

8.8.1.4 Medical Treatment

Symptoms of SD frequently improve on sedatives such as alcohol and benzodiazepines. Generally, oral drug treatment might be considered as an additional option, however, without expecting significant benefit. Baclofen is a GABA receptor agonist; there are no controlled studies to guide recommendations for its use, but retrospective studies and anecdotal experience suggest it is most often useful in childhood-onset dystonias, especially those with concomitant spasticity. Some adults also enjoy benefits from oral treatment, although most do not. The use of anticholinergics is often limited by peripheral and central side effects. Further medications that showed positive results include diphenhydramine, benztropine, and antiparkinson agents. To summarize, no pharmacological agent provides significant relief of SD. Even when success is noticed, their use is often limited due to side effects.

8.8.1.5 Surgical Therapy

A definitive surgical approach for adductor-type SD is microlaryngoscopic resection of both thyroarytenoid muscles. Significant improvement has been reported in seven Japanese patients [27] and later with longer follow-up in further 15 patients [28]. Moderate and marked vocal improvement after 31 months of follow-up has been reported in up to 90% of the patients in a larger sample [29]. Earlier, TA muscle removal together with partial removal of the lateral cricoarytenoid muscle under local anesthesia has been reported with favorable outcome [30]. Laser vaporization of TA muscle has recently been reported with good results after 48 months of follow-up [31].

Type II thyroplasty, also called lateralization thyroplasty, has been proposed for treatment of SD in six patients by Isshiki and coworkers [32]. The authors later reported successful treatment in 41 patients after implanting a titanium bridge with 70% of the patients judging their voice as excellent and the remaining patients as improved to good or fair. Advantages of thyroplasty are reported to be unlikely recurrence, reversibility, no damage to the function of phonation, and the ability to perform readjustments [33]. High rates of early and late failures after 1-year follow-up later (only one-third of patients with marked improvement after 1-year follow-up) led to questioning of thyroplasty by a different group of surgeons [34]. Recently, myectomy and widening thyroplasty have been compared in a retrospective study in 35 patients. The authors reported that myectomy led to better voice quality in line with increased breathiness after the surgery [35].

Recurrent laryngeal nerve surgery is a third reported option. Transection of one recurrent nerve has been reported early [36]. Later, selective laryngeal adductor denervation combined with ansa cervicalis transfer and anastomosis to prevent total atrophy of TA muscles has been reported with good results [37, 38]. Chronic breathiness has been reported to be more likely in men. Adjuvant removal of TA muscle therefore has been recommended in women in case of recurrence [39].

Surgery for SD has even been reported to even result in better voice in comparison to BT treatment; however, the BT sample was small and the study design was retrospective [40]. To summarize, voice breaks can be effectively reduced by surgery, although severe hoarseness may result and long-term results are not yet predictable. Follow-up is crucial since there is a high risk of symptom recurrence within 5 years. Currently, surgery might therefore be considered in patients that cannot be provided with BT, refuse BT treatment, or are refractory to BT.

8.8.1.6 Adjuvant Therapy

SD is a chronic dystonia; a clear delineation from functional voice disorders can be difficult. Voice disorders frequently include or interfere with psychological disorders [41], and functional voice disorders can respond to voice or behavioral therapies; hence, a trial of voice therapy might be recommended before or in line with BT injections. However, dystonia of the larynx does normally not respond to voice therapy, a fact that also has been demonstrated in a prospective controlled trial [42]. One study addressed the role of behavioral (speech) therapy in combination with BT injections with suggestion that behavioral treatment may enhance the effectiveness of BT injections [43]. Recently, five subjects were implanted with electrical implant into the TA muscle with promising immediate results [44]. Targeting the interventions proximal to the TA muscle are promising future research projects.

8.9 Follow-Up and Evaluation of Treatment

A large number of articles have described the effectiveness of BT for the improvement of vocal symptoms in SD. However, the applied methods for outcome measurements are extremely variable in the literature. Measured variables include perceptual analysis and electroglottographic-myographic, acoustic, endoscopic, and stroboscopic evaluation. Further variables are duration of benefit, aerodynamics, and subjective ratings [17]. A telephone screening tool with standardized utterances with high interrater reliability can be used during follow-up. Outcome measures as possible should include acoustic function via computerized analysis, perception analysis, as well as aerodynamic function (Table 8.1). Literature with comparison of treatment versus no treatment is rare. Improvement of fundamental frequencies, self-ratings of improvement, and spectrographic ratings were documented in one placebo-controlled trial [45]. In a longitudinal study of adductor-type SD, an initial breathy phase could be distinguished from a late declining phase during a mean duration of one injection cycle of 26 weeks [46].

Table 8.1 Recommended outcome measurements for the treatment of SD

Acoustic measurements	• Fundamental frequency • Frequency and amplitude perturbation • Signal-to-noise ratio
Perception	• Subjective voice improvement • VHI • Spectrographic ratings of normalcy
Aerodynamic function	• Mean airflow • Coefficient of airflow variation • Air pressure • Phonation time

Conclusions

Adductor-type SD is a voice disorder of idiopathic neurogenic origin. Symptoms include mild to profound "strain and strangle" sensations during speech tasks. Two main clinical presentations exist: abductor- and adductor-type SD. The diagnosis is mainly based on perceptual analysis of speech. Treatment approaches have evolved from behavioral attempts at voice modification to surgical treatment with BT. By chemically denervating the TA muscle with BT, symptoms get better in up to 90% of the patients. Repeated injections are necessary because symptoms of SD always reappear after BT treatment within months. Surgery should only be considered as second-line treatment.

References

1. Van Pelt F, Ludlow CL, Smith PJ. Comparison of muscle activation patterns in adductor and abductor spasmodic dysphonia. Ann Otol Rhinol Laryngol. 1994;103:192–200.
2. Biller HF, Som ML, Lawson W. Laryngeal nerve crush for spastic dysphonia. Ann Otol Rhinol Laryngol. 1983;92:469.
3. Schweinfurth JM, Billante M, Courey MS. Risk factors and demographics in patients with spasmodic dysphonia. Laryngoscope. 2002;112:220–3.
4. Nutt JG, Muenter MD, Aronson A, Kurland LT, Melton LJ III. Epidemiology of focal and generalized dystonia in Rochester, Minnesota. Mov Disord. 1988;3:188–94.

5. Butler AG, Duffey PO, Hawthorne MR, Barnes MP. An epidemiologic survey of dystonia within the entire population of northeast England over the past nine years. Adv Neurol. 2004;94:95–9.
6. Blitzer A, Brin MF, Stewart CF. Botulinum toxin management of spasmodic dysphonia (laryngeal dystonia): a 12-year experience in more than 900 patients. Laryngoscope. 1998;108:1435–41.
7. Marras C, Lohmann K, Lang A, Klein C. Fixing the broken system of genetic locus symbols: Parkinson disease and dystonia as examples. Neurology. 2012;78:1016–24.
8. Tanner K, Roy N, Merrill RM, et al. Risk and protective factors for spasmodic dysphonia: a case-control investigation. J Voice. 2011;25:e35–46.
9. Perlmutter JS, Mink JW. Dysfunction of dopaminergic pathways in dystonia. Adv Neurol. 2004;94:163–70.
10. Cohen LG, Ludlow CL, Warden M, et al. Blink reflex excitability recovery curves in patients with spasmodic dysphonia. Neurology. 1989;39:572–7.
11. Simonyan K, Ludlow CL. Abnormal activation of the primary somatosensory cortex in spasmodic dysphonia: an fMRI study. Cereb Cortex. 2010;20:2749–59.
12. Childs L, Rickert S, Murry T, Blitzer A, Sulica L. Patient perceptions of factors leading to spasmodic dysphonia: a combined clinical experience of 350 patients. Laryngoscope. 2011;121:2195–8.
13. Sataloff RT, Mandel S, Mann EA, Ludlow CL. Practice parameter: laryngeal electromyography (an evidence-based review). Otolaryngol Head Neck Surg. 2004;130:770–9.
14. Van Houtte E, Claeys S, D'Haeseleer E, Wuyts F, Van Lierde K. An examination of surface EMG for the assessment of muscle tension dysphonia. J Voice. 2013;27:177–86.
15. Yang Q, Xu W, Li Y, Cheng L. Value of laryngeal electromyography in spasmodic dysphonia diagnosis and therapy. Ann Otol Rhinol Laryngol. 2015;124(7):579–83.
16. Watts C, Nye C, Whurr R. Botulinum toxin for treating spasmodic dysphonia (laryngeal dystonia): a systematic Cochrane review. Clin Rehabil. 2006;20:112–22.
17. Watts CR, Truong DD, Nye C. Evidence for the effectiveness of botulinum toxin for spasmodic dysphonia from high-quality research designs. J Neural Transm. 2008;115:625–30.
18. Simpson DM, Blitzer A, Brashear A, et al. Assessment: Botulinum neurotoxin for the treatment of movement disorders (an evidence-based review): report of the Therapeutics and Technology Assessment Subcommittee of the American Academy of Neurology. Neurology. 2008;70:1699–706.
19. Bielamowicz S, Squire S, Bidus K, Ludlow CL. Assessment of posterior cricoarytenoid botulinum toxin injections in patients with abductor spasmodic dysphonia. Ann Otol Rhinol Laryngol. 2001;110:406–12.
20. Garcia Ruiz PJ, Cenjor Espanol C, Sanchez Bernardos V, Astarloa R, Sanabria J, Garcia de Yebenes J. Botulinum toxin treatment for spasmodic dysphonia: percutaneous versus transoral approach. Clin Neuropharmacol. 1998;21:196–8.
21. Kim JW, Park JH, Park KN, Lee SW. Treatment efficacy of electromyography versus fiberscopy-guided botulinum toxin injection in adductor spasmodic dysphonia patients: a prospective comparative study. Sci World J. 2014;2014:327928.
22. Stong BC, DelGaudio JM, Hapner ER, Johns MM III. Safety of simultaneous bilateral botulinum toxin injections for abductor spasmodic dysphonia. Arch Otolaryngol Head Neck Surg. 2005;131:793–5.
23. Holden PK, Vokes DE, Taylor MB, Till JA, Crumley RL. Long-term botulinum toxin dose consistency for treatment of adductor spasmodic dysphonia. Ann Otol Rhinol Laryngol. 2007;116:891–6.
24. Holzer SE, Ludlow CL. The swallowing side effects of botulinum toxin type A injection in spasmodic dysphonia. Laryngoscope. 1996;106:86–92.
25. Novakovic D, Waters HH, D'Elia JB, Blitzer A. Botulinum toxin treatment of adductor spasmodic dysphonia: longitudinal functional outcomes. Laryngoscope. 2011;121:606–12.
26. Venkatesan NN, Johns MM, Hapner ER, DelGaudio JM. Abductor paralysis after botox injection for adductor spasmodic dysphonia. Laryngoscope. 2010;120:1177–80.
27. Nakamura K, Muta H, Watanabe Y, Mochizuki R, Yoshida T, Suzuki M. Surgical treatment for adductor spasmodic dysphonia–efficacy of bilateral thyroarytenoid myectomy under microlaryngoscopy. Acta Otolaryngol. 2008;128:1348–53.
28. Tsuji DH, Takahashi MT, Imamura R, Hachiya A, Sennes LU. Endoscopic laser thyroarytenoid myoneurectomy in patients with adductor spasmodic dysphonia: a pilot study on long-term outcome on voice quality. J Voice. 2012;26:666 e7–12.
29. Su CY, Lai CC, Wu PY, Huang HH. Transoral laser ventricular fold resection and thyroarytenoid myoneurectomy for adductor spasmodic dysphonia: long-term outcome. Laryngoscope. 2010;120:313–8.
30. Koufman JA, Rees CJ, Halum SL, Blalock D. Treatment of adductor-type spasmodic dysphonia by surgical myectomy: a preliminary report. Ann Otol Rhinol Laryngol. 2006;115:97–102.
31. Gandhi S, Remacle M, Mishra P, Desai V. Vocal outcome after endoscopic thyroarytenoid myoneurectomy in patients with adductor spasmodic dysphonia. Eur Arch Otorhinolaryngol. 2014;271:3249–54.
32. Isshiki N, Haji T, Yamamoto Y, Mahieu HF. Thyroplasty for adductor spasmodic dysphonia: further experiences. Laryngoscope. 2001;111:615–21.
33. Sanuki T, Isshiki N. Overall evaluation of effectiveness of type II thyroplasty for adductor spasmodic dysphonia. Laryngoscope. 2007;117:2255–9.
34. Chan SW, Baxter M, Oates J, Yorston A. Long-term results of type II thyroplasty for adductor spasmodic dysphonia. Laryngoscope. 2004;114:1604–8.
35. Nomoto M, Tokashiki R, Hiramatsu H, et al. The comparison of thyroarytenoid muscle myectomy and

type II thyroplasty for spasmodic dysphonia. J Voice. 2015;29(4):501–6.
36. Dedo HH. Recurrent laryngeal nerve section for spastic dysphonia. Ann Otol Rhinol Laryngol. 1976;85:451–9.
37. Berke GS, Blackwell KE, Gerratt BR, Verneil A, Jackson KS, Sercarz JA. Selective laryngeal adductor denervation-reinnervation: a new surgical treatment for adductor spasmodic dysphonia. Ann Otol Rhinol Laryngol. 1999;108:227–31.
38. Allegretto M, Morrison M, Rammage L, Lau DP. Selective denervation: reinnervation for the control of adductor spasmodic dysphonia. J Otolaryngol. 2003;32:185–9.
39. Chhetri DK, Mendelsohn AH, Blumin JH, Berke GS. Long-term follow-up results of selective laryngeal adductor denervation-reinnervation surgery for adductor spasmodic dysphonia. Laryngoscope. 2006;116:635–42.
40. Mendelsohn AH, Berke GS. Surgery or botulinum toxin for adductor spasmodic dysphonia: a comparative study. Ann Otol Rhinol Laryngol. 2012;121:231–8.
41. Willinger U, Volkl-Kernstock S, Aschauer HN. Marked depression and anxiety in patients with functional dysphonia. Psychiatry Res. 2005;134:85–91.
42. Silverman EP, Garvan C, Shrivastav R, Sapienza CM. Combined modality treatment of adductor spasmodic dysphonia. J Voice. 2012;26:77–86.
43. Murry T, Woodson GE. Combined-modality treatment of adductor spasmodic dysphonia with botulinum toxin and voice therapy. J Voice. 1995;9:460–5.
44. Pitman MJ. Treatment of spasmodic dysphonia with a neuromodulating electrical implant. Laryngoscope. 2014;124:2537–43.
45. Troung DD, Rontal M, Rolnick M, Aronson AE, Mistura K. Double-blind controlled study of botulinum toxin in adductor spasmodic dysphonia. Laryngoscope. 1991;101:630–4.
46. Paniello RC, Barlow J, Serna JS. Longitudinal follow-up of adductor spasmodic dysphonia patients after botulinum toxin injection: quality of life results. Laryngoscope. 2008;118:564–8.

Non-cosmetic Botulinum Toxin Treatments in the Head and Neck

9

Lyndsay L. Madden and Clark A. Rosen

Abstract

Treatment of dystonias in the head and neck can be challenging for even the most experienced otolaryngologist. Available oral therapeutic options often fail to provide improvement in many patients and oftentimes come with intolerable systemic side effects that limit their use. With the introduction of botulinum toxin (BTX) to the treatment armamentarium for patients with dystonias, patients would have the chance for treatment by targeting only focal areas. With the use of BTX, treating physicians can focus treatment to only areas affected by the dystonia. This greatly minimizes the occurrence of systemic side effects. In this chapter, we will present a review of the history of the medical applications of BTX and discuss its role in the treatment of various dystonias of the head and neck.

9.1 Introduction

9.1.1 History

Botulinum toxin is the most powerful neurotoxin used by humans to date [1]. It is a large complex protein from the anaerobic, spore-forming bacillus *Clostridium botulinum* which forms spores that germinate, reproduce, and produce toxin under appropriate conditions. The prospect for medical applications of BTX was not recognized until early 1980 by Scott [2], who used small doses of the BTX to alter spastic muscles for strabismus. This study generated a successful, safe, and effective treatment algorithm, using BTX for strabismus without any significant local or systemic side effects. This study and a series of other clinical reports [3–6] led to the Food and Drug Administration (FDA) approval of BTX for ophthalmologic and neurologic uses in strabismus, blepharospasm, and hemifacial spasm in 1989.

Today, several brands of BTX have been approved for therapeutic use in cervical dystonia, strabismus, blepharospasm, hyperhidrosis, overactive bladder, chronic migraine, and upper limb spasticity and cosmetically for temporary improvement in vertical glabellar rhytids and lateral canthal lines. Although "off-label," the clinical use of BTX has been expanded widely to include the treatment of many other conditions,

L.L. Madden • C.A. Rosen (✉)
Department of Otolaryngology, University of Pittsburgh Voice Center, Building D.Suite 2100, 1400 Locust Street, Pittsburgh, PA 15219, USA
e-mail: rosenca@upmc.edu

C. Sittel, O. Guntinas-Lichius (eds.), *Neurolaryngology*,
https://doi.org/10.1007/978-3-319-61724-4_9

including bruxism, Frey syndrome, other types of facial hyperkinetic lines, muscle tension dysphonia, torticollis, spasmodic dysphonia, and bilateral masseteric hypertrophy, to name a few.

Seven separate antigenic BTXs produced by *C. botulinum* have been described (BTX-A, BTX-B, BTX-C, BTX-D, BTX-E, BTX-F, BTX-G) [7]. The human nervous system has been found to be reactive to only five of the toxin serotypes (BTX-A, BTX-B, BTX-E, BTX-F, BTX-G) and unaffected by two (BTX-C, BTX-D) [8].

9.1.2 Mechanism of Action

Botulinum toxin acts by blocking the release of acetylcholine from cholinergic nerve endings, causing inactivity of muscles or glands. In order to wield its clinical action, BTX has to gain entry into the presynaptic neuronal and terminal thru its translocation domain via endocytosis, and this binding causes disruption to SNARE proteins (soluble *N*-ethylmaleimide-sensitive factor attachment protein receptors) [9]. Without an active SNARE protein, the neurotransmitter vesicle can no longer fuse with the cell membrane, effectively preventing the exocytotic release of acetylcholine. BTX-A binds to and cleaves the 25 kD SNARE protein "SNAP-25" (synaptosomal-associated protein), while BTX-B binds to and cleaves the "VAMP" (vesicle-associated membrane protein) [9]. Flaccid paralysis that follows injection with BTX is temporary. Chemodenervation from BTX is followed by regrowth and sprouting of axonal collaterals, which establish new connections at the muscle's motor end plates. At close to 3 months, neural transmission through the initial nerve terminal is reestablished, and collateral axons regress. This correlates to regaining of muscle function at around 3–4 months postinjection [10].

BTX has also been shown to block efferent autonomic fibers to exocrine glands and smooth muscle [11], which accounts for its use in hyperhidrosis and gustatory sweating (Frey's syndrome). SNARE proteins have also been shown to play a role in C-fiber nociceptive neurons that release glutamate and substance P. Those substances result in vasodilation with the release of bradykinin, prostaglandins, histamine, and serotonin, all of which promote inflammation [12]. Since BTX-A inhibits these pro-inflammatory factors, this may account for treatment possibilities in chronic pain disorders such as migraine headache and various neuralgias.

9.1.3 Immunogenicity/Allergy/ Resistance of Botulinum Toxin

Botulinum toxin has the potential to trigger an immunogenic response postinjection that can result in the formation of neutralizing antibodies. These antibodies may render BTX ineffective at the next injection. Studies suggest that a larger neurotoxin complex, as with certain formulations of BTX, could lead to a higher possibility of development of neutralizing antibodies [13]. Protein loads in current commercially available preparations are much lower than in earlier formulations (prior to 1998), leading to a decrease in antibody formation. However, immunogenic responses still occur with more contemporary formulations, predominantly with the utilization of larger doses of BTX in therapeutic, non-cosmetic applications [14]. Certain measures and precautions can be taken to avoid this response, including using the lowest effective dose, avoiding booster injections, and not injecting patients prior to a 3-month postinjection waiting period [1]. If immunogenic resistance to BTX-A occurs, the use of BTX-B may prove beneficial [15].

Allergic responses to BTX are extremely rare and have sparsely been reported in the literature. Allergic reactions that have been reported range from mild skin rashes to severe skin rashes with granuloma formation and systemic even anaphylactic reactions [16–18]. It is unknown and untested if the allergic responses are related to the BTX itself or the solvent used for reconstitution.

9.1.4 Commercially Available Botulinum Toxin

There are several brands of commercially available BTX [19]. Each formulation possesses characteristics that are neither identical nor interchangeable, and each has different potencies and indications. For a comparison and overview of current commercially available preparations of BTX, see Table 9.1.

Table 9.1 Comparison of BTX preparations

	OnabotulinumtoxinA	AbotulinumtoxinA	IncobotulinumtoxinA	RimabotulinumtoxinB	CBTX-A	Bonta
Commercial name	Botox®, Botox Cosmetic®, Vistabel®, Vistabex®	Dysport®, Reloxin®, Azzalure®	Xeomin®/Bocouture®	Myobloc®, NeuroBloc®	Prosigne®, Lantox®	Neuronox®
Company	Allergan Inc.	Medicis Pharmaceutical Group	Merc Pharmaceuticals	Solstice Neurosciences Inc.	Lanzhou Institute of Biological Products, China	Medy-Tox Inc., South Korea
Type	A	A	A	B	A	A
Strength (BTX-A: product)	1:1	1:2–1:4	1:1	1:50–1:100		
FDA approval	*Botox*®: cervical dystonia, severe primary axillary hyperhidrosis, blepharospasm, neurogenic detrusor overactivity, chronic migraine, upper limb spasticity, strabismus, blepharospasm *Botox Cosmetic*®: glabellar lines (moderate-severe), lateral canthal lines (moderate-severe)	Cervical dystonia, glabellar lines (moderate-severe)	Blepharospasm, cervical dystonia, glabellar lines	Cervical dystonia	None (risk of prion infection)	None
Units/vial	100 or 200	300 or 500	50 or 100	2500; 5000; 10,000	50 or 100	100
Reconstitution	Preservative-free 0.9% NaCl	Preservative-free 0.9% NaCl	Preservative-free 0.9% NaCl	Not necessary		
Countries available	Worldwide, including the USA and Canada	>65 countries, including the USA and Canada	The USA since 2011, Germany, other European countries, Mexico, Argentina, Brazil	The USA and some European countries	>10 countries, not in the USA or Canada	South Korea, India, South America, not in the USA or Canada

Botox®/Botox Cosmetic® is the trade name for onabotulinumtoxinA and is approved for over 20 indications in more than 75 countries [20]. It comprises 85% of the worldwide BTX market, and most scientific articles on BTX are about Botox® [20]. This product was initially purified by Shantz and later used clinically by Scott in San Francisco [2].

Dysport®, Reloxin®, and Azzalure® are the trade names for abotulinumtoxinA [21] which was first approved by the FDA in 2009 for the treatment of cervical dystonia and temporary improvement of moderate to severe glabellar lines [22]. Although the same neurotoxin, BTX-A, is used in both Botox® and Dysport®, the difference lies in the purification process. Botox® is purified with repetitive precipitation and redissolution, and Dysport® is purified using a column separation method [20]. Postinjection, Dysport® has been shown to have a greater spreading effect, leading to a more diffuse distribution clinically. Dose ratios between the two toxins have been greatly debated. The literature suggests a dose ratio, in clinical practice, to be approximately 3:1 when compared to Botox® [23].

Xeomin®/Bocouture®, the trade name for incobotulinumtoxinA, is licensed in Germany. In this product, the complexing proteins are stripped from the active toxin. In 2011, Xeomin® was FDA approved in the USA for temporary improvement of moderate to severe glabellar lines in adults. It exhibits a dose ratio with Botox® that is 1:1 [20]. No significant differences in safety and efficacy have been found in studies comparing Botox® and Xeomin®. Xeomin® has been formulated to be free of therapeutically unnecessary complexing proteins, as aforementioned. This is suggested to lead to greater efficacy and reduced risk of antibody formation and sensitization [24] but has yet to be clinically determined. It is also of note that storage of an unopened vial of this product may be stored at room temperature, 20–25 °C (68–77 °F).

Neuronox®, Prosigne®, CBTX-A, and Lantox® are other commercially available BTX-A from other countries but are not FDA approved in the USA [20, 25]. It is worth noting that CNBTX-A is a BTX-A that is not approved or licensed in any country. It should not be confused with CBTX-A or other BTX-A preparations. CNBTX-A has been found to contain much higher levels of neurotoxin than listed on its package insert and could lead to severe health risk if administered to humans [26].

Myobloc® and NeuroBloc® are the trade names associated with rimabotulinumtoxinB. It is the only botulinum toxin type B commercially available in the USA indicated for cervical dystonia and associated neck pain and was the first FDA-approved treatment for cervical dystonia in the USA. Myobloc®/NeuroBloc® has a more rapid onset and greater area of diffusion in clinical use [27]. It is a liquid preparation with a pH of 5.5–6.5, which leads to increased discomfort at the injection site. When compared to Botox®, it is significantly less effective per unit in a rate of 50:1–100:1 [27, 28].

9.2 The Injection Procedure

9.2.1 Reconstitution

OnabotulinumtoxinA (Botox®) is the most studied neurotoxin. From this point forward, the reader should know that we will only discuss treatments using this product. Initially, BTX was thought to be a fragile substance [29], but later studies have dismissed this initial belief and proven the activity of BTX in different preparatory situations. Various other studies have shown that reconstitution of onabotulinumtoxinA (Botox®) with preserved saline, which contains benzyl alcohol, does not affect the neurotoxin's potency [30, 31]. In 2004 a consensus panel stated that preserved saline is the preferable method for the reconstitution of onabotulinumtoxinA (Botox®) [32]. It is also of note that a second panel reported that the benzyl alcohol component acts as a local anesthetic at low volumes [33]. Other products have also been studied for the reconstitution of BTX, including unpreserved saline [29], lidocaine with epinephrine [34–37], bupivacaine [26], and sterile water [38].

9.2.2 Dilution

The package insert of Botox® recommends dilution of 100 units with varying amounts of saline to achieve a wide range of concentrations. For injection into the vocal folds, accepted doses range from concentrations of 0.625–10 U/0.1 mL. Many physicians believe that the higher the volume of diluted BTX, the greater the chance of diffusion to unwanted sites and the shorter the duration of effect, leading to suboptimal results [39]. Preferably, 0.1 mL of solution is used for injection into a single vocal fold; however, a volume of 0.2 mL is also acceptable. At that volume, there is little to virtually no risk of airway obstruction from vocal fold engorgement. A needle larger than a 21 gauge should be used for reconstitution, dilution, and transfer from vial to injection syringe. This allows for multiple uses of one vial of toxin. Despite the FDA's recommendation to use Botox® as a single-dose vial, Barrow et al. looked at 743 subjects receiving Botox® using single-dose vials in a multidose fashion with no reported evidence of infection [40]. After the correct dose is sterilely prepared, the appropriate injection needle, which depends on the route of administration, is attached to the syringe.

9.2.3 Storage

FDA-approved product labeling for Botox® recommends intramuscular administration within 4 h of reconstitution [41]. Because a single 100-MU vial may be sufficient to treat more than one patient and administration is limited to a 4-h window, a few issues arise: waste of an expensive product if multiple patients are unable to be treated within this very restricted time limit and inconvenience to patients who are faced with limited or restricted time intervals to receive treatment. Consequently, many physicians have adopted the off-label practice of refrigeration (4 °C) or freezing (−20 °C) of the product in storage. Studies have shown that effectiveness of fresh vs. stored BTX is comparable [29, 42–46]. Storage for up to 30 days is adequate.

9.2.4 Botulinum Toxin Injection Approaches

There are a variety of approaches to delivering botulinum toxin to the larynx, including percutaneous injection with EMG guidance (most traditional), percutaneous injection with laryngoscopic guidance, supraglottic injection with laryngoscopic guidance, and a combined approach using both EMG and laryngoscopic guidance. Distinct advantages and disadvantages exist for the above approaches. The surgeon, equipment availability, patient's disease characteristics, and preference determine selection of the most advantageous approach. It is important to note that BTX is not FDA approved, and patients should be counseled on its off-label usage, but the American Academy of Otolaryngology-Head and Neck Surgery (AAO-HNS) endorses the use of EMG-guided BTX injection into targeted laryngeal musculature for the primary treatment of laryngeal dystonias [47]. The literature also suggests that EMG-guided BTX injection is the gold standard for spasmodic dystonia (SD)/laryngeal dystonias, and its efficacy of treatment has been supported in double-blind placebo-controlled trials [48, 49].

Percutaneous injection under EMG guidance is the quickest and most precise method of botulinum toxin delivery into the larynx and other areas of the head and neck, including muscles involved in oromandibular dystonias and blepharospasm. This technique does, however, have a learning curve and requires skill, training, and EMG equipment. Given these barriers, some surgeons choose to use an alternate method, which includes a percutaneous or peroral technique under laryngoscopic (visual) guidance or "blind" percutaneous injection. These techniques are less precise and often require a higher dose of BTX than the EMG-guided percutaneous injection technique, and they are suboptimal.

Supraglottic BTX injection for adductor SD (ADSD) with laryngoscopic guidance offers the advantage of a more gradual onset of action, smoothing of vocal "peaks and troughs" associated with true vocal fold injection, less-severe breathy voice, and preservation of singing voice/pitch control in many patients. This approach's disadvantages include a shorter duration, less-predictable voice results, and a more involved and timely injection procedure. This unreliability most likely occurs from variable anatomy of the supraglottis with variable needle location during the injection. This procedure may be preferred by the professional voice user stricken with ADSD due to the reduced number of days with a soft, breathy, or weaker voice. This same approach can be used for treating the false vocal folds in laryngeal essential tremor (ET).

Treatment of the interarytenoid muscle is accomplished using a combined approach. This muscle is treated by both percutaneous EMG guidance and visualization accomplished via flexible transnasal laryngoscopy.

9.2.5 Equipment

Equipment needed for BTX injection via an EMG-guided percutaneous approach:

- EMG machine
- Botulinum toxin
- Reconstitution solution of choice
- Insulated 26 g EMG needle (both 37 mm and 50 mm in length)
- Ground and reference electrodes
- Tuberculin syringe
- Local anesthetic for the skin (1% lidocaine with 1:100,000 epinephrine) (optional)

Additional equipment necessary for percutaneous injection with laryngoscopic guidance and/or peroral supraglottic injection with laryngoscopic guidance:

- Flexible laryngoscope (with working channel or EndoSheath® with channeled sheath)
- C-Mount camera to attach to flexible laryngoscope (unless using a distal chip flexible laryngoscope)
- Video monitor for visualization
- Three to 6 mL of 4% plain lidocaine
- 27 g needle, 37 mm in length (percutaneous injection with laryngoscopic guidance)
- Orotracheal injector device for peroral injection approach
- Benzocaine topical spray (optional)
- Curved Abraham cannula
- Fine-gauge injection needle for use with working channel in flexible laryngoscope

9.3 Hyperkinetic Disorders of the Head and Neck and Treatment Techniques

9.3.1 Dystonia

Dystonia is a chronic neurologic disorder of central motor processing within the basal ganglia (extrapyramidal system). Characteristic symptoms of a patient with dystonia include involuntary sustained muscle contractions of agonist and antagonist muscles, which cause twisting and repetitive movements or abnormal postures. Oftentimes, sedatives may mitigate the movements; anxiety will aggravate the movements; and posturing disappears during sleep. Dystonias may be focal, as in spasmodic dysphonia or cervical dystonia; segmental, as in Meige's syndrome; multifocal when two or more noncontiguous body regions are involved; or generalized and can be secondary to a wide variety of causes or simply idiopathic. Treatment of dystonic conditions of the head and neck commonly involves a multidisciplinary treatment team including the primary care physician, neurologist, and otolaryngologist.

Laryngeal dystonia, also known as spasmodic dystonia (SD), is a focal, task-specific, action-induced spasm of the laryngeal musculature. It is usually classified into adductor (ADSD), abductor (ABSD), and mixed forms via hallmark clinical features. ADSD, the far more common form, is characterized by inappropriate, excessive glottic closure and, as a result, produces strangled breaks in connected speech. ABSD, in contrast, causes inappropriate glottal opening that produces breathy breaks and hypophonia. Classification of SD into ADSD and ABSD is imperative to treatment: ADSD is treated with injection of BTX into the thyroarytenoid/lateral cricoarytenoid (TA/LCA) muscles and/or the interarytenoid (IA) muscle and in ABSD. BTX is injected into the posterior cricoarytenoid (PCA) muscle.

9.3.2 Essential Tremor of the Vocal Tract

Essential tremor of the vocal tract (ETV) is a benign, commonly age-related, and likely inherited voice disorder consisting of involuntary muscle contractions, which can affect the voice to a debilitating extent in some patients [50]. Rhythmic head titubation and shaking of the hands are most commonly seen. These oscillatory movements can also be seen, in varying degrees, along all portions of the respiratory tract (i.e., velum, base of the tongue, pharynx, larynx, vocal folds) and can be graded on laryngoscopy using the Vocal Tremor Scoring System (VTSS) [51]. Although aggravated by anxiety, public speaking, and telephone use and mitigated by alcohol and benzodiazepines, ETV differs from SD with its rhythmic nature and presence across all speaking tasks. Patients with ET are treated with medicinal, systemic agents such as propranolol and primidone; however, in our experience, ETV does not respond as readily as with axial-based tremor disease. BTX treatment has been effective at symptomatic relief for ETV by injecting the false vocal folds, TA/LCA complex, PCA, CT, IA, FVF, strap muscles, etc. [52].

9.3.3 Percutaneous EMG-Guided Botulinum Toxin Injection

a. Connecting EMG electrodes: A ground and reference electrode is attached to a patient's skin near the injection site. The insulated injection needle, which serves as a monopolar sampling electrode during the injection, is attached to an EMG recording device.
b. *TA/LCA muscle complex localization and injection*: The patient is placed in semirecumbent position with the mentum elevated and occiput or the head back. The headpiece of an ENT chair can be positioned to allow neck extension (Fig. 9.1). The patient is asked not to swallow and breathe quietly. With all of the following techniques, the skin is anesthetized with local anesthetic. The author uses a 30 g needle and 3 cc syringe with 1% lidocaine with 1:100,000 epinephrine and sodium bicarbonate. The EMG needle electrode is inserted into the cricothyroid space 2–3 mm off of the midline toward the side to be injected and advanced superiorly and laterally (Fig. 9.2). An off-the-midline entry point is used to attempt to avoid the airway, which is very stimulating to a patient. Entry into the airway produces a characteristic sound in the EMG

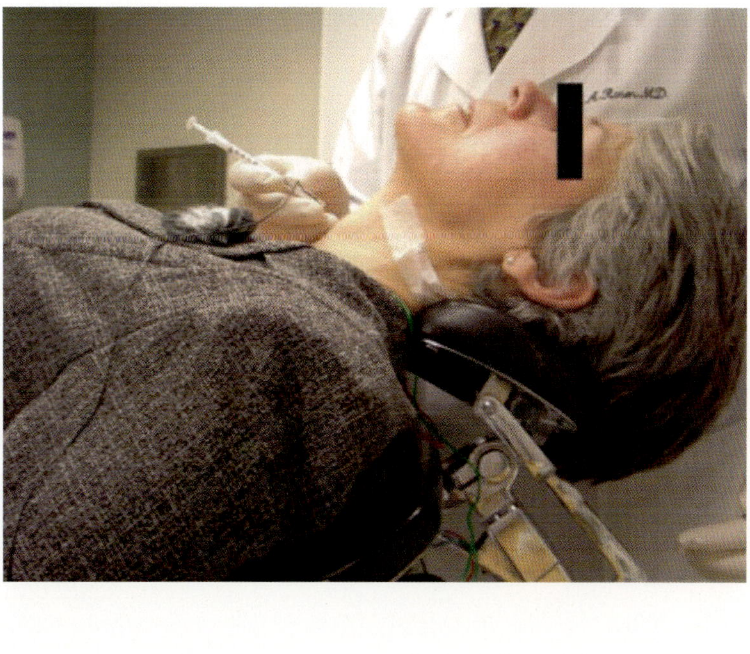

Fig. 9.1 Position of the patient for percutaneous TA/LCA muscle botulinum toxin injection [Reprinted from Ref. [53], with permission from Springer-Verlag]

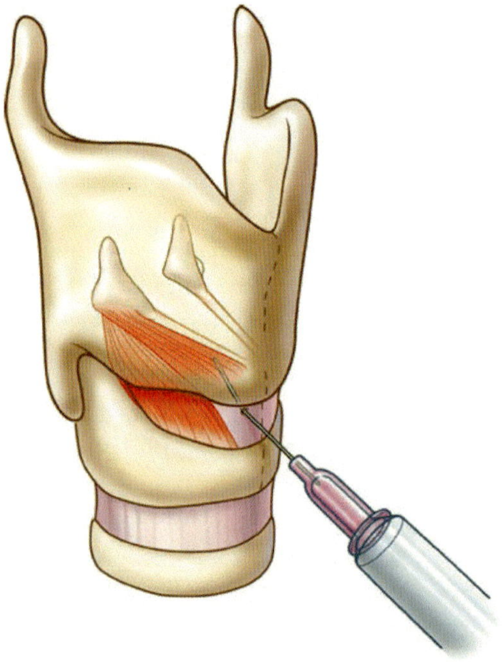

Fig. 9.2 Insertion of needle through cricothyroid membrane into the TA/LCA muscle complex for botulinum toxin injection [Reprinted from Ref. [53], with permission from Springer-Verlag]

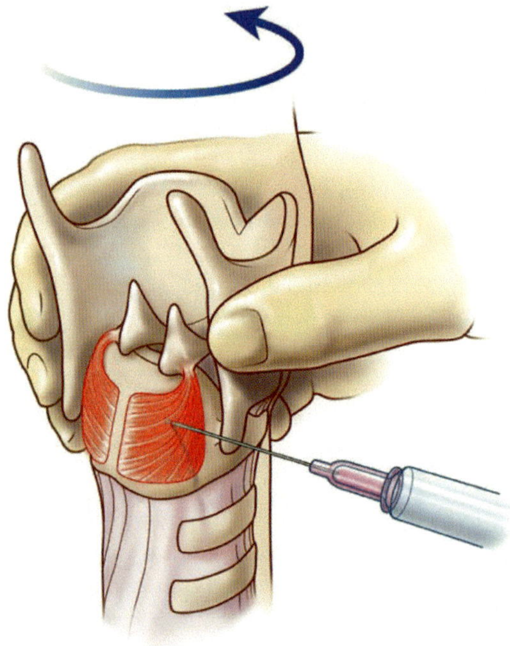

Fig. 9.3 Placement of EMG needle into the posterior cricoarytenoid muscle, using a retrolaryngeal approach [Reprinted from Ref. [53], with permission from Springer-Verlag]

signal, which should alert the physician to redirect the needle more laterally. Once the needle has been inserted through the cricothyroid membrane, it is maneuvered within the tissues until the tip lies in an area of crisp motor unit potentials. The patient is asked to phonate or perform a Valsalva maneuver, a brisk recruitment and a full interference pattern confirm placement, and the BTX is injected. A characteristic prephonatory burst on EMG is of benefit for optimal injection localization.

c. *PCA muscle localization and injection*: A retrolaryngeal or a translaryngeal approach can be taken to inject the PCA. If using the *retrolaryngeal technique*, the patient is seated upright, and the physician places his or her thumb at the posterior border of the thyroid cartilage on the side to be injected. Using counterpressure on the opposite side of the thyroid cartilage from the other four fingers, the larynx is gently rotated to expose its posterior aspect. An adequate amount of anesthetic is then used. The needle pierces the skin along the lower half of the posterior border of the thyroid cartilage and is advanced until it stops against the posterolateral surface of the cricoid. The needle is then pulled back slightly, and the patient is asked to sniff for confirmation of placement (Fig. 9.3). When the sniff is initiated and a brisk recruitment is initiated, the BTX is injected. If using the *translaryngeal approach*, the needle must cross the endolaryngeal mucosa so an intratracheal injection of 4% plain lidocaine is useful to prevent coughing and discomfort. After this, the needle is inserted through the cricothyroid membrane in the midline and directed posteriorly across the glottis lumen and angled toward the side to be injected. Using gentle pressure, it is pushed through the lamina of the cricoid cartilage until the opposite side is reached (this may be difficult in a very calcified cricoid cartilage in an older adult). The first electrical signal encountered on the far side represents the PCA muscle. Confirmation, again, is achieved using a sniff task. Once the physician finds an area with brisk recruitment, the BTX is injected (Fig. 9.4).

d. *IA muscle localization and injection*: The IA muscle is injected using a translaryngeal injection with flexible transnasal laryngoscopic guidance technique. Local anesthesia is applied to the endolarynx. The nasal cavity is anesthetized (50/50 mix of oxymetazoline and 4% lidocaine), and an assistant inserts a flexible laryngoscope, attached to a video monitor through the nasal cavity. After this, the needle is inserted through the cricothyroid membrane in the midline across the glottic lumen and directed straight posterior and slightly cephalad toward the IA muscle, which lies on the inner surface of the cricoid cartilage. The patient is asked to phonate, placement is confirmed with brisk recruitment, and the BTX is injected (Figs. 9.5 and 9.6).

e. *Supraglottic injection with laryngoscopic guidance*: As mentioned earlier, supraglottic BTX injection with laryngoscopic guidance is effective for treatment of ADSD as well as ETV involving the supraglottis. Two different injection approaches can be employed: (1)

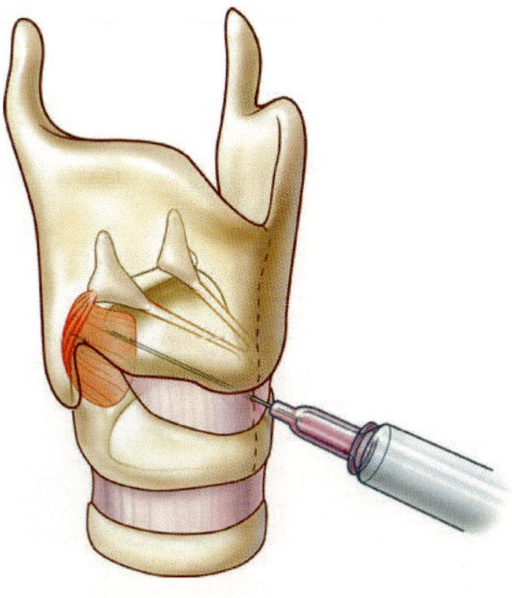

Fig. 9.4 Placement of EMG needle into the posterior cricoarytenoid muscle using a translaryngeal approach [Reprinted from Ref. [53], with permission from Springer-Verlag]

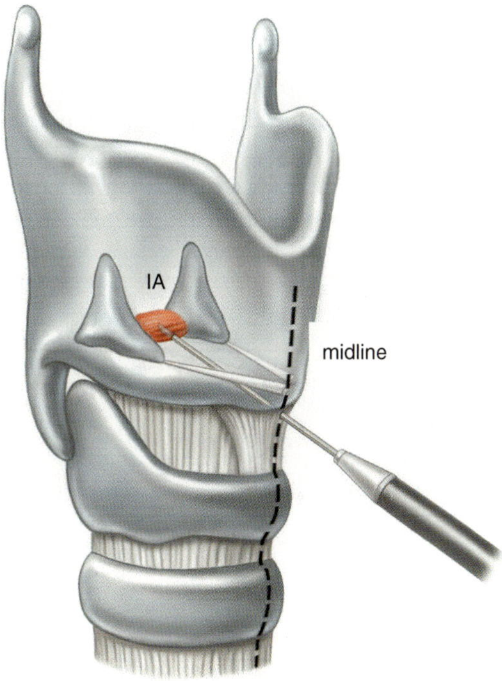

Fig. 9.5 Translaryngeal injection of the interarytenoid muscle (IA)

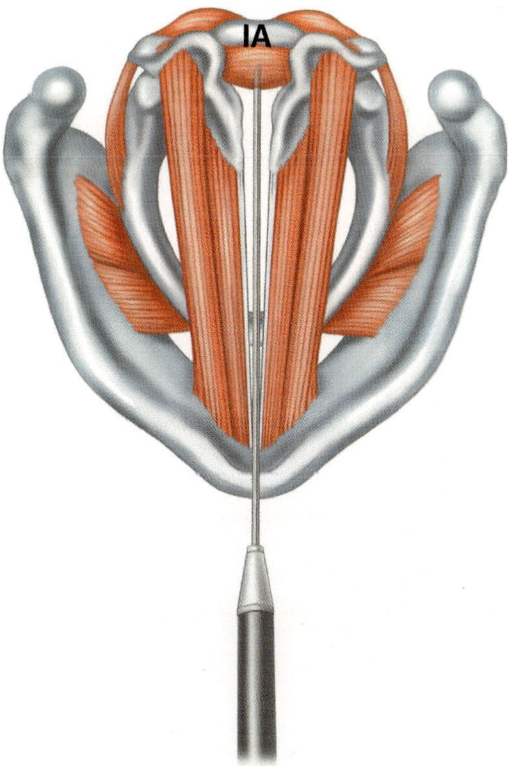

Fig. 9.6 Endoscopic-guided view of translaryngeal injection of the interarytenoid muscle (IA)

peroral injection and (2) an approach using a working channel of a flexible laryngoscope (Fig. 9.7). Each of these two approaches is efficacious, and the chosen technique is chosen by the physician. Patients tend to tolerate injection through a working channel of a flexible laryngoscope more than using the peroral route. When using the *laryngoscopic technique*, the nose is anesthetized (50/50 mix of oxymetazoline and 4% lidocaine) as well as the oropharynx and larynx (nebulized 3 cc of 4% lidocaine). The flexible scope attached to a video monitor is then passed through the nasal cavity. At this point, additional 4% lidocaine can be "dripped" onto the larynx through the channel on the laryngoscope (care should be taken not to give a patient more lidocaine than necessary as toxic doses can be easily reached. Maximum dose of lidocaine should not exceed 4 mg/kg). The patient is bent forward at the waist with the neck extended into a "sniffing" position to maximize laryngeal exposure. An injector needle device is placed through the channel in the scope, and BTX can be injected into the false vocal folds. The plane of injection needs to ideally be into a superficial/submucosal area, forming a characteristic "bleb" (Fig. 9.8). When using the *peroral technique with laryngoscopic guidance*, the flexible scope is passed through the nasal passage as in the technique above with the same positioning of the patient. After this BTX is drawn up into a 1-mL syringe and secured into a curved injector device (orotracheal injection device, Xomed, Jacksonville,

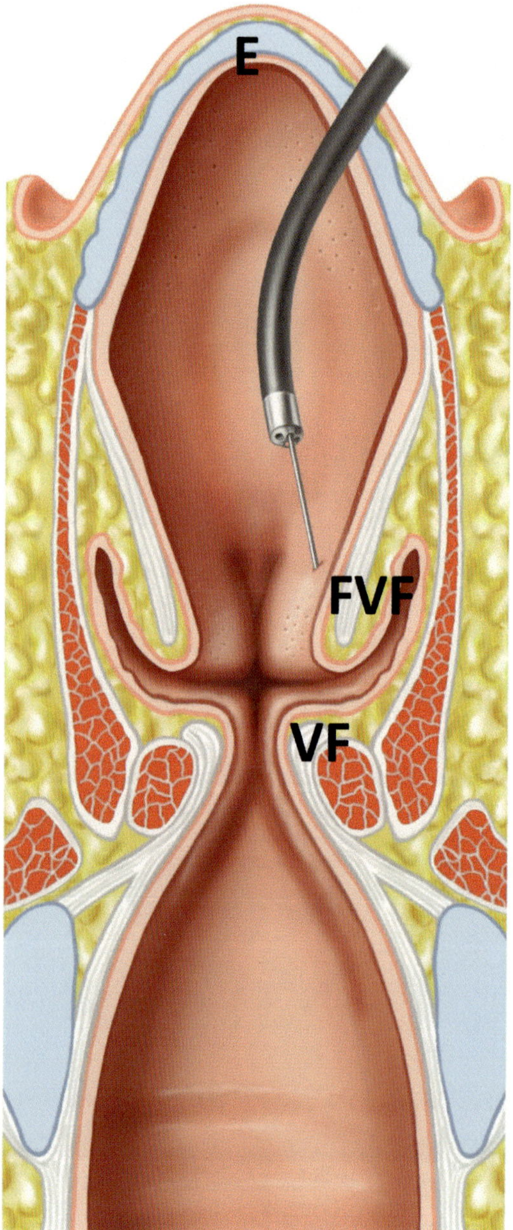

Fig. 9.7 False vocal fold (FVF) injection with the transnasal, endoscopic technique. *VF* vocal fold, *E* epiglottis

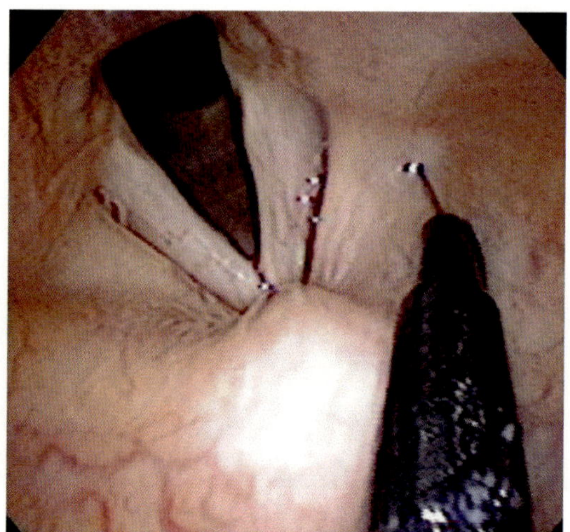

Fig. 9.8 False vocal fold site(s) for transoral botulinum toxin injection [Reprinted from Ref. [53] with permission from Springer-Verlag]

Fl). The needle is advanced into the oropharynx under direct visualization through the laryngoscope (a Hopkins rod-lens telescope, 70° or 90°, can also be used). The patient is instructed to phonate as the needle enters the oral cavity, which elevates the soft palate, clearing a path into the oropharynx. The assistant should position the flexible scope just above the palate until the needle is visualized in the oropharynx. The needle is then advanced to the false vocal folds with the assistant following behind with the laryngoscope. Injection is carried out, again, in the submucosal plane forming a bleb (Fig. 9.9).

f. *Post procedure care*: Patients may be discharged immediately after the injection. Patients receiving TA/LCA injections should be advised that they may have a period of breathiness and dysphagia. Patients receiving topical anesthesia to their larynx should be warned to not drink or eat for 2 h to prevent aspiration.

Systemic medical treatments are occasionally used for hyperkinetic disorders of the head and neck. Medications such as carbidopa/levodopa [49], trihexyphenidyl [54], benztropine [55], baclofen [56], clonazepam [57], and tetrabenazine [58] have been used but come with a high incidence of intolerance and a wide side effect profile when compared to BTX treatment. Patients with debilitating symptoms refractory to treatment with medication and/or BTX can be considered for deep brain stimulator placement [59].

Summary slide for laryngeal injections is shown in Table 9.2.

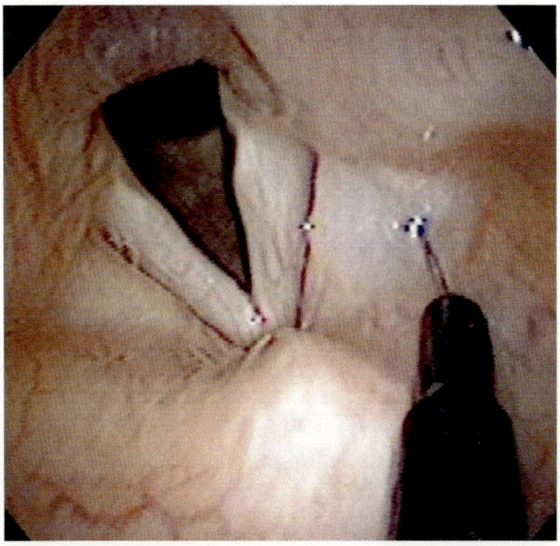

Fig. 9.9 Characteristic submucosal bleb immediately after transoral botulinum toxin injection [Reprinted from Ref. [53], with permission from Springer-Verlag]

9.3.4 Sites of Injections for Other Head and Neck Focal Dystonias

The authors also use BTX as an adjunctive therapy for other focal dystonias of the head and neck. These are also completed under EMG guidance with tasks specific to each muscle group, for engagement and determination of correct area of administration of BTX. These are summarized in Tables 9.3 and 9.4.

Table 9.2 Botox® administration site, indication, dose range, and technique for laryngeal hyperkinetic disorders

Site	Indication	Dose range	Technique
TA/LCA	ADSD, ETV	0.625–2.5 U	EMG percutaneous
PCA	ABSD, ETV	1.25–10 U	EMG percutaneous
CT	ETV	0.625–5 U	EMG percutaneous
IA	ADSD, ETV	0.625–5 U	Combined endoscopic and EMG percutaneous
FVF	ETV	0.625–5 U	Endoscopic

Table 9.3 Botox® administration site and dose range for blepharospasm used by the author

Muscle	Botox dosage
Orbicularis oculi (pretarsal fibers)	1–2.5 units/site
Frontalis	2.5–7.5 units/site
Corrugators	2.5–5 units/site
Procerus	2.5–5 units/site

Table 9.4 Botox® administration sites of oromandibular dystonias used by the author

Dystonia	Involved muscle
Jaw-closing dystonia	Masseters
	Temporalis
Jaw-opening dystonia	Lateral pterygoids
	Digastric
	Omohyoid
	Geniohyoid
Lingual dystonia	Genioglossus
	Hypoglossus
Jaw deviation	Lateral pterygoids (contralateral to the side of deviation
Orofacial dystonias (dyskinesias)	Orbicularis oris
	Mentalis
	Platysma
	Nasalis
	Depressor labii
	Risorius
	Zygomaticus

9.4 Other Uses of Botulinum Toxin in the Head and Neck

9.4.1 Cervical Dystonia and Torticollis

Cervical dystonia is the most commonly occurring cervical dystonia, and BTX types A and B have been approved for the treatment of cervical dystonia since 2000 [60]. Botulinum toxin has been shown to improve both the abnormal posture and the pain associated with cervical dystonia [61–63]. A combination of torticollis, laterocollis, anterocollis, and retrocollis is frequently observed, and knowledge of the muscles involved for each subtype and/or presentation is indispensable for the formation of a treatment plan using EMG-guided injection of BTX.

9.4.2 Frey's Syndrome

Frey's syndrome is an autonomic condition that typically occurs after parotidectomy and is caused by aberrant regeneration of postganglionic parasympathetic fibers innervating sympathetic cholinergic sweat glands resulting in sweating, flushing, and piloerection while eating (gustatory sweating) [64]. Several case series have documented the effectiveness of BTX in Frey's syndrome [65–69]. With the use of BTX in Frey's syndrome, the area of gustatory sweating is identified by an iodine-starch test or simply by patient report of the involved area.

9.4.3 First Bite Syndrome

First bite syndrome (FBS) is a complication of parapharyngeal space surgical procedures. Patients with FBS oftentimes present with pain in the parotid and jaw, with radiation to the ear lasting a few seconds that improves with each bite, and is typically worst at the first meal of the day [70, 71]. It was proposed by Netterville et al. [72] that FBS involves a loss of sympathetic nerve function to the parotid, causing a denervation supersensitivity of salivary gland myoepithelial cells. Studies suggest that with BTX treatment of the parotid gland, in FBS, blockade of cholinergic innervations on the affected gland may minimize the contraction of myoepithelial cells and salivation, in turn decreasing the severity of FBS [73]. The affected parotid gland is typically treated with 30 units of Botox®, with three injections of 10 units each in the area of the parotid gland.

9.4.4 Cricopharyngeus/TEP Failure

In most cases, tracheoesophageal puncture (TEP) in laryngectomy patients allows excellent speech quality. The procedure involves cricopharyngeal (CP) myotomy and placement of a speaking valve. Failure of the TEP can be caused directly by CP spasm leading to dysphagia and difficulty with speech [74]. This has traditionally been treated with serial esophageal dilations, pharyngeal myotomy, or pharyngeal neurectomy [75]. BTX injection to the CP muscle under EMG guidance has been reported to improve dysphagia. Several retrospective [76–79] and one prospective studies [80] have examined the efficacy of BTX in treating TEP failure and associated dysphagia. These studies have shown promising results.

9.4.5 Recurrent Vocal Fold Granuloma

Vocal fold granulomas are notoriously recalcitrant to surgical therapy and are commonly exacerbated by LPR. Most vocal fold granulomas are located in the posterior 1/3 of the vocal fold, either unilaterally or bilaterally at or near the vocal process of the arytenoid cartilage. Treatment of LPR often leads to resolution of the granuloma. One study found that of patients with LPR, up to 75% responded to clinical treatment with PPI therapy; however, 21% demonstrated recurrence [41]. A treatment option for these recalcitrant granulomas involves voice therapy in combination with BTX injection into the TA/LCA muscle complex. This reduces extensive interarytenoid contact by causing a temporary paresis of the vocal fold. BTX in this patient population causes significant dysphonia; the patient should be prepared for this vocal limitation.

References

1. Huang W, Foster JA, Rogachefsky AS. Pharmacology of botulinum toxin. J Am Acad Dermatol. 2000;43(2pt1):249–59.
2. Scott AB. Botulinum toxin injection into extraocular muscles as an alternative to strabismus surgery. Ophthalmology. 1980;87:1044–9.
3. Scott AB. Botulinum toxin injection of eye muscles to correct strabismus. Trans am Ophthalmol Society. 1981;79:734–70.
4. Scott AB, Kennedy RA, Stubbs HA. Botulinum a toxin injection as a treatment for blepharospasm. Arch Ophthalmol. 1985;103:347–50.
5. Dutton JJ, Buckley EG. Long-term results and complications of botulinum A toxin in the treatment of blepharospasm. Ophthalmology. 1988;95:1529–34.
6. Savino PJ, Sergott RC, Bosley TM, Schatz NJ. Hemifacial spasm treated with botulinum A toxin injection. Arch Ophthalmol. 1985;103:1305–6.
7. Shon CC. Clostridium botulinum neurotoxins, their structures and modes of action. In: Watson ED, editor. Natural toxicants in foods. Chichester: Ellis Harwood, Ltd.; 1986. p. 11–57.
8. Coffield JA, Bakry N, Zhang RD, Carlson J, Gomella LG, Simpson LL. In vitro characterization of botulinum toxin types A, C, and D action on human tissues: combined electrophysiologic, pharmacologic, and molecular biologic approaches. J Pharmacol Exp Ther. 1997;280:1489–98.
9. Binz T, Rummel A. Cell entry strategy of clostridial neurotoxins. J Neurochem. 2009;109:1584–95.
10. Alderson K, Holds JB, Anderson RL. Botulinum-induced alteration of nerve-muscle interactions in the human orbicularis oculi following treatment for blepharospasm. Neurology. 1991;41:1800–5.
11. Dressler D, Saberi AF. Botulinum toxin: mechanisms of action. E Neurol. 2005;53:3–9.
12. McMahon SB, Bennett DLH, Bevan S. Inflammatory mediators and modulators of pain. In: McMahon SB, Koltzenberg M, editors. Wall and Melzack's textbook of pain. 5th ed. Philadelphia, PA: Churchill Livingstone; 2005.
13. Jankovic J, Vuong KD, Ahsan J. Comparison of efficacy and immunogenicity of original versus current botulinum toxin in cervical dystonia. Neurology. 2003;60(7):1186–8.
14. Mejia NI, Vuong KD, Jankovic J. Long-term botulinum toxin efficacy, safety and immunogenicity. Mov Disord. 1997;20:592–7.
15. Kim EJ, Ramirez AL, Reeck JB, et al. The role of botulinum toxin type B (Myobloc) in the treatment of hyperkinetic facial lines. Plast Reconstr Surg. 2003;112:88S–93S.
16. Li M, Goldberger BA, Carolyn H. Fatal case of Botox® -related anaphylaxis? J Forensic Sci. 2005;50:169–72.
17. LeWitt PA, Trosch RM. Idiosyncratic adverse reactions to intramuscular botulinum toxin type a injection. Mov Disord. 1997;12:1064–7.
18. Ahbib S, Lachapelle JM, Marot L. Sarcoidal granulomas following injections of boltulic toxin a (Botox®) for corrections of wrinkles. Ann Dermatol Venereol. 2006;133:43–5. (in French)
19. Nettar K, Maas C. Neuromodulators: available agents, physiology and anatomy. Facial Plast Surg. 2011;27(6):517–22.
20. Carruthers J, Carruthers A. The evolution of botulinum neurotoxin type a for cosmetic applications. J Cosmetic Laser Ther. 2007;9(3):186–92.
21. Matarasso A, Shafer D. Botulinum neurotoxin type A-ABO (Dysport®): clinical indications and practice guide. Aesthet Surg J. 2009;29(6 Suppl):S72–9.
22. Kane MA. The effects of botulinum toxin injections on the nasolabial fold. Plast Reconstr Surg. 2003;112(Suppl 5):66S–72S. (discussion 73S–74S)
23. Kranz G, Haubenberger D, Voller B, et al. Respective potencies of Botox® and Dysport® in a human skin model: a randomized, double blind study. Mov Disord. 2009;24:231–6.
24. Jost WH, Blumel J, Grafe S. Botulinum neurotoxin type A free of complexing proteins (XEOMIN®) in focal dystonia. Drugs. 2007;67:669–83.

25. Rieder CR, Schestatsky P, Socal MP, et al. A double-blind randomized, crossover study of Prosigne® vs. Botox ® in patients with blepharospasm and hemifacial spasm. Clin Neuropharmacol. 2007;30(1):39–42.
26. Hunte T, Clarke K. Potency of the botulinum toxin product CNBTX-A significantly exceeds labeled units in standard potency test. J Am Acad Dermatol. 2008;58(3):517–8.
27. Spencer JM, Gordon M, Goldberg DJ. Botulinum B treatment of the glabellar and frontalis regions: a dose response analysis. J Cosmet Laser Ther. 2002;4:19–23.
28. Jacob CI. Botulinum neurotoxin type-B—a rapid wrinkle reducer. Semin Cutan Med Surg. 2007;22(2):131–5.
29. Klein AW. Dilution and storage of botulinum toxin. Dermatol Surg. 1998;24:1179–80.
30. Kwiat DM, Bersani TA, Bersani A. Increased patient comfort utilizing botulinum toxin A reconstituted with preserved versus nonpreserved saline. Ophthal Plast Reconstr Surg. 2004;20:186–9.
31. Sarifakioglu N, Sarifakioglu E. Evaluating effects of preservative-containing saline solution on pain perception during botulinum toxin type A injections at different locations: a prospective, single-blinded, randomized controlled trial. Aesth Plast Surg. 2005;29:113–5.
32. U.S. Food and Drug Administration. Information for Healthcare Professionals: OnabotulinumtoxinA (marketed as Botox®), AbobotulinumtoxinA (marketed as Dysport®) and RimabotulinumtoxinB (marketed as Myobloc®). http://www.fda.gov/Drugs/Drugsafety/PostmarketDrugSafetyInformationforPatientsandProviders/DrugSafetyInformationforHealthcareProfessionals/ucm174949.htm. Accessed Nov 2014.
33. Carruthers J, Carruthers A. The evolution of botulinum neurotoxin type A for cosmetic applications. J Cosmet Laser Ther. 2007;9(3):186–92.
34. Gassner HG, Sherris DA. Addition of an anesthetic agent to enhance the predictability of the effects of botulinum toxin type a injections: a randomized controlled study. Mayo Clin Proc. 2000;75:701–4.
35. Haubner F. Simultaneous injection of lidocaine improves predictability of effect of botulinum toxin. Laryngorhinootologie. 2009;88:764.
36. Kenner JR. Hyaluronic acid filler and botulinum neurotoxin delivered simultaneously in the same syringe for effective and convenient combination aesthetic rejuvenation therapy. J Drug Dermatol. 2010;9:1135–8.
37. Vadoud-Seyedi J, Simonart T. Treatment of axillary hyperhidrosis with botulinum toxin type a reconstituted in lidocaine or in normal saline: a randomized side-by-side, double-blind study. Br J Dermatol. 2007;156:986–9.
38. Moore P, Naumann M. General and clinical aspect of treatment with botulinum toxin. In: Moore P, Naumann M, eds. Handbook of botulinum toxin treatment, 2nd ed., 3. Massachusetts: Blackwell Science; 2003:41.
39. Trindade De Almeida AR, Secco LC, Carruthers A. Handling botulinum toxins: an updated literature review. Dermatol Surg. 2011;37(11):1553–65.
40. Barrow EM, Rosen CA, Hapner ER, Smith S, Hatcher JL, Simpson B, Johns MM III. Safety and efficacy of multiuse botulinum toxin vials for intralaryngeal injection. Laryngoscope. 2015;125(5):1149–54.
41. Cosmetic B. Botox (package insert). Irvine, CA: Allergan, Inc.; 2000.
42. Gartlan MG, Hoffman HG. Crystalline preparation of botulinum toxin type A (Botox): degradation of potency with storage. Otolaryngol Head Neck Surg. 1993;108(2):135–40.
43. Greene P. Potency of frozen/thawed botulinum toxin type A in the treatment of torsional dystonia. Surg. 1993;109(5):968–9.
44. Sloop RR, Cole BA, Escutin RO. Reconstituted botulinum toxin type A does not lose potency in humans if it is refrozen or refrigerated for 2 weeks before use. Neurology. 1997;48(1):249–53.
45. Thomas JP, Slupinskiene N. Frozen versus fresh reconstituted Botox for laryngeal dystonia. Otolaryngol Head Neck Surg. 2006;135(2):204–8.
46. Yang GC, Chiu RJ, Gillman GS. Questioning the need to use botox within 4 hours of reconstitution. Arch Facial Plast Surg. 2008;10(4):273–9.
47. Blitzer A, Crumley RL, Dailey SH, et al. Recommendations of the neurolaryngology study group on laryngeal electromyography. Otolaryngol Head Neck Surg. 2009;140(6):782–93. doi:10.1016/j.otohns.2009.01.026.
48. Blitzer A, Brin MF, Stewart CF. Botulinum toxin management of spasmodic dysphonia (laryngeal dystonia): a 12-years experience in more than 900 patients. Laryngoscope. 1998;108:1435–41.
49. Nygaard TG, Trugman JM, de Yebenes JG, Fahn S. Dopa-responsive dystonia: the spectrum of clinical manifestations in a large North American family. Neurology. 1990;40:66–9.
50. Pahwa R, Lyons KE. Essential tremor: differential diagnosis and current therapy. Am J Med. 2003;115:134–42.
51. Bové M, Daamen N, Rosen C, Wang CC, Sulica L, Gartner-Schmidt J. Development and validation of the vocal tremor scoring system. Laryngoscope. 2006;116(9):1662–7.
52. Gurey LE, Sinclair CF, Blitzer A. A new paradigm for the management of essential vocal tremor with botulinum toxin. Laryngoscope. 2013;123(10):2497–501. doi:10.1002/lary.24073.
53. Simpson CB, Rosen CA. Botulinum toxin injection of the larynx. In: Simpson CB, Rosen CA, editors. Operative techniques in laryngology. Heidelberg: Springer Verlag; 2008. p. 221–7.
54. Burke RE, Fahn S, Marsden CD. Torsion dystonia: a double-blind, prospective trial of high-dosage trihexyphenidyl. Neurology. 1986;36:160–4.

55. Fahn S. Generalized dystonia: concept and treatment. Clin Neuropharmacol. 1986;9:S37–48.
56. Greene P. Baclofen in the treatment of dystonia. Clin Neuropharmacol. 1992;15:276–88.
57. Jankovic J, Ford J. Blepharospasm and orofacial-cervical dystonia: clinical and pharmacological findings in 100 patients. Ann Neurol. 1983;13:402–11.
58. Jankovic J. Treatment of hyperkinetic movement disorders with tetrabenazine: a double-blind crossover study. Ann Neurol. 1982;11:41–7.
59. Rodriguez RL, Fernandez HH, Haq I, Okun MS. Pearls in patient selection for deep brain stimulation. Neurologist. 2007;13:253–60.
60. Nutt JG, Muenter MD, Aronson A, Kurland LT, Melton LJ III. Epidemiology of focal and generalized dystonia in Rochester, Minnesota. Mov. Disord. 1988;3(3):188–94.
61. Brashear A, Lew MF, Dykstra DD, et al. Safety and efficacy of NeuroBloc (botulinum toxin type B) in type A-responsive cervical dystonia. Neurology. 1999;53(7):1439–46.
62. Comella CL, Jankovic J, Brin MF. Use of botulinum toxin type A in the treatment of cervical dystonia. Neurology. 2000;55(12 suppl 5):S15–21.
63. Pappert EJ, Germanson T. Botulinum toxin type B vs. type A in toxin naïve patients with cervical dystonia: randomized, double blind, noninferiority trial. Mov Disord. 2008;23(4):510–7.
64. Neumann A, Rosenberger D, Vorsprach O, Dazert S. The incidence of Frey syndrome following parotidectomy: results of a survey and follow up. HNO. 2011;59:173–8.
65. Beerens AG, Snow GB. Botulinum toxin a in the treatment of patients with Frey syndrome. Br J Surg. 2002;89:116–9.
66. Cantarella G, Berlusconi A, Mele V, Cogiamanian F, Barbieri S. Treatment of Frey's syndrome with botulinum toxin type B. Otolaryng Head Neck Surg. 2010;143:214–8.
67. de Bree R, Duyndam JE, Kuik DJ, Leemans CR. Repeated botulinum toxin type a injections to treat patients with Frey syndrome. Arch Otolaryngol Head Neck Surg. 2009;135:287–90.
68. Drobik C, Laskawi R. Frey's syndrome: treatment with botulinum toxin. Acta Otolaryngol. 1995;115:459–61.
69. Pomprasit M, Chintrakarn C. Treatment of Frey's syndrome with botulinum toxin. J Med Assoc Thail. 2007;90:2397–402.
70. Haubrich WS. The first-bite syndrome. Henry Ford Hospit Med J. 1986;34:275–8.
71. Chiu AG, Cohen JI, Burningham AR, Andersen PE, Davidson VJ. First bite syndrome: a complication of surgery involving the parapharyngeal space. Head Neck. 2002;24:996–9.
72. Netterville JL, Jackson CG, Miller FR, Wanamaker JR, Glasscock ME. Vagal paraganglioma: a review of 46 patients treated during a 20-year period. Arch Otolaryngol Head Neck Surg. 1998;124:1133–40.
73. Lee BJ, Lee JC, Lee YO, Wang SG, Kim HJ. Novel treatment of first bite syndrome using botulinum toxin type a. Head Neck. 2008;31(8):989–93. doi:10.1002/hed.21054.
74. Chao SS, Graha SM, Hoffman HT. Management of pharyngoesophageal spasm with botox. Otolaryngol Clin N Am. 2004;37:559–66.
75. Blitzer A, Komisar A, Baredes S, Brin MF, Stewart C. Voice failure after tracheoesophageal puncture: management with botulinum toxin. Otolaryng Head Neck Surg. 1995;113:668–70.
76. Bartolomei L, Zambito Marsala S, Pighi GP, et al. Botulinum toxin type a: an effective treatment to restore phonation in laryngectomized patients unable to voice. Neurol Sci. 2011;32:443–7.
77. Lewis JS, Bishop-Leone JK, Forman AD, Diaz EM Jr. Further experience with botox injection for tracheoesophageal speech failure. Head Neck. 2001;23:456–60.
78. Meleca RJ, Dworkin JP, Zormeier MM, Simpson ML, Shibuya T, Mathog RH. Videostroboscopy of the pharyngoesophageal segment in laryngectomy patients treated with botulinum toxin. Otolaryngol Head Neck Surg. 2000;123:38–43.
79. Zormier MM, Meleca RJ, Simpson ML, et al. Botulinum toxin injection to improve tracheoesophageal speech after total laryngectomy. Otolaryngol Head Neck Surg. 1999;120:314–9.
80. Hamaker C, Blom ED. Botulinum neurotoxin for pharyngeal constrictor muscle spasm in tracheoesophageal voice restoration. Laryngoscope. 2003;113:1479–82.

Phonosurgery: Transoral Endoscopic Techniques

10

Christian Sittel

Abstract

Injection laryngoplasty is a transoral technique of vocal fold augmentation in order to close or reduce glottic insufficiency. Unilateral vocal fold paralysis is the most important indication. The technique is an alternative to thyroplasty in many cases, an adjuvant treatment in some. Both options should be offered to the patient and should be considered complementary. Technically, the injection can be done under general anaesthesia or office based in the awake patient. Advantages and disadvantages of both approaches are discussed. There is a variety of injection materials with significant differences in characteristics, mode of application and indication. A review of substances available and used in clinical routine is performed. With proper patient and material selection, injection laryngoplasty plays a major role in the treatment of many patients with dysphonia.

10.1 Introduction

From a neurolaryngologist's perspective, glottic insufficiency due to lower motor neuron-type injury of the recurrent or vagal nerve is the most frequent and most important application for phonosurgical techniques. There are two main strategies to improve this condition: restitution of vocal fold mobility and closure of the glottic gap by bringing the paralysed fold into a more median position. Theoretically, reinnervation techniques as well as laryngeal pacing are treatment options also for cases of unilateral vocal fold immobility of neurogenic origin. Reinnervation is a complex procedure which is mastered by only few surgeons, therefore lacking reproducibility so far. As a consequence, it is reserved for cases of bilateral paralysis. Laryngeal pacing as an innovative tool is under investigation only for the treatment of bilateral vocal fold palsy for the time being. It may be speculated that there is a role for treating unilateral paresis in the future, once there is convincing evidence of efficiency and efficacy for the device as a modality for bilateral vocal fold

Electronic Supplementary Material The online version of this chapter (doi:10.1007/978-3-319-61724-4_10) contains supplementary material, which is available to authorized users.

C. Sittel
Department of Otorhinolaryngology/Head and Neck Surgery, Klinikum Stuttgart, Stuttgart, Germany
e-mail: c.sittel@klinikum-stuttgart.de

C. Sittel, O. Guntinas-Lichius (eds.), *Neurolaryngology*,
https://doi.org/10.1007/978-3-319-61724-4_10

paresis, which should be transferable to a significant extent. Both approaches are discussed in detail elsewhere in the book.

Surgical options aiming at closing a glottic gap can be divided in open (thyroplasty, arytenoid adduction) and transoral endoscopic techniques. As a general rule, transoral vocal fold augmentation is working best in smaller gaps of up to 3 mm, while thyroplasty is more suitable for marked glottic insufficiency and, in combination with arytenoid rotation, posterior gaps. A combination of techniques is an option for severe cases, using thyroplasty to close the glottic gap as much as possible and to bring the arytenoid into an appropriate position, followed by injection laryngoplasty to correct a persisting insufficiency in a sense of "fine-tuning" for an optimal result. With indications overlapping both approaches can accomplish convincing results and should be considered as complementary more than competitive [1]. Neither injection laryngoplasty nor thyroplasty should be labelled as "superior" in general compared to each other. Nevertheless, a variety of parameters should be analysed in detail prior to making a choice in order to tailor surgical voice rehabilitation to the specific patient's needs.

The term "injection laryngoplasty" comprises all techniques aiming at adding bulk to one vocal fold by injecting some kind of augmenting substance in order to correct a glottic insufficiency. Since its first description by Brünings [2] well over 100 years ago, a great variety of different materials have been used for this purpose, with some showing unfavourable results or significant complications [3, 4].

Over the decades, only minor achievements have been made in finding a perfect material for vocal fold augmentation. In recent years, the application of injection laryngoplasty techniques for managing unilateral vocal fold paralysis has regained popularity. Nowadays a number of injectable substances are available, which have been tested in the clinical setting of glottic insufficiency. Basically almost every filler substance having been tested and used in facial plastic surgery has also been utilized in laryngology at some point.

10.2 Application Techniques

In contrast to thyroplasty requiring an external incision, injection laryngoplasty as a transoral endoscopic procedure may be considered as minimally invasive. There are several factors influencing the setting in which the injection can be performed, like surgeon's and patient's preference, individual anatomy, exact goal of the procedure and type of material, which may require overcorrection or, in contrast, needs to be injected meticulously to fill the defect precisely. It is the laryngologist's responsibility to choose from these multiple options, which requires comprehensive knowledge of these technical details as well as personal experience and expertise.

Suspension microlaryngoscopy is the classic approach. By using an operation microscope, the view of the glottis is magnified. The patient can be positioned optimally and is not moving. Exposure can be modified repeatedly and with ample time. Multiple injections in every vocal fold segment are possible, and instruments can be used to adjust the final localization of materials like Vox Implants. Subglottic overfilling (Video 10.2) as complication of particular importance, which can be almost impossible to correct, can still occur in the hand of less experienced surgeons but can be controlled more effectively in comparison to other techniques. For all these reasons, suspension microlaryngoscopy definitively remains the most precise, accurate and versatile way to perform vocal fold injection. This is of paramount importance for materials which do not resorb, since malpositioning cannot be corrected. Typically, these non-resorbable substances need to be deposited in the lateral paraglottic space, which can be controlled effectively under suspension microlaryngoscopy only. It seems to be safe to say that all materials with these characteristics have to be injected under suspension microlaryngoscopy without exception. On the other hand, also for resorbable materials, the highest standards of precision and accuracy should be respected for medical purposes. Even though due to dissipation over time malpositioning has less drastic consequences, it still may seem odd that a less meticulous approach may be sufficient for these substances, as it is put by some authors [5].

Main argument against the use of suspension microlaryngoscopy is the lack of feedback from the patient, who cannot phonate during the intervention. Hence, there is no functional control available guiding the surgeon through the injection process. While admittedly there is some truth to this objection, it should not be overestimated. Basically all resorbable substances are requiring substantial overcorrection, which is questioning the concept of functional feedback. For the reasons discussed above, possible risks clearly outweigh the benefits of office-based procedures whenever using non-resorbable materials.

Depending on healthcare peculiarities in different countries, there may be contrasting incentives to avoid or to prefer interventions requiring general anaesthesia. In many instances, this may seem to be a biasing factor, which is not discussed openly, but has a potential to influence surgeon's preference. Without any doubt the need for general anaesthesia is increasing total costs, requires a more sophisticated setup and is more time-consuming [6].

Ventilation in suspension microlaryngoscopy can be maintained in several ways: infraglottic jet ventilation using a small-bore catheter is offering a good compromise between technical effort and undistorted view and is therefore the option being used most frequently, probably. More sophisticated jet ventilation techniques require special equipment: the twin-stream device (Carl Reiner, Austria) delivers a combination of high- and low-frequency jet streams over customized laryngoscopes allowing for a completely unobstructed view. In combination with air humidification, interventions of more than 1 h length with unmatched exposure of the glottis are possible.

More recently, a completely tubeless system of apnoea oxygenation has become available (Optiflow, Fisher & Paykel Healthcare Ltd., New Zealand), which is delivering high-flow oxygen at up to 70 l/min via a nasal mask. With the laryngoscope in place, apnoeic periods of well over 30 min can be accomplished (personal experience). CO_2 retention is usually the limiting factor in this setting.

If none of these options should be available, an endotracheal ventilation tube can be used as well. It should be chosen as small as possible to remain in the posterior aspect of the glottis without blocking the view on the vocal folds. Even for male adults, a short-term ventilation using an ET tube of not more than 5.5 mm outer diameter is usually possible. As an alternative the laryngoscope can be positioned in apnoea first, and then the ET tube is positioned through the channel of the laryngoscope into the trachea. After preoxygenation usually an apnoeic period of sufficient length for injection laryngoplasty is available before reinserting the ET tube becomes necessary.

Office-based transoral techniques in the sitting, awake patient have become more and more common in the recent years. This development has been fuelled primarily by technical innovations like chip-on-the-tip flexible endoscopes allowing for excellent visualization of the larynx with less discomfort compared to conventional indirect laryngoscopy. Obviously there is a benefit in having a patient being able to phonate during the procedure, thus giving an immediate functional feedback. This may allow for more precise placement of smaller amounts of injection material [7]. Voice outcomes, as measured by standardized patient-based voice surveys, seem to be similar to injection performed under general anaesthesia when performed by an experienced laryngologist [8, 9]. Even in patients tolerating the procedure well, some movement is inevitable, which may lead to inaccurate substance delivery. There are a significant number of patients in which any awake endolaryngeal intervention is not possible. This is the main limitation of the concept. The technical challenge is remarkable and requires laryngological expertise and training. Actual time requiring the presence of the surgeon may well be longer than for suspension microlaryngoscopy in general anaesthesia. In summary, office-based injection laryngoplasty deserves an important role but is not right away superior to conventional suspension microlaryngoscopy. Many laryngologists including the author still find there are more and better arguments for performing injection laryngoplasty in suspension microlaryngoscopy than office-based in the awake patient. With general anaesthesia at nowadays' standards being a safe routine approach very rarely causing any complications, it makes sense to leave the final decision to the patient. In many centres, however, there is only one approach established in clinical routine.

There are several descriptions on how to perform injection laryngoplasty in an awake patient [10–12]. Typically, surface anaesthesia is applied to the hypopharynx first. In a second step, a curved applicator is used to target the anaesthetic agent under direct vision to the epiglottis, the false vocal folds and the glottis. Sufficient anaesthesia of the laryngeal aspect of the epiglottis is necessary to allow for contact of the injection device in order to retract the epiglottis [13]. Uncritical overuse of anaesthetic agents in the whole upper respiratory tract is contraindicated, since it may cause oversecretion as well as aspiration and pooling of secretions, adding significantly to patient's discomfort.

In patients not lending themselves for the transoral approach, but still willing to avoid general anaesthesia, transcutaneous techniques may be a good alternative. This approach seems to be of increasing popularity, since it is possible even in the presence of a significant gag reflex. Therefore, patient selection is less critical. The procedure is described as being painless in general [5]. Major disadvantage is limited access to the vocal folds. Several anatomical trajectories have been described to direct the injection needle, either using a straight pathway through the thyroid cartilage or a more angled approach from below (through the cricothyroid membrane) or above (through the preepiglottic space) the level of the vocal folds [14].

10.3 Injection Materials

A basic distinction can be made between resorbable and non-resorbable substances, with the former having a temporary effect, though with considerable differences in longevity, and the latter providing a permanent effect. In the heterogeneous and bigger group of resorbable materials, a further classification between biological origins will be made. For the smaller group of non-resorbable substances, the term "injectable implants" has been coined; they are of non-biological origin.

10.4 Resorbable Substances

10.4.1 Xenogeneic Origin

These substances are derived from animals, with bovine collagen being the most popular due to its long record in facial plastic surgery. The first description on collagen use for vocal fold augmentation is dating back to 1986 [15, 16]. The variety of preparations is mainly differing in concentration of the solution that comes in prefilled syringes ready for injection. Collagen is providing a temporary augmentation between 3 and 12months, according to several authors. With about 3% of human beings carrying preformed antibodies against collagen, hypersensitivity skin testing is considered mandatory prior to its use. Collagen is a fluid of low viscosity, making application possible via small-bore injection devices with mild pressure. For these reasons it is an obvious choice for office-based interventions. Foreign body reactions seem to be minimal to non-existent. Although FDA approved, there is no formal approval in Europe for using collagen in the human larynx, but it has been probably the most widely used injection material for many years. For reasons not communicated, bovine collagen has not been available for medical use any more since a couple of years now.

Similar to collagen in many aspects, hyaluronic acid is a polysaccharide, which is not species specific and does not elicit humoral or cell-mediated immune response. It can be derived from different animals or can be produced by biological engineering techniques. Therefore, hypersensitivity skin testing is not necessary. Viscoelastic properties could be shown to be quite similar to vocal fold lamina propria [17].

This is making hyaluronic acid the material of choice for aligning vocal fold irregularities like in sulcus vocalis or vocal fold scarring. An optimal indication for hyaluronic acid seems to be a unilateral paresis with supposedly good prognosis in a patient wishing for transient voice improvement. Injection may and should be superficial within Reinke's space. Deep injection into the paraglottic space seems to increase speed of resorption, leading to augmentation effects of some weeks only. This can be used intentionally, however, to offer a trial intervention to patients in doubt without any significant risk profile ("test-drive"). There is an increasing amount of publications on the use of hyaluronic acid in the human larynx [18–25].

10.4.2 Allogenic Origin

An alternative to bovine collagen is human collagen, made of cadaveric dermal tissue. It has been FDA approved for skin augmentation, but not injection laryngoplasty, so it is used off-label in the USA. It is not distributed in Europe. During the production process, all cellular components are removed without altering the collagen and elastin matrix. The final material is a micronized acellular compound which is freeze-dried into powder form (Life Cell Corp., Branchburgh, NJ, USA), which needs to be reconstituted for injection. So far, no infectious transmission has been documented. Viscosity and injection characteristics are similar to bovine collagen. Information on longevity after injection are quite contradictory: Pearl [26] reported stable parameters like laryngeal airflow and subjective voice assessment (VHI) at 1 and 3 months, although some absorption was noted on follow-up laryngoscopy. In sharp contrast Karpenko et al. report no significant improvement at 1 month in patient perceptual voice quality and aerodynamic measurements [27]. In addition, there are first reports on substance-associated complications like locoregional migration [28]. As a consequence, Cymetra seems to have lost ground to other materials in the USA over the recent years.

10.4.3 Autogenic Origin

In the early 1990s of the last century, autogenic fat has been described as material for augmentation [29]. Harvesting of the graft material is being performed at the same time as injection laryngoplasty, usually by needle aspiration or through a periumbilical incision. Survival of adipocytes after transplantation is most likely depending on a correct harvesting procedure [30]. The obvious advantages of excellent biocompatibility, simple acquisition and low cost have made this approach rapidly popular throughout the world. Before the turn of the millennium, autogenic fat has probably been the substance used most frequently in many countries. Information on extent and time course of resorption is quite different. By using magnetic resonance tomography, permanent longevity as well as complete resorption could be found [31, 32]. The unpredictable rate and degree of resorption are the main disadvantage of fat injection, limiting significantly the predictability of long-term voice outcomes. Overcorrection is recommended in general, but it remains unclear at large to which extent. Repeat injection procedures may be necessary to maintain adequate vocal fold bulk. Lacking reproducibility in combination with the advent of new materials avoiding these shortcomings has continuously diminished the role of fat as injection material [33].

Originally described by a Finnish group [34, 35], fascia lata is another source of autogenic material. The tissue harvested is minced at the table by the surgeon in order to form an injectable preparation, requiring an injection cannula with great needle bore. Initial reports have suggested greater longevity compared to fat, which could not be reproduced by other authors [36]. Actual use in clinical routine seems to be limited to a few centres only.

10.5 Non-resorbable Substances

Polytetrafluoroethylene, better known as Teflon, has been the mainstay of treatment for vocal fold augmentation between 1960 and 1980. Apparently, it is still available in the USA, although it has fallen out of favour because of significant substance-associated complications. Teflon has a tendency to elicit foreign body reactions with occasional formation of hardly resectable and potentially airway-obstructing granuloma, even if applicated in flawless technique [3]. In addition, migration to distant organs could be shown [37]. In Europe, Teflon is being considered as obsolete for these reasons.

Polydimethylsiloxane elastomers (PDMS), introduced in 1989, have been used in plastic surgery for the treatment of soft tissue deficiencies [38] as well as in paediatric urology for the treatment of vesicoureteral reflux and in adults for the treatment of male and female urinary stress incontinence [39]. First systematic use in the human larynx has been published in 2000 [40].

PDMS particles used for injection purposes consist of textured elastomers, mean particle size being 200 μm approximately, with a minimum size of 100 μm. Earlier studies [41] suggest a particle size of less than 65 μm to be critical for the risk of local and distant migration via lymphatic pathways. Particle size combined with surface texture prevents mechanical dislodgement or migration, thus warranting greater anchorage and stability [42, 43]. PDMS elastomers have been in use for medical applications like insulation for pacemaker leads, catheters, hydrocephalic shunts and others for many years. It should be noted that controversies regarding the safety of silicone implants were aimed exclusively at silicone oil and gel, not silicone elastomers [44]. In contrast to silicone oil and gel, an elastomer is a rubbery solid made of fully polymerized PDMS molecules. The textured implants are held in place at the implantation site when host fibroblasts subsequently deposit collagen around the particles. PDMS are commercially available under the brand name Vox Implants™ (manufactured by Bioplasty BV, Hofkamp 2, 6161 DC Geleen, the Netherlands, distributed by Medtronic Europe, Route du Molliau, CH-1131 Tolochenaz, Switzerland). It is a thick yellow paste shipped in 1.0 cc polypropylene syringes that becomes tacky on exposure to air. In 2001 Vox Implants™ have been approved for injection laryngoplasty in humans within all member states of the European Union. In 1991, the FDA declared the use of injectable silicone illegal. Although this ban was aimed at silicone oil, a completely different material sharing almost no characteristics with PDMS particles, Vox Implants have no FDA approval so far.

For injection a malleable needle with sufficient needle bore is supplied with the injection material as a set to make sure that also bigger particles of up to 500 μ size are passing through. A considerable pressure needs to be applied during injection, since the material has a high viscosity. To ensure high accuracy and perfect control during the injection process, the use of an administration gun incorporating a ratchet mechanism allowing for precise placement of the microimplants in portions of 0.03 cc is mandatory. The correct application site for PDMS particles is deep lateral to the thyroarytaenoid muscle (Figs. 10.1 and 10.2). This is basically the region in which thyroplasty implants are localized; hence, the term "injectable microimplants" seems to be justified. It is important to keep in mind that Vox Implants are put into motion as chain of particles following the principle of elastic coupling. As a result it takes some seconds for the row of particles to start actually moving as well as to come to a complete halt, making it necessary to keep the injection needle steady at the puncture site for about 10 s after having released the pressure on the syringe. Typically, a total volume of 0.5–0.7 cc in 2–3 injections is sufficient to augment a paralysed vocal fold (Video 10.1). Subglottic overfilling needs to be avoided carefully (Video 10.2). Building up of a sufficient bulk is usually well possible (Figs. 10.3 and 10.4). Injecting too superficial into Reinke's space leads to stiffening of the vocal fold due to the high viscoelasticity and the corpuscular character of the material. Positioning of the material can be difficult with injecting alone, but immediate correction is well possible: using a closed cup forceps the mass of injected PDMS can be distributed in the paraglottic space, allowing for precise remodelling of the augmented vocal fold (Video 10.3). Taking into account these characteristics, it may seem self-explaining why suspension

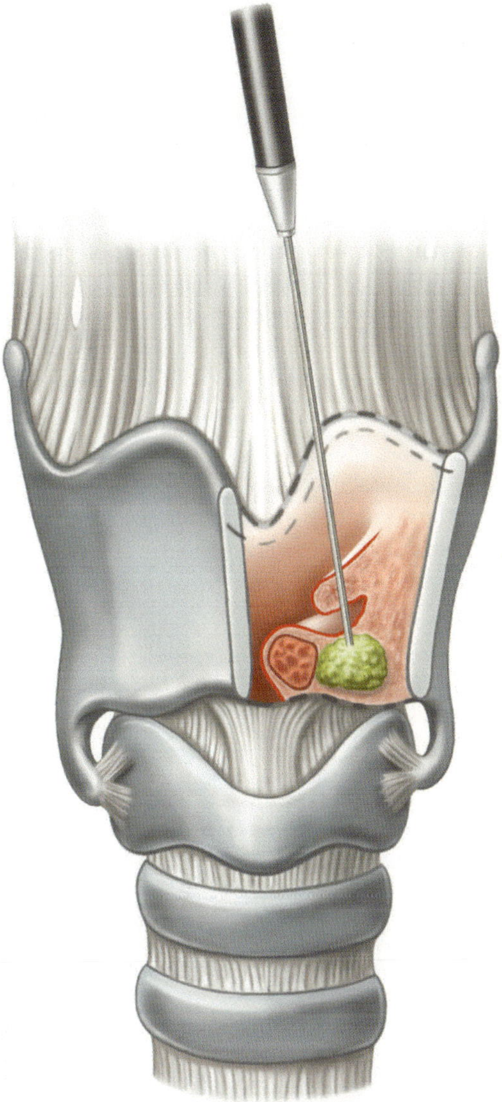

Fig. 10.1 The optimal injection site for Vox Implants is the deep paraglottic space, between the thyroarytenoid muscle and the inner perichondrium of the thyroid cartilage

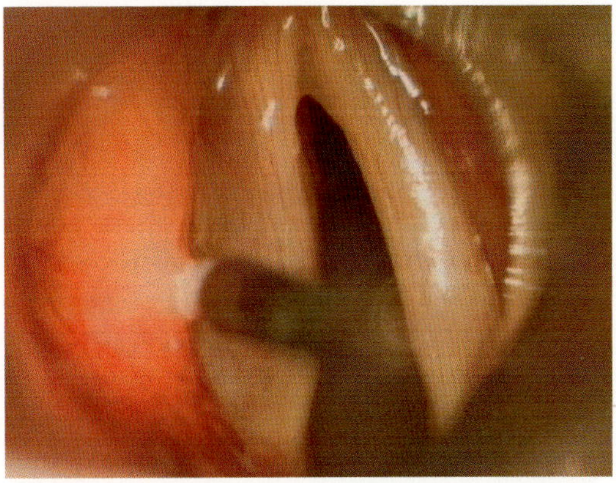

Fig. 10.2 Microlaryngoscopic view of the augmentation process (Vox Implants)

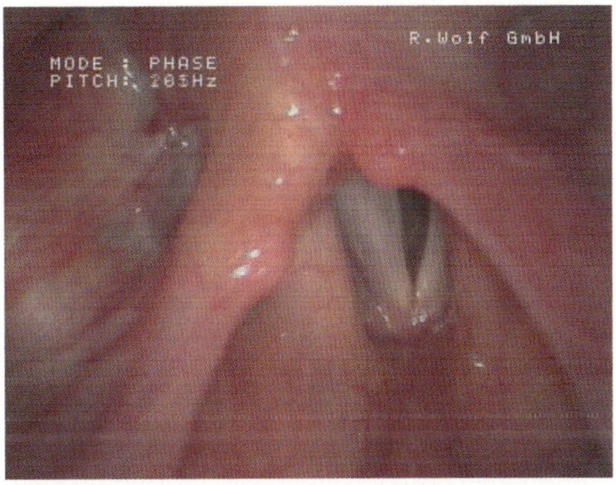

Fig. 10.3 Left recurrent nerve palsy with glottic gap, preoperative videostroboscopic view

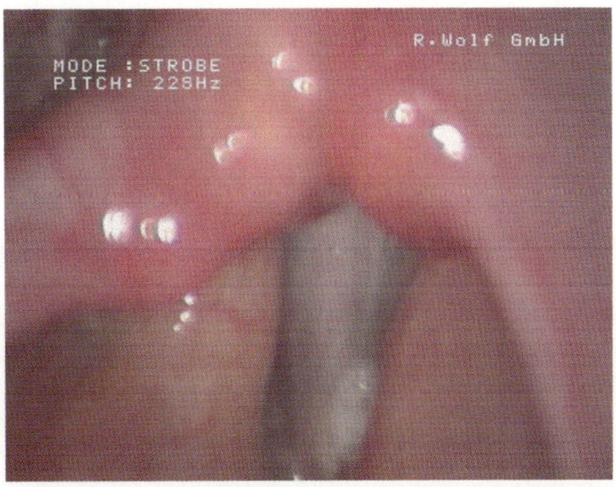

Fig. 10.4 Same patient as in Fig. 10.3, 6 weeks post injection: note complete glottic closure

microlaryngoscopy is highly advocated for PDMS injection into the human larynx.

Animal studies show an excellent biocompatibility of PDMS particles [45]. Hypersensitivity is not an issue for subcutaneously located PDMS elastomers, neither in animals nor in humans [46], so skin testing is not required prior to injection. Particle size prevents the material from being phagocytosed. Hence, it does not serve as an antigen.

Several studies show favourable results in terms of voice restoration (Videos 10.4, 10.5, 10.6, and 10.7) similar to thyroplasty [1, 47–50]. PDMS particles provide a long-term augmentation with documented follow-up of 6 years in average [51]. Substance-associated complications seem to be a rare exception and can be difficult to separate from adverse findings as a consequence of malpositioning, i.e. by injecting to superficial, which may happen more frequently. As a last resort, surgical removal of displaced PDMS particles is technically feasible to a certain degree, though a marked stiffness of the erroneously injected subepithelial space cannot be restored completely [52, 53].

In the group of permanent, non-resorbable substances, longevity, safety and efficacy in terms of voice improvement are best documented for PDMS particles. Therefore, Vox Implants™ are most suitable for deep injection laryngoplasty addressing mild to moderate glottic insufficiency in unilateral vocal fold paralysis. Thus, PDMS particles are offering a true alternative to open thyroplasty for patients preferring an endoscopic approach.

Calcium hydroxylapatite (CaHA) is a calcium phosphorus compound found as basic component in the bone and teeth. There is a commercially available material consisting of CaHA microspheres and a carrier gel marketed under the brand name Radiesse that can be injected through a fine needle (25–27 gauge). Once injected, the carrier gel is replaced by fibrosis with the CaHA microspheres remaining in place.

The substance has been studied in both animal and human studies. In an in vivo canine vocal fold model, it has been shown that CaHA injection provided adequate medialization of the canine vocal fold up to 12 months follow-up without migration or resorption and a giant cell reaction without appreciable chronic inflammation [54]. A recent multi-institutional clinical trial revealed excellent results of 80% improvement at 12-month follow-up Rosen 2009 [55]. It is intended as a permanent implant, but resorption occurs to some degree. There are data [56] on longevity showing a loss of benefit in 64% of patients, with an average length of benefit of 18, 6 months (ranging from 8 to 36 months). Therefore, Radiesse is more appropriately labelled as slowly resorbable than non-resorbable. In many aspects similar to collagen, CaHA can be used for the same indications; also the technical process of injection is basically identical. Versatility and ease of use have made it a very popular substance for injection laryngoplasty in the office as well as in the operating room.

There is FDA approval for potentially long-term vocal fold injection. Nevertheless, some substance-associated complications have been described [57, 58]. Voice results seem to be well comparable to those accomplished using thyroplasty type I [59].

References

1. Koelmel JC, Sittel C. Stimm- und Lebensqualitat nach Injektionslaryngoplastik mit VOX-Implants(R) (Polydimethylsiloxan). Laryngorhinootologie. 2014; 93(5):316–20.
2. Brünings W. Über eine neue Behandlungsmethode der Rekurrenslähmung. Ver Deutsch Laryng. 1911;18:58.
3. Rubin HJ. Misadventures with injectable polytef (Teflon). Arch Otolaryngol. 1975;101(2):114–6.
4. Varvares MA, Montgomery WW, Hillman RE. Teflon granuloma of the larynx: etiology, pathophysiology, and management. Ann Otol Rhinol Laryngol. 1995;104(7):511–5.
5. O'Leary MA, Grillone GA. Injection laryngoplasty. Otolaryngol Clin N Am. 2006;39(1):43–54.
6. Hillel AT, Ochsner MC, Johns MM III, Klein AM. A cost and time analysis of laryngology procedures in the endoscopy suite versus the operating room. Laryngoscope. 2016;126(6):1385–9.
7. Ford CN, Roy N, Sandage M, Bless DM. Rigid endoscopy for monitoring indirect vocal fold injection. Laryngoscope. 1998;108(10):1584–6.
8. Bove MJ, Jabbour N, Krishna P, Flaherty K, Saul M, Wunar R, et al. Operating room versus office-based injection laryngoplasty: a comparative analysis of reimbursement. Laryngoscope. 2007;117(2):226–30.
9. Mathison CC, Villari CR, Klein AM, Johns MM III. Comparison of outcomes and complications between awake and asleep injection laryngoplasty: a case-control study. Laryngoscope. 2009;119(7):1417–23.
10. Clary MS, Milam BM, Courey MS. Office-based vocal fold injection with the laryngeal introducer technique. Laryngoscope. 2014;124(9):2114–7.

11. Mayerhoff RM, Kuo C, Meyer T. A novel approach to the challenging injection laryngoplasty. Ann Otol Rhinol Laryngol. 2016;125(5):415–20.
12. Sardesai MG, Merati AL, Hu A, Birkent H. Impact of patient-related factors on the outcomes of office-based injection laryngoplasty. Laryngoscope. 2016; 126(8):1806–9.
13. Hoffman H, McCabe D, McCulloch T, Jin SM, Karnell M. Laryngeal collagen injection as an adjunct to medialization laryngoplasty. Laryngoscope. 2002;112(8 Pt 1):1407–13.
14. Verma SP, Dailey SH. Office-based injection laryngoplasty for the management of unilateral vocal fold paralysis. J Voice. 2014;28(3):382–6.
15. Ford CN, Bless DM. Clinical experience with injectable collagen for vocal fold augmentation. Laryngoscope. 1986;96(8):863–9.
16. Remacle M, Marbaix E, Hamoir M, Bertrand B, van den Eeckhaut J. Correction of glottic insufficiency by collagen injection. Ann Otol Rhinol Laryngol. 1990;99(6 Pt 1):438–44.
17. Dahlqvist A, Garskog O, Laurent C, Hertegard S, Ambrosio L, Borzacchiello A. Viscoelasticity of rabbit vocal folds after injection augmentation. Laryngoscope. 2004;114(1):138–42.
18. Hallen L, Dahlqvist A, Laurent C. Dextranomeres in hyaluronan (DiHA): a promising substance in treating vocal cord insufficiency. Laryngoscope. 1998;108(3):393–7.
19. Hallen L, Johansson C, Laurent C. Cross-linked hyaluronan (Hylan B gel): a new injectable remedy for treatment of vocal fold insufficiency--an animal study. Acta Otolaryngol. 1999;119(1):107–11.
20. Chan RW, Titze IR. Hyaluronic acid (with fibronectin) as a bioimplant for the vocal fold mucosa. Laryngoscope. 1999;109(7 Pt 1):1142–9.
21. Branco A, Rodrigues SA, Fabro AT, Fonseca-Alves CE, Martins RH. Hyaluronic acid behavior in the lamina propria of the larynx with advancing age. Otolaryngol Head Neck Surg. 2014;151(4):652–6.
22. Dorbeau C, Marmouset F, Lescanne E, Bakhos D, Moriniere S. Functional assessment of glottal insufficiency treated by hyaluronic acid injection: retrospective 20-case series. Eur Ann Otorhinolaryngol Head Neck Dis. 2016;134(3):145–9.
23. Heris HK, Daoud J, Sheibani S, Vali H, Tabrizian M, Mongeau L. Investigation of the viability, adhesion, and migration of human fibroblasts in a hyaluronic acid/gelatin microgel-reinforced composite hydrogel for vocal fold tissue regeneration. Adv Health Mater. 2016;5(2):255–65.
24. Kim YS, Choi JW, Park JK, Kim YS, Kim HJ, Shin YS, et al. Efficiency and durability of hyaluronic acid of different particle sizes as an injectable material for VF augmentation. Acta Otolaryngol. 2015;135(12):1311–8.
25. Young VN, Gartner-Schmidt J, Rosen CA. Comparison of voice outcomes after trial and long-term vocal fold augmentation in vocal fold atrophy. Laryngoscope. 2015;125(4):934–40.
26. Pearl AW, Woo P, Ostrowski R, Mojica J, Mandell DL, Costantino P. A preliminary report on micronized alloderm injection laryngoplasty. Laryngoscope. 2002;112(6):990–6.
27. Karpenko AN, Dworkin JP, Meleca RJ, Stachler RJ. Cymetra injection for unilateral vocal fold paralysis. Ann Otol Rhinol Laryngol. 2003;112(11): 927–34.
28. Bock JM, Lee JH, Robinson RA, Hoffman HT. Migration of Cymetra after vocal fold injection for laryngeal paralysis. Laryngoscope. 2007;117(12):2251–4.
29. Brandenburg JH, Kirkham W, Koschkee D. Vocal cord augmentation with autogenous fat. Laryngoscope. 1992;102(5):495–500.
30. Shaw GY, Szewczyk MA, Searle J, Woodroof J. Autologous fat injection into the vocal folds: technical considerations and long-term follow-up. Laryngoscope. 1997;107(2):177–86.
31. Bauer CA, Valentino J, Hoffman HT. Long-term result of vocal cord augmentation with autogenous fat. Ann Otol Rhinol Laryngol. 1995;104(11):871–4.
32. Brandenburg JH, Unger JM, Koschkee D. Vocal cord injection with autogenous fat: a long-term magnetic resonance imaging evaluation. Laryngoscope. 1996;106(2 Pt 1):174–80.
33. McCulloch TM, Andrews BT, Hoffman HT, Graham SM, Karnell MP, Minnick C. Long-term follow-up of fat injection laryngoplasty for unilateral vocal cord paralysis. Laryngoscope. 2002;112(7 Pt 1):1235–8.
34. Reijonen P, Lehikoinen-Soderlund S, Rihkanen H. Results of fascial augmentation in unilateral vocal fold paralysis. Ann Otol Rhinol Laryngol. 2002;111(6):523–9.
35. Rihkanen H, Reijonen P, Lehikoinen-Soderlund S, Lauri ER. Videostroboscopic assessment of unilateral vocal fold paralysis after augmentation with autologous fascia. Eur Arch Otorhinolaryngol. 2004;261(4):177–83.
36. Duke SG, Salmon J, Blalock PD, Postma GN, Koufman JA. Fascia augmentation of the vocal fold: graft yield in the canine and preliminary clinical experience. Laryngoscope. 2001;111(5):759–64.
37. Ellis JC, McCaffrey TV, DeSanto LW, Reiman HV. Migration of Teflon after vocal cord injection. Otolaryngol Head Neck Surg. 1987;96(1):63–6.
38. Ersek RA, Gregory SR, Salisbury AV. Bioplastique at 6 years: clinical outcome studies. Plast Reconstr Surg. 1997;100(6):1570–4.
39. Guys JM, Simeoni-Alias J, Fakhro A, Delarue A. Use of polydimethylsiloxane for endoscopic treatment of neurogenic urinary incontinence in children. J Urol. 1999;162(6):2133–5.
40. Sittel C, Thumfart WF, Pototschnig C, Wittekindt C, Eckel HE. Textured polydimethylsiloxane elastomers in the human larynx: safety and efficiency of use. J Biomed Mater Res. 2000;53(6):646–50.
41. Groff GD, Schned AR, Taylor TH. Silicone-induced adenopathy eight years after metacarpophalangeal arthroplasty. Arthritis Rheum. 1981;24(12):1578–81.

42. Caballero M, Bernal-Sprekelsen M, Calvo C, Farre X, Quinto L, Alos L. Polydimethylsiloxane versus polytetrafluoroethylene for vocal fold medialization: histologic evaluation in a rabbit model. J Biomed Mater Res B Appl Biomater. 2003;67(1):666–74.
43. Sittel C. Polydimethylsiloxane particles are not experimental in the human larynx. J Biomed Mater Res B Appl Biomater. 2004;69(2):251.
44. Marotta JS, Widenhouse CW, Habal MB, Goldberg EP. Silicone gel breast implant failure and frequency of additional surgeries: analysis of 35 studies reporting examination of more than 8,000 explants. J Biomed Mater Res. 1999;48(3):354–64.
45. Beisang AA 3rd, Ersek RA. Mammalian response to subdermal implantation of textured microimplants. Aesthet Plast Surg. 1992;16(1):83–90.
46. Allen O. Response to subdermal implantation of textured microimplants in humans. Aesthet Plast Surg. 1992;16(3):227–30.
47. Duruisseau O, Wagner I, Fugain C, Chabolle F. Endoscopic rehabilitation of vocal cord paralysis with a silicone elastomer suspension implant. Otolaryngol Head Neck Surg. 2004;131(3):241–7.
48. Alves CB, Loughran S, MacGregor FB, Dey JI, Bowie LJ. Bioplastique medialization therapy improves the quality of life in terminally ill patients with vocal cord palsy. Clin Otolaryngol Allied Sci. 2002;27(5):387–91.
49. Sittel C, Echternach M, Federspil PA, Plinkert PK. Polydimethylsiloxane particles for permanent injection laryngoplasty. Ann Otol Rhinol Laryngol. 2006;115(2):103–9.
50. Hagemann M, Seifert E. The use of polydimethylsiloxane for injection laryngoplasty. World J Surg. 2008;32(9):1940–7.
51. Mattioli F, Bettini M, Botti C, Busi G, Tassi S, Malagoli A, et al. Polydimethylsiloxane injection laryngoplasty for unilateral vocal fold paralysis: long-term results. J Voice. 2017; doi:10.1016/j.jvoice.2016.12.017.
52. Leuchter I, Giovanni A. Description of complications after injection laryngoplasty with polydimethylsiloxane. Rev Laryngol Otol Rhinol (Bord). 2009;130(1):69–72.
53. Echternach M, Delb W, Wagner M, Sittel C, Verse T, Richter B. Polydimethylsiloxane in the human vocal fold: description of partial explantation. Laryngoscope. 2008;118(2):375–7.
54. Chhetri DK, Jahan-Parwar B, Hart SD, Bhuta SM, Berke GS. Injection laryngoplasty with calcium hydroxylapatite gel implant in an in vivo canine model. Ann Otol Rhinol Laryngol. 2004;113(4):259–64.
55. Rosen CA, Gartner-Schmidt J, Casiano R, Anderson TD, Johnson F, Remacle M, et al. Vocal fold augmentation with calcium hydroxylapatite: twelve-month report. Laryngoscope. 2009;119(5):1033–41.
56. Carroll TL, Rosen CA. Long-term results of calcium hydroxylapatite for vocal fold augmentation. Laryngoscope. 2011;121(2):313–9.
57. DeFatta RA, Chowdhury FR, Sataloff RT. Complications of injection laryngoplasty using calcium hydroxylapatite. J Voice. 2012;26(5):614–8.
58. Cohen JC, Reisacher W, Malone M, Sulica L. Severe systemic reaction from calcium hydroxylapatite vocal fold filler. Laryngoscope. 2013;123(9):2237–9.
59. Shen T, Damrose EJ, Morzaria S. A meta-analysis of voice outcome comparing calcium hydroxylapatite injection laryngoplasty to silicone thyroplasty. Otolaryngol Head Neck Surg. 2013;148(2):197–208.

Laryngoscopic Techniques and Office-Based Phonosurgery in Neurolaryngological Disorders

11

Markus M. Hess and Susanne Fleischer

Abstract

Neurolaryngological diseases and disorders can affect voice function, swallowing, and breathing. With comprehensive office-based laryngoscopy procedures, mostly performed transnasally, the biomechanics needed for voice production, breathing, and effective swallowing can be assessed in almost all cases. With ambulatory phonosurgical interventions under topical anesthesia such as vocal fold augmentation and botulinum toxin injections, patients can be helped by improving vocal loudness, voice quality, durability, and stabilizing vocal function significantly. Concerning aspiration of liquid and solid food due to glottic insufficiency as one of the most severe problems, office-based vocal fold augmentation may effectively improve swallowing function.

11.1 Introduction

The aim of this chapter is to delineate the possibilities of office-based diagnoses by visual assessment of the larynx and to encompass options for surgical interventions in neurolaryngological disorders. Our focus will be on indications and techniques for a practical use of laryngoscopy with specific tips and tricks as well as presenting surgical interventions in the ambulatory office setting. All statements made in this chapter represent the authors' opinion and are based on many years of experience in performing office-based diagnostics and ambulatory surgery in the awake patient [1–4].

Neurolaryngological disorders are most frequently encountered as unilateral/bilateral arytenoid movement disturbances. The muscular "problem" is primarily affecting arytenoid cartilage movements and their position. The ligamentous parts of the vocal folds may–secondarily–cause a phonatory or a respiratory problem.

The neurolaryngologist therefore has to assess and judge on the basis of a profound knowledge of the biomechanical properties of the larynx.

M.M. Hess (✉)
Deutsche Stimmklinik,
Martinistrasse 64, Hamburg 20251, Germany
e-mail: hess@stimmklinik.de

S. Fleischer
Department of Voice, Speech and Hearing Disorders,
University Medical Center Hamburg-Eppendorf,
Hamburg, Germany

C. Sittel, O. Guntinas-Lichius (eds.), *Neurolaryngology*,
https://doi.org/10.1007/978-3-319-61724-4_11

This includes the muscular pulling vectors of all muscles as well as degrees of freedom of all anatomic components (cartilages, tissues) and especially the corresponding movements allowed by the cricothyroid and cricoarytenoid joints.

Neurolaryngological disorders reveal themselves in pathophysiologic movements of endolaryngeal structures [5]. Thus, a comprehensive and systematic visual inspection during relaxed breathing periods (sometimes up to 10 s!) as well as during induced (voluntary) vegetative and phonatory tasks plays a crucial role in diagnostics. Furthermore, specific muscular diagnostics including laryngeal electromyography (LEMG) will add to the diagnostic process.

11.2 Laryngoscopic Techniques and Typical Findings

Patients with neurolaryngological disorders mostly have endolaryngeal movement disorders that can be seen during office-based laryngoscopy. However, because many muscles are involved, the clinical picture can be quite complex, depending on the degree of activity or total muscular inactivity of the laryngeal muscles involved. Interpretation is facilitated by a combination of online examination and scrutinized offline assessment, specifically when easy review is enabled with computer-based archiving and retrieving software for selected video sequences. Although image resolution plays an important role in diagnostics of benign mass lesions of the vocal folds, image resolution is not the most essential feature for the diagnostic process within neurolaryngological disorders. The most important assessment is to view the entire larynx during a series of specifically selected tasks while eliciting movements that usually prove physiologic (and not compromised) laryngeal function [6]. Within these tasks, it is of crucial importance to compare left and right sides with each other, which gives very helpful information about the individual laryngeal (neuro) muscular function.

When examining patients with neurolaryngological disorders, we primarily prefer flexible transnasal endoscopy, because this enables more "natural" laryngeal movements in running speech, phonatory tasks, relaxed breathing, forced inspiratory nasal breathing, and swallowing. Furthermore, having said that exposure and laryngeal visibility plays a crucial role, it is clear that thin, flexible endoscopes with high-resolution tip-chip cameras offer best chances to visualize the larynx without eliciting too much of a disturbing gag response (Fig. 11.1).

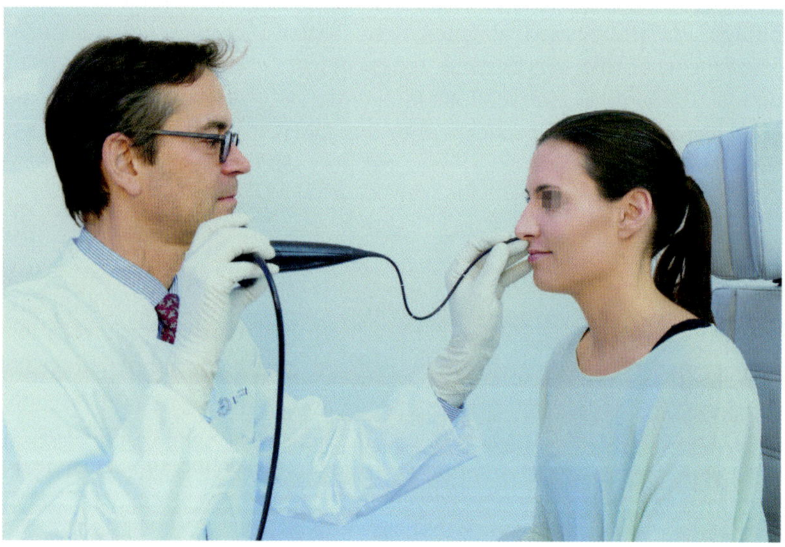

Fig. 11.1 Flexible transnasal endoscopy is the preferred approach to assess neuromuscular movement disorders within clinical diagnostics [Courtesy of Olympus Europe SE & Co. KG, Hamburg, Germany]

11.2.1 Testing of Motor Function

An uncompromised efferent vagal innervation within the larynx is visually assessed by asking the patient to perform a series of tasks. In the following, we will describe these tests according to assessment of spontaneous and/or pathologic movements of the entire larynx in an overview endoscopic position with either (1) uni- and/or bilateral recurrent laryngeal nerve (RLN) function or (2) superior laryngeal nerve (SLN) function.

11.3 Whole-Larynx Movements

Positioning the tip of a flexible, transnasally routed endoscope at the height of the uvula enables an overview of the larynx, hypopharynx, and base of tongue. It also allows for assessment of bolus/saliva retentions in the piriform sinuses and valleculae. Assessment of quiet breathing, phonation, vegetative maneuvers such as throat clearing and coughing, quick diadochokinetic adduction-abduction tasks such as laughing, and swallowing of fluid/solid bolus gives an overview of biomechanical function of all structures in this region. Focus is always on anatomical structures, left-right symmetry, range of motion of arytenoids and of vocal folds, ability of tensioning vocal folds, and speed of motion within tasks, including special attention targeted at unilateral "lagging" of movements (reduced speed or latency differences). A key point is immobility or hypomobility in contrast to normally expected mobility of any of the aforementioned structures. For diagnostic assessment of neurolaryngological disorders, it is of crucial importance to also look for tremor, myoclonus, paradoxical movements, etc. [5].

11.4 Vocal Fold and Arytenoid Movements: RLN-Related Disorders

The most common neurolaryngological disorder is motor RLN paresis or paralysis which leads to hypomobility or immobility of the affected side. RLN-related disorders are frequently unilateral, but of course they can be bilateral. While it is in most cases rather easy to visualize a unilateral paralysis with immobility of one side, a slight unilateral hypomobility may be difficult to detect and requires a comprehensive examination. A slight bilateral hypomobility can also be hard to verify because the comparison with the contralateral side is unreliable.

Checking for adduction-abduction diadochokinesis while asking for rapid changes of forced nasal sniffing and hard onset phonation of /eee/ (e.g., using an /eee/–sniff test) can reveal impaired range of motion and lagging of the arytenoids. Phonation of /eee/ in chest and falsetto voice, each for at least 5 s, while keeping the sound as stable as possible, should enable assessment for tremor as well as provide enough time for stroboscopy. Inspiratory phonation facilitates visualization of true vocal folds in cases of overlying ventricular folds in chest voice phonation, because inspiratory phonation induces adduction of vocal folds and abduction of ventricular folds.

When checking vocal folds for underlying neurolaryngological disorders, keep in mind that motor branches of the RLN affect muscular actions that primarily move the arytenoid cartilage. Thus, comprehensive assessment of actively inducible arytenoid movements for rocking, gliding, and tilting is the primary target for neurolaryngological diagnostics. The cartilage's most easily visible part is the vocal process, and thus this prominent structure should be inspected first (and not only the arytenoid hump or the membranous part of the vocal fold). Examiners should look for active abductory and adductory movements of the vocal process, its range of motion and symmetry of motion when compared with the contralateral side, movement lagging, and level differences. In cases of side asymmetry, it goes without saying that the hypomobile side is the affected side.

Arytenoid Mobility Test To exclude unilateral arytenoid dislocation or fixation in unilateral movement disorders, an office-based procedure for assessment of active and passive arytenoid mobility is very helpful. Under topical anesthesia

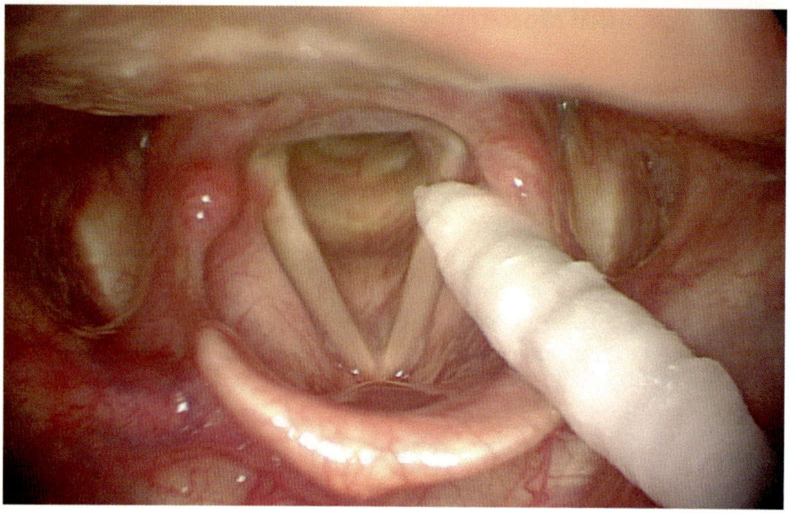

Fig. 11.2 With a transorally routed bent wire with a soft cotton at its tip, passive arytenoid mobility testing is possible in topical anesthesia. This is a valuable alternative to check for cricoarytenoid joint fixation without having the patient in general anesthesia. Here, the instrument is just about to lateralize the arytenoid cartilage [Courtesy of Deutsche Stimmklinik Management GmbH]

and using a blunt, cotton-coated probe, transoral passive arytenoid mobility testing with the cotton probe is a rapid, safe, and easy method for differential diagnosis. In our experience, arytenoid dislocation and joint fixation could be ruled out in almost all cases of immobile arytenoids, suggesting that recurrent nerve paresis or paralysis was most likely. Joint fixation is – statistically seen – very unlikely (Fig. 11.2).

In bilateral hypomobility, a posterior glottic stenosis is an important differential diagnosis one has to keep in mind. In most cases it can be seen with special laryngoscopic techniques such as flexible endoscopy with intralaryngeal tip position (use the “dipping maneuver” to inspect the posterior inferior part of the endolarynx at the level of the vocal processes). In some cases an examination in general anesthesia can be necessary for exclusion of posterior glottic stenosis.

11.5 Vocal Fold Elongation: Motor SLN-Related Disorders

Within differential diagnosis of vagal lesions, the assessment of superior laryngeal nerve (SLN) impairment is mandatory. The quickest way to examine the motor function of the SLN is to ask for a glissando (gliding sound like a siren within a few seconds) of an /eee/ vowel from low-pitch phonation in chest voice up to the highest notes in falsetto voice and then gliding back down. Impairment of SLN function should be audible as inability of performing this task, inability to phonate in falsetto register, inability to perform a glissando without sound breaks, or when more roughness is audible while increasing pitch. Visually, the vocal folds show failure in getting elongated (unilaterally or bilaterally – due to impairment of the cricothyroid muscle to contract).

11.6 Laryngeal Electromyography (LEMG)

When assessing uni- or bilateral impairment of the motor function of the SLN or RLN, the use of laryngeal electromyography (LEMG) is very helpful. Because details are provided in a special chapter in this book, we just mention the different ways of needle placement in this chapter. Needles can be positioned indirect transorally or percutaneously, (e.g., with monopolar and bipolar needles or hooked wire electrodes). With special techniques, all laryngeal muscles can be assessed with LEMG [7]. Although the CT muscle is the most superficial muscle, it is a very thin muscle, and therefore needle positioning can be quite challenging. But by far the most difficult muscle to reach is the posterior cricoarytenoid (PCA) muscle.

11.7 Testing of Sensitivity During Laryngoscopy

Although we mostly associate neurolaryngological disorders with motor deficits, we must not forget that afferent deficits may be present in a substantial number of patients and can be the cause of significant problems, not only food aspiration.

Many publications have addressed the assessment of sensitivity testing within in-office procedures. In this chapter we can only briefly touch upon the most important assessment techniques. The etiology of impairment of supraglottal sensitivity is caused by an affection of the supralaryngeal nerve, where nerve problems can be located in the neck, or being part of an upper vagal problem, including all kinds of possible central or peripheral nervous system etiologies. In contrast to calibrated air puff stimulation supplied by a machine through an instrument channel during flexible endoscopy, we propose that soft touching of mucosal surfaces with the tip of the endoscope can also provide a good estimate of surface sensitivity and will suffice in many cases to enable a reliable diagnosis. The most important regions to test are arytenoid humps, epiglottis, and aryepiglottic folds – the so-called aditus ad laryngis. Indirect signs of reduction or loss of mucosal sensitivity can be seen in silent aspiration during swallowing assessment with bolus leakage and retentions and of course as reduced response to touching during flexible endoscopy.

11.8 Office-Based Interventions

As pointed out before, neurolaryngological disorders mostly result in phonatory impairment due to vocal fold motion and position alterations. Of course, breathing and swallowing will also be affected in more severe conditions, for example, with bilateral vagal paresis or paralysis. Although bilateral disorders are mostly affecting functions more dramatically, *office-based* surgery is more of a therapeutic option in unilateral vocal fold disorders.

Anesthesia We usually administer lidocaine 4% for topical anesthesia in the nose, the pharynx, and the larynx. Tetracaine can even lead to better numbing of the mucosal surface. Special swabbing and spraying techniques are helpful to access the endolarynx. Furthermore, we consider sufficient "verbal anesthesia" of utmost importance conveying an atmosphere of confidence, trust, and reassurance. This comforts patients, helps to calm them down, and finally reduces gag response – thus making interventions easier for the surgeon. We do not routinely administer midazolam nor atropine; however, we recommend to continuously monitor oxygen saturation and pulse rate (Fig. 11.3).

11.8.1 Voice and Swallowing: Therapeutic Options with Office-Based Interventions

As stated at the beginning of this chapter, office-based surgery in patients with voice and swallowing disorders has only a few but nevertheless vital

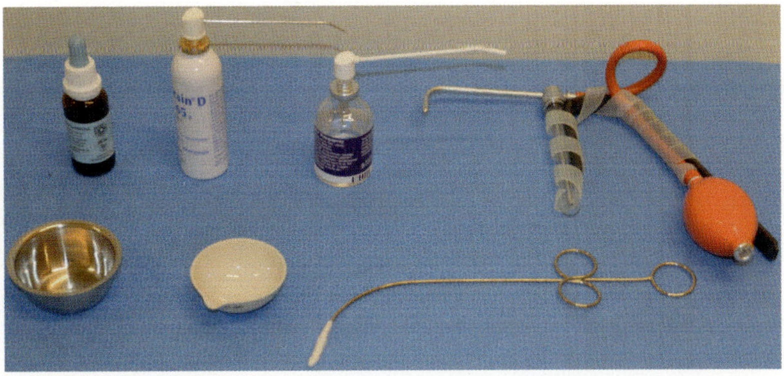

Fig. 11.3 Instrument table: One-handed spraying device (*upper right*), different kinds of anesthetics (*upper left*), cups for lidocaine 2% and lidocaine 4% and cotton swab (*center*) [Courtesy of Deutsche Stimmklinik Management GmbH]

indications. Mostly, breathy voice as well as aspiration in patients with RLN disorders can be alleviated when performing augmentations of the vocal folds. Glottal closure is a main component of achieving a louder voice and to effectively improve pharyngoesophageal bolus transport. Furthermore, it supports an effective cough by enabling higher subglottal pressure build-up. Many clinical cases are recognized where patients suffer more from aspiration than from voice problems [8]. Thus, the examiner who is assessing vocal function should also keep swallowing function in mind.

11.9 Office-Based Interventions in Glottic Insufficiency: Injections Laryngoplasty (Augmentation with Fillers)

The overall worldwide number of office-based injection laryngoplasties, i.e., vocal fold augmentations with fillers, is increasing rapidly. With good injection techniques, the augmentation can be easily performed in the office, either indirect transorally, transnasally, or percutaneously [9]. Although the cannula placement into the vocal fold is not too difficult, manual skills are required for finding the adequate position and dosage of the injectate (Fig. 11.4).

This chapter cannot go into full detail on how and when to perform office-based augmentations. However, the authors look back at more than 25 years and many hundreds of augmentations in the past and try to focus on the main prerequisites. We prefer transoral indirect injections because of best control of needle placement, but as soon as there is a significant gag response, we switch over to a transnasally controlled percutaneous approach. In females with high larynx position, we favor the cricothyroid approach; in males with very low larynges, the thyrohyoid technique may be preferable.

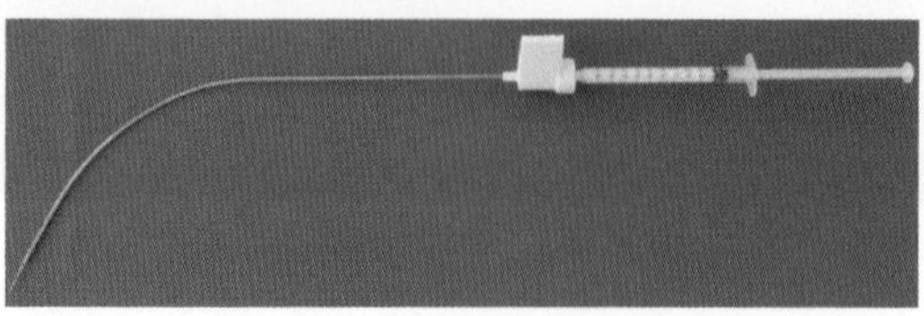

Fig. 11.4 Injectable implant attached to a bent cannula ready for transoral vocal fold augmentation [Courtesy of Deutsche Stimmklinik Management GmbH]

Transoral Augmentation The technique of transoral interventions is 150 years old, and the first augmentation was performed more than 100 years ago. However, injections for augmentation are widely used only since approximately 20 years. The technique is quite straightforward and can be performed by one surgeon alone. The patient has to hold his own tongue. The surgeon's non-dominant hand holds the 70° rigid endoscope, and the dominant hand advances a bent cannula transorally and places the needle in a position lateral to the tip of the vocal process, lateral to the superior arcuate line and approx. 5 mm into the vocalis muscle, or even further lateral into the paraglottic tissue. Injected materials are preferably resorbable (hyaluronic acid, calcium hydroxylapatite, carboxymethylcellulose, or other materials). Approx. 0.1 ml up to 1.0 ml are injected, including slight overcorrection considering that resorption of the fluid (lubricant) component of the filler will be resorbed within days after the operation.

Transnasal Augmentation This route can only be used when a long flexible cannula in combination with a high-pressure pumping device is used. The technique is not frequently used because of the need of specially designed instruments for this procedure.

Percutaneous Augmentation Separation of injection cannula access (here percutaneous) and laryngeal endoscopic monitoring (transnasal with flexible endoscope) is used more and more in office-based procedures. Advantages are that the surgeon has two hands for surgery and can more easily handle the intervention, but this technique needs a second person as endoscopist who is cooperating well coordinated with the surgeon.

Three pathways can be chosen for percutaneous augmentation: the trans-cricothyroid, the trans-cartilage (through the thyroid ala), and the trans-thyrohyoid approach. For most females it seems easiest to choose the cricothyroid approach for passing the injection cannula (20G–25G and >30 mm long, angled up 45°) into a vocal fold. The patient is lying supine on a plinth with the neck overextended. To avoid eliciting of cough reflex, the cannula should be inserted ipsilaterally and approx. 5 mm paramedian, thus avoiding intraluminal passage. In some cases it may help to apply topical anesthesia onto the endolaryngeal mucosa.

In males with a low larynx position, the thyrohyoid approach is the most promising approach to reach the vocal folds. The patient sits in a chair for this injection technique. Cannulas can be of the same diameter as for cricothyroid injections but have to be slightly longer (>40 mm, 20G–23G cannula). Thinner cannulas (25G–27G) may be too flexible for some male patients (Figs. 11.5 and 11.6).

11.10 Possible Complications in Office-Based Augmentation

In general, after thousands of interventions in the office, including all kinds of biopsies and excisions, we have not encountered any severe complications. In patients with pronounced gag reflexes, we realized that at a second trial in another visit, there is almost always a habituation for the patients considering the tolerance of instruments within the upper airway – facilitating an easier access to the larynx in the following interventions. We avoid office-based surgery when patients are under coumarin medication, but we do surgery when patients are on acetylsalicylic acid medication. We have never seen severe bleeding forcing us to move the patient onto an emergency operation or having the patient be hospitalized, but we always have to be able to cope with those potential risks of airway compromising swelling of the larynx after injection laryngoplasty.

No severe cardiovascular reactions nor significant bradycardia have been encountered by us in the past 25 years when performing office-based procedures. Vasovagal reactions were seen and handled by supine positioning with legs up and monitoring of the patient. We dropped our preoperative administration of subcutaneous atropine since more than 10 years now – without any negative side effect. Sedation is used in less than 5% of augmentations. Laryngospasm from topical sprays is rapidly and effectively treated with breathing techniques and reassurance.

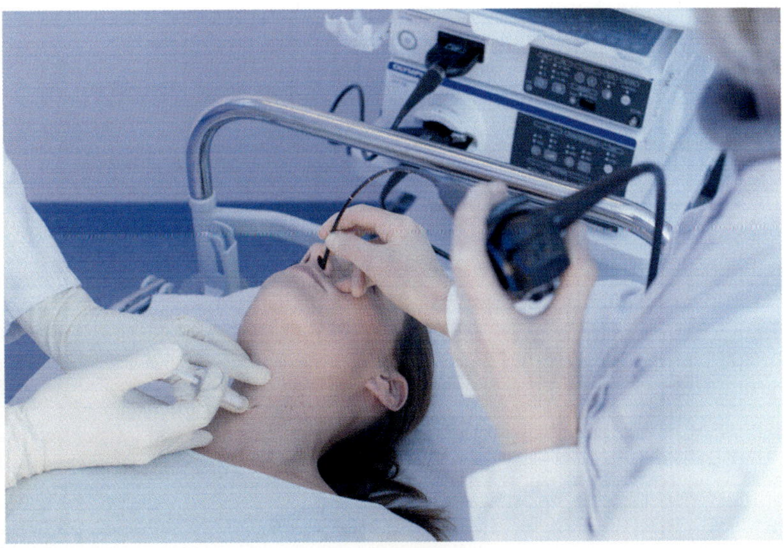

Fig. 11.5 Percutaneous, cricothyroid approach for vocal fold augmentation. An assistant is needed for transnasal endoscopy, visualizing the vocal folds during injection laryngoplasty. Here, the patient is lying on a plinth. The procedure can also be performed in a sitting position [Courtesy of Olympus Europe SE & Co. KG, Hamburg, Germany]

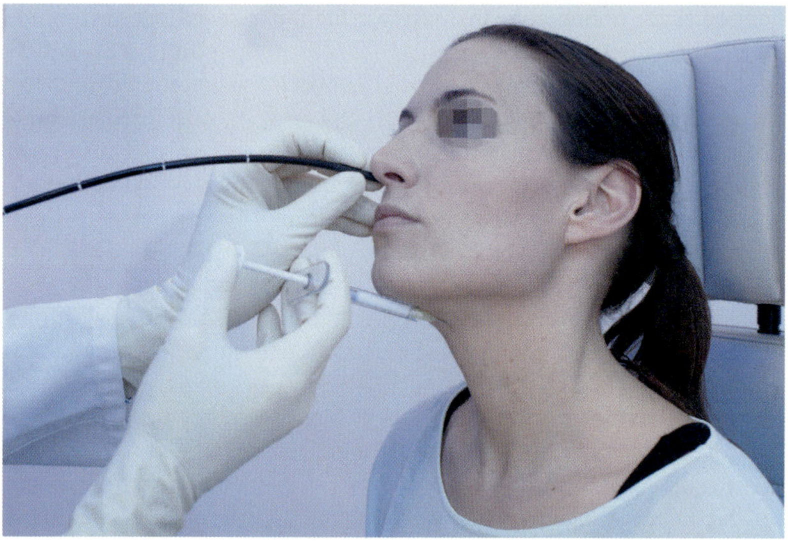

Fig. 11.6 Percutaneous, thyrohyoid approach for vocal fold augmentation. Again, an assistant is needed for transnasal endoscopy, visualizing the vocal folds during injection laryngoplasty. In this example, the procedure is performed with the patient in a sitting position. The procedure could also be performed with the patient lying on a plinth [Courtesy of Olympus Europe SE & Co. KG, Hamburg, Germany]

11.11 Injection with Botulinum Neurotoxin

Injections of botulinum neurotoxin (BoNT) can be easily performed in the office, either in an indirect transoral approach, percutaneously (with LEMG control), or transnasally (transnasal endoscopic approach via endoscope channel). Special injection cannulas provide the possibility to perform simultaneous LEMG for better positioning of the needle tip during injections. In most neurolaryngological casesv, the indication is spasmodic dysphonia (SD), a focal dystonia affecting the larynx. Other indications might be breathing problems where bilateral relaxation of adductory muscles in bilateral RLN paralysis or paresis, in cases of paradoxical vocal fold movement disorder, and in central nervous disorders with stridor. BoNT injections may avoid major surgery of vocal folds or even tracheostomy for these patients when inspiratory airflow is increased in a favorable manner by keeping the vocal folds from a paramedian position (Fig. 11.7).

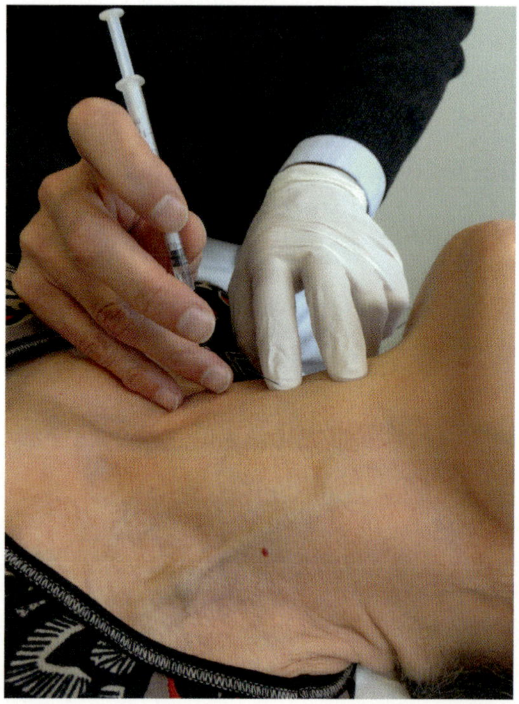

Fig. 11.7 The percutaneous, cricothyroid approach is an easy technique to inject botulinum toxin injection into the vocal folds, especially in patients with adductor spasmodic dysphonia. [Courtesy of Deutsche Stimmklinik Management GmbH]

Acknowledgments Special thanks go to Olympus Europe SE & Co. KG, Hamburg, Germany, and to the Deutsche Stimmklinik Management GmbH for permission to reprint several images from the "office-based laryngoscopy" manual.

Financial Support and Sponsorship None.

Conflicts of Interest None.

References

1. Fleischer S, Hess M. Systematic investigation technique in videolaryngoscopy and stroboscopy. HNO. 2003;51(2):160–7.
2. Fleischer S, Hess M. Durch Augmentation wieder gut bei Stimme. HNO Nachrichten. 2016;46(2):2–6.
3. Fleischer S, Hess M. Office based laryngoscopy. KG Hamburg: Olympus Europe SE & Co; 2016.
4. Fleischer S, Pflug C, Hess M. High-sensitivity FEES with NBI-illumination. Laryngoscope. 2017;127(5):1140–2.
5. Rosen CA, Mau T, Remacle M, Hess M, Eckel HE, Young VN, Hantzakos A, Yung KC, Dikkers FG. Nomenclature proposal to describe vocal fold motion impairment. Eur Arch Otorhinolaryngol. 2016;273(8):1995–9.
6. Rosen CA, Amin MR, Sulica L, Simpson CB, Merati AL, Courey MS, Johns MM III, Postma GN. Advances in office-based diagnosis and treatment in laryngology. Laryngoscope. 2009;119(Suppl 2):S185–212.
7. Volk GF, Hagen R, Pototschnig C, Friedrich G, Nawka T, Arens C, Mueller A, Foerster G, Finkensieper M, Lang-Roth R, Sittel C, Storck C, Grosheva M, Kotby MN, Klingner CM, Guntinas-Lichius O. Laryngeal electromyography: a proposal for guidelines of the European laryngological society. Eur Arch Otorhinolaryngol. 2012;269(10):2227–45.
8. Cates DJ, Venkatesan NN, Strong B, et al. Effect of vocal fold medialization on dysphagia in patients with unilateral vocal fold immobility. Otolaryngol Head Neck Surg. 2016;155(3):454–7.
9. Friedrich G, Remacle M, Birchall M, Marie JP, Arens C. Defining phonosurgery: a proposal for classification and nomenclature by the Phonosurgery Committee of the European Laryngological Society (ELS). Eur Arch Otorhinolaryngol. 2007;264(10):1191–200.

12 Framework Surgery

Rebecca J. Howell and Gregory N. Postma

Abstract

Framework surgery is a widely accepted treatment for vocal fold paralysis; however indications have expanded over time to include other forms of glottal insufficiency. Vocal fold paralysis is the clinical entity that frames our understanding and the historical concepts of what is today known as framework surgery. Over many years adjunct procedures, modifications, and improved clinical evaluation have benefited clinical outcomes. Furthermore, vocal patients can be compared in a number of different measures including visual (videostroboscopy), acoustic (noise-to-harmonic ratio, jitter, shimmer, etc.), and quality of life (voice handicap index, etc.). Initially shaped by our gross anatomic knowledge, fine-tuned by the cover-body theory of vocal fold vibration, and finally research-driven changes based on the biomechanical model will allow us to further improve vocal outcomes in glottal insufficiency with respect to framework surgery.

12.1 Introduction

In order to produce a "pure" tone, four physical properties of the vocal fold must be met: (1) inertia (or mass), (2) elasticity (or stiffness), (3) resistance, and (4) symmetry [1]. Unilateral vocal fold paralysis results in a change of all four characteristics. Unilateral vocal fold paralysis can be treated in many ways including voice therapy, reinnervation procedures, injection laryngoplasty, and laryngeal framework surgery. The indications for framework surgery have expanded beyond vocal fold paralysis to include laryngeal paresis and vocal fold atrophy. However, it is vocal fold paralysis that frames our understanding and the historical concepts of these procedures.

R.J. Howell
Otolaryngology, Head and Neck Surgery, University of Cincinnati, 231 Albert Sabin Way, ML # 0528, Cincinnati, OH 45267-0528, USA

G.N. Postma (✉)
Otolaryngology, Medical College of Georgia at Augusta University, 1120, 15th Street, Augusta, GA 30912, USA
e-mail: thegpostma@gmail.com

C. Sittel, O. Guntinas-Lichius (eds.), *Neurolaryngology*,
https://doi.org/10.1007/978-3-319-61724-4_12

12.2 Historical

Laryngology was "born" in the mid-1800s with Garcia's invention of the laryngeal mirror. Shortly thereafter, Legallois and Longet described laryngeal paralysis [2, 3]. At the time, there was a divergence in medical illustration with the only commonality the "famous wavy or even serpentine cords" demonstrating laryngeal paralysis [2]. In 1881, Semon began to publish his research explaining a sequence of paralytic vocal cords later known as Semon's law: (1) isolated abductor paralysis, (2) midline position as a result of spastic contracture of adductors, (3) cadaveric position in the stage of complete paralysis of all muscles innervated by the recurrent nerve, and (4) compensation of the paralytic condition by the healthy cord crossing over the midline [2]. In 1857, Grossman describes his concept of laryngeal paralysis as the "median position in complete recurrent paralysis while intermediary position is combined paralysis of both laryngeal nerves" [2]. In 1921, the German Otolaryngological Society entrusted a special commission to study laryngeal paralysis, a detailed questionnaire was published, and many began to reject the validity of Semon's law, while accepting the greater vulnerability of the abductor fibers based on clinical observation [2].

In 1911, Brünings first developed a method to narrow the glottis using a paraffin injection. This was subsequently abandoned due to adverse side effects of paraffin [4, 5]. Payr in 1915 was the first to describe laryngeal framework surgery using an anteriorly based rectangular thyroid cartilage flap for vocal cord medialization [5]. Meurman in 1952 was the next to utilize a cartilage implant designed from costal rib. Later described were variations of thyroid cartilage by Opheim (1955), Sawashima (1968), and Kramer and Som (1972) [2, 5]. Beginning in 1957, Arnold (innovator of Teflon injection laryngoplasty) described the debate regarding laryngeal paralysis, neural innervation, and clinical signs subsequently writing one of the early comprehensive reviews on laryngeal vocal fold paralysis [2].

These surgeons laid the foundation for Isshiki's landmark article in 1974 for what is now known as laryngeal framework surgery [4]. Isshiki initially described four types of framework surgery called thyroplasty: type 1 lateral compression, type 2 lateral expansion, type 3 shortening, and type 4 lengthening [4]. Most notable and still most commonly used today for laryngeal paralysis is the type 1 thyroplasty, also known as medialization laryngoplasty (ML). Type 2 was occasionally used in patients with hyperfunctional dysphonia such as plica ventricularis. Type 3 thyroplasty was designed as a relaxation or shortening procedure for abnormally high-pitched voices as in "mutational voice disorder or sulcus vocalis" [4]. Finally, there was type 4 described to recreate the stretching or lengthening for high vagal paralysis, typically in combination with type 1 [4].

Later, Isshiki also described the successful use of an alloplastic implant material (silastic) for medialization laryngoplasty [6]. The adjustability and reversibility of ML was popularized in North America by Koufman and Netterville as they demonstrated highly reproducible voice outcomes in which implants could be adjusted and replaced as necessary [7, 8].

However, the shortcomings of medialization laryngoplasty for unilateral vocal fold paralysis were recognized early on by Isshiki [9]. He described the large posterior glottal chink and vertical height difference, which were not corrected for by ML. In 1978, Isshiki details the first surgery to change the position of the arytenoid cartilage in order to improve vocal outcomes beyond that of medialization laryngoplasty [9]. Over the years, this arytenoid adduction (AA) procedure has undergone several modifications including the posterior anchoring suture [10], cricothyroid subluxation [11], and adduction arytenopexy [12].

Today, framework surgery is the workhorse in surgical management for unilateral vocal fold paralysis. Over time the indications have expanded as we have gained further insight into not only the structural anatomy but also the biomechanical properties of the larynx to further improve vocal outcomes.

12.3 Structural Anatomy

Just as there are gender differences in the vocal folds, not surprisingly, there are also gender differences in the laryngeal cartilaginous framework. The thyroid cartilage diameter in males is thicker than females [13]. The angle of the thyroid ala is greater in the female group (i.e., more obtuse), and the dimension of male larynges is larger on average by 11.4 mm [13]. When measuring the anterior commissure, however, both male and females are consistently in the midline just below the midpoint measuring from the thyroid notch to the inferior border of the thyroid cartilage within 1 mm in both superior and inferior directions [13].

The muscular process of the arytenoid cartilage is located halfway between the roots of the superior and inferior cornu of the thyroid lamina [14]. The recurrent laryngeal nerve is always located deep and medial to the cricothyroid joint and lateral and at the same level of the posterior cricoarytenoid muscle, with no other nerves in this vicinity [14].

The posterior cricoarytenoid muscle is the only abductor; it has two separate identifiable medial and lateral bellies [15]. The medial belly courses superolaterally at an angle of 41° before inserting on the medial aspect of muscular process of the arytenoid [15]. The axis of rotation with horizontal pull has a stronger vertical component compared to the lateral belly with a stronger anterior-posterior component. The lateral belly is at a 33° angle inserting on lateral surface of the muscular process [15]. The motion of the arytenoid rotates about a nearly vertical axis, which allows the vocal process to move more medial without much medial displacement of the arytenoid body [15]. Additionally the arytenoid undergoes a forward tilting motion, which changes the vertical height appreciated clinically in vocal paralysis and corrected post-procedure after arytenoid adduction surgery [15]. Posterior glottic closure improves vocalization following arytenoid adduction by increased subglottic airflow resistance [15].

12.4 Neural Anatomy

Pressman and Kelemen demonstrated the recurrent laryngeal nerve supplies unilaterally all intrinsic muscles of the larynx, while the external branch of the superior laryngeal nerve supplies the external cricothyroid muscle. Both recurrent laryngeal nerves innervate the interarytenoid muscles bilaterally. Hofer and Jeschek demonstrated the internal branch as a purely sensory nerve to reach the mucosa of the aryepiglottic folds [2]. This is a simplistic version of neural anatomy; it is widely accepted that there exists a large variability in cross innervation between left, right, and RLN and SLN differences [16–18].

Laryngeal electromyography (EMG) studies have documented that laryngeal muscles become reinnervated after recurrent laryngeal nerve (RLN) section but rarely after vagus nerve injury [19]. EMG of the thyroarytenoid (TA) and posterior cricoarytenoid (PCA) muscles with vagal injury show denervation and no spontaneous respiratory activation. Woodson also demonstrated both histologic and EMG evidence indicating reinnervation of the TA muscle greater than PCA and showing synkinetic activity especially with respiration. This suggests nerve fibers supposed to supply the PCA had instead synkinetic reinnervation to the TA muscle [19]. This is consistent with clinical observation that patients with vagus nerve injury often demonstrate that the paralyzed vocal fold lies more laterally and with less improvement over time compared to a RLN injury [19]. In unilateral paralysis, preferential reinnervation of adductor muscles is favorable because it enhances glottic closure. Whereas in bilateral paralysis, sustained adduction is unfavorable resulting in airway narrowing during inspiration and therefore more respiratory symptoms despite an acceptable voice [19].

Both clinical experience and animal models demonstrate a spontaneous regeneration of the RLN with a predominance of reinnervation to adductor muscles [19, 20]. This explains the classic observation that over time many vocal folds move medially after RLN injury yielding an acceptable voice [19, 20].

12.5 Mechanics of Voice Production

Van den Berg's "myoelastic-aerodynamic" model in 1959 was based on experiments of excised larynges; the variables described are initial glottal size, tension of the vocal folds, and subglottal pressure [21]. This model was the first to discover a certain minimal flow was required to vibrate the vocal folds and if the lateral force was too small (persistent glottal gap), the larynges did not respond, i.e., did not vibrate and did not create an acoustic sound [21]. Furthermore, glottal gap was the most important factor to decide the voice quality [22]. When the glottal gap is too small or excessively tight, the voice can be abnormal, rough, or strained. When the stiffness of the vocal folds increases, the range for a normal voice narrows, requiring a higher subglottal pressure [22].

When a paralyzed vocal fold is adequately reconstructed, the stroboscopic findings will reflect improvement in efficient translation of aerodynamic force into an acoustic signal [12]. The stroboscopy may even show normal phase symmetry despite the presence of vocal folds with radically different viscoelastic properties [12]. With uncorrected unilateral paralysis, patients intuitively adjust for glottal incompetence with varying hyperfunctional muscular behaviors [12]. Although static reconstruction realigns the vocal fold to gain aerodynamic competence, the residual perturbation in vocal quality is the result of differential viscoelasticity between the vocal folds [12].

The two biomechanical subunits of the vocal fold can be considered as an anterior and posterior component [23]. By medializing and stiffening the anterior membranous vocal fold of patients with unilateral vocal fold paralysis, glottal efficiency improves [23]. The posterior subunit is the anatomic cartilaginous vocal fold; changes made to this component adjust the position and tension of the vocal process. A midline vocal process results in a better valve to resist airflow leakage, allowing better buildup of subglottic pressure, therefore better acoustic power [23].

The force necessary to lateralize the vocal fold is much less than the force needed to lateralize the vocal process. In Noordizj's canine model, tension remained relatively unchanged at the mid-membranous region of the vocal fold as suture tension increased [23]. However at the vocal process, vocal fold tension increased with suture tension until 100 g [23]. Suture tensions greater than 100 g did not further increase vocal fold tension at the vocal process. This model helps to explain the suboptimal vocal outcomes with both hypo- and hyper-adduction, clinically experienced during arytenoid adduction surgery [23].

12.6 Patient Evaluation

Glottal incompetence is a common disorder causing both phonatory and swallowing impairments. The voice may be described as weak, breathy with a restricted pitch range [24]. Patients can be virtually asymptomatic or can have a variety of symptoms of glottal insufficiency such as liquid dysphagia, cough, shortness of breath, or exercise intolerance. Clearly, dysphonia is the most common reason for seeking treatment but can present as insufficient loudness, vocal fatigue, globus sensation, effortful voice, impaired singing, etc. [25].

The more specific form of glottal insufficiency, vocal fold paralysis, also varies in clinical presentation. Flaccid paralysis results in altered glottic configuration and arytenoid position [9, 10]. Unilateral vocal fold paralysis can present with structural asymmetries of the membranous folds, vocal fold height, length, and or tension. The arytenoid of the flaccid vocal fold may be rotated so that the vocal process is displaced rostrally and laterally [10]. Because of the angle between the cartilaginous and membranous vocal fold, the patient cannot approximate the vocal folds yielding incomplete glottic closure.

Isshiki's arytenoid adduction was developed specifically for those patients with a "posterior glottal gap" [9]. Successful AA surgery can increase the apparent length of the paralyzed vocal fold by rotating it toward the visual plane [10]. Another characteristic of laryngeal paralysis is an "anterior tipping" of the arytenoid partially obscuring the vocal fold which is often more severe in complete denervation [10]. This likely occurs by loss of support from the PCA muscles and contributes to inferior displacement of the vocal fold [10]. Contraction of the PCA results in rotation on an axis perpendicular to the AA with posterior "rocking."

Results of EMG data in laryngeal paralysis may also be beneficial to help guide decision-making. This can come in three general categories: (1) no spontaneous activity and normal recruitment (good prognosis), (2) spontaneous activity in the absence of normal recruitment (poor prognosis), and (3) markedly reduced recruitment with no evidence of denervation (equivocal) [5].

The preoperative videostroboscopy demonstrates the position of the paralyzed vocal fold. According to Netterville, if during phonation the mobile vocal processes contact the immobile side, then medialization alone will be successful [7]. If on the other hand, there is a wide posterior glottic gap then the patient will do better with both ML and AA combined [7, 22].

Improved posterior glottic closure and vocal height discrepancy are two of the most common reasons offered why AA may be considered. However, ML and AA + ML both close the glottal gap with significant improvements in voice quality, but those differences are unique to various independent studies, and no definitive significance has been found looking at vocal outcomes [24, 26, 27]. In reality, the decision based on what surgery is performed is often a function of the physician's preference and experience [26]. Furthermore, the success of laryngoplastic voice surgery is based on several critical factors, first being the proper patient selection and, second, surgical expertise [22]. Isshiki's policy for dysphonia second to glottal insufficiency was described as "rough tuning by laryngeal framework surgery and fine tuning by voice therapy" which is an acceptable practice even today [22].

12.7 Indications

According to Netterville, beyond voice outcomes, the second major benefit of medialization laryngoplasty is an improvement in dysphagia with a decrease in aspiration [7]. However, dysphagia is often multifactorial, and improved glottic closure often does not result in better swallowing even with improved voice and a more effective cough [28].

Medialization laryngoplasty with or without arytenoid adduction is useful for narrowing the glottis, especially in the case of a paralyzed vocal cord but is also useful in vocal fold bowing, presbylaryngis, and paresis [29]. Koufman and Postma have described bilateral ML for vocal fold bowing/atrophy [30]. Important considerations for bilateral ML include the following: (1) Overcorrection anteriorly can cause harsh, strained voice. (2) The posterior flange must not contact the arytenoid; otherwise, there is risk of restricting arytenoid motion [30]. Furthermore, ML can be used for a variety of complex anatomic soft tissue deficiencies as a result of cancer resection, trauma, atrophy, and sulcus vocalis. A large prospective study by Zeitels demonstrated the expanded indications for ML, also describing Gore-Tex as a versatile implant ideal for phonosurgical reconstruction [31].

Managing patient expectations is always important. In the case of ML, a consistent pattern of vocal improvement occurs where immediate intraoperative vocal improvements quickly deteriorate as perioperative edema ensues. This needs to be explained to the patient and family so that a somewhat rough immediate postoperative result is expected particularly with the overcorrection required with Gore-Tex ML. Edema is dependent on procedural time and collateral trauma to surrounding soft tissue [12].

12.8 Medialization Laryngoplasty

Generally, framework surgery is recommended and performed under local anesthesia with IV sedation [7]. The size of the implant or degree of adduction is mainly determined by intraoperative voice quality [7]. It is not necessary to use transnasal flexible laryngoscopy with video monitoring; however, it is generally advisable and provides excellent visual feedback during the procedure [7].Intermittent visualization of the larynx by surgeon or assistant can be equally beneficial [7]. If continuous monitoring is used, it is advisable for the patient to receive both topical nasal anesthesia and atropine, an anticholinergic and drying agent [7].

The patient's head is placed in neutral position, and a 4–5 cm horizontal incision is centered at the mid-thyroid ala, extending just across the midline. Skin is incised, subplatysmal flaps are raised, and the median raphe of the strap muscles is divided. Almost the entire hemilarynx on the involved side is exposed from the thyroid notch superiorly to the cricothyroid membrane inferiorly and midline laterally to the posterolateral border of the thyrohyoid muscle [8]. The perichondrium is elevated from the paralyzed side.

12.8.1 Silastic Implant

The next steps in Isshiki's type 1 thyroplasty using a silastic implant are as follows. The thyroid window is fashioned. Koufman describes window size in proportion to laryngeal size where men are 5–6 mm high and 12–15 mm wide and women are typically 4–5 mm high and 10–12 mm wide [8]. Half the distance of the thyroid cartilage measured at the thyroid notch determines the position of the upper horizontal window incision [8]. The window is placed parallel to the lower border of the thyroid cartilage, paying close attention to the variability of the anterior third and identifying instead the lower anterior edge and the portion behind the muscular process [7]. This line is angled slightly cephalad (2–4 mm) posteriorly [8]. The window should be as inferior as possible, while still leaving a stable inferior strut [7]. The distance from the anterior commissure to the anterior edge of the window is determined by the shape of the cartilage, which often is a function of gender. More commonly, the laryngeal angle is more obtuse in women (5 mm from the anterior commissure) so more anterior compared to the acute angle in men where the window should be positioned more posteriorly (7 mm from the anterior commissure) [7]. Alternatively or in addition, a pilot hole can be created with an 18G catheter. Next, a 27G needle can be used to gently apply lateral to medial pressure at the suspected level of the true vocal fold. Under direct visual laryngoscopic guidance, the surgeon can verify the position of the glottis prior to creation of the window. Typically the cartilage is calcified, and a 2–3 mm cutting burr using an otologic drill is used to create the window (as an alternative to sharp dissection) and subsequently remove the cartilage island or fragments [7]. The inner perichondrium is widely elevated using a short laryngeal or Penfield elevator. Isshiki's original description kept the inner perichondrium intact for fear of extrusion of the implant [4]. However, Netterville later described microscopically incising the inner perichondrium to improve medialization without increased rates of extrusion [7]. Thyroarytenoid fascia and distal branches of superior laryngeal vessels are left intact throughout this part of the dissection. Even with the violation of inner perichondrium, a capsule forms around the implant [7]. Next, a blunt instrument or depth gauge is used with vocal feedback from the patient and laryngeal video monitoring to establish the anterior, middle, and posterior depths of the window [7].

Many different variations have been described in carving a silastic implant, first described by Isshiki but further modified by Koufman, Netterville, Bielamowicz, and Montgomery [6–8, 24, 32]. The implant is carved such that the point of maximal medialization is at the inferior edge of the window and away from the ventricle and false vocal folds [7]. Again, because of laryngeal gender differences, the point of maximal medialization measured from the anterior aspect of the window is approximately 10 mm in women and 13–14 mm in men [7]. A 5–6 mm posterior extension can be considered [7]. According to Netterville, the implant can be divided into two pieces to allow a more gentle insertion [7]. Bielamowicz describes a posterior locking flange [24]. Silastic implants are also commercially available as Netterville PhonoForm® Silicone Blocks (Medtronic ENT Jacksonville, FL).

In order to address lengthy intraoperative time and posterior glottic incompetency, Montgomery developed his standardized prosthesis for ML surgery [32, 33]. Available since 1993, the Montgomery® Thyroplasty Implant System is available in 6, 7, 8, 9, and 10 mm female implants and 8, 9, 10, 11, and 12 mm male sizing (Boston Medical Products, Inc., Westborough, MA) [33].

12.8.2 Expanded Polytetrafluorethylene (ePTFE) Implant

Alternatively, the use of expanded polytetrafluoroethylene (ePTFE) or Gore-Tex (W.L. Gore and Associates, Flagstaff, AZ) implants has also been described [34, 35]. This was used to simplify the technique itself and allow incremental adjustment of vocal fold position [34].

Hoffman first described the use of a Gore-Tex cardiovascular patch as an ML implant in 1998 [34]. The incision is approached the same as described above. After the thyroid cartilage has been exposed, a window is planned paralleling the projection of the vocal fold; next a 4 mm burr is used to drill a single hole through the cartilage. This mini-thyrotomy is usually much smaller than the windows for silastic block implants. Next, the inner cartilage edge is removed, and inner perichondrium is elevated almost 3 mm in all directions. This may be incised, as most surgeons prefer. The implant material comes from the ePTFE cardiac patch (5 × 7.5 × 0.6 cm) cut to 5–7 mm wide ribbon [34]. Prior to implantation, the ePTFE ribbon is soaked in antibiotic solution [34]. To allow for stabilization, it can be wrapped once or twice around the inferior strut [34]. The medialization is fine-tuned by folding the ePTFE ribbon onto itself with a micro-alligator and annulus elevator; each fold is approximately 1.2 mm thick. Material is inserted to achieve a sufficient prolongation in maximum phonation time, and intraoperative assessment of the patient's vocal quality is acceptable to the operating surgeon [34]. Overcorrection with a mildly pressed voice should be done when using ePTFE [36].

Stasney adapted the technique using mini-fenestration, ePTFE, and a thyroid ala perichondrium flap for medialization thyroplasty in 2001 [35]. A posteriorly based apron flap is designed using the outer perichondrium of the thyroid ala elevated widely inferior and lateral on the surgical side. Next, the window and minifenestration is performed as described above. Two smaller holes are drilled using a very fine drill bit superior and inferior to the minifenestration, large enough to allow a 4-0 monofilament suture to anchor the implant [35]. After enough ePTFE has been implanted, the suture is secured to the thyroid ala (bolstering the implant), and the outer perichondrium can be sutured back into place and the remaining incision closed in the usual fashion [35].

12.9 Arytenoid Adduction

As initially described by Isshiki, the patient is positioned supine with the neck slightly extended and head turned away from the operative site [8, 9]. A horizontal incision is planned similar to the medialization thyroplasty (level of the midpoint between the thyroid notch and lower margin of the thyroid cartilage); however it is longer and extends laterally 1–2 cm to anterior border of the sternocleidomastoid [8, 9]. Again, subplatysmal flaps are elevated. As opposed to ML, the posterior aspect of the thyroid cartilage can be approached by dissecting lateral to the strap muscles [7, 8]. Alternatively, continued elevation of the outer perichondrium might be done until the entire ala is visible from medial to lateral (as in the approach for ML). A portion of the posterior rim of thyroid cartilage can be removed to expose the muscular process of the arytenoid cartilage [7]. Next, the inferior constrictor is sharply dissected to expose the cartilage inferiorly to the tip of the inferior cornu. Elevation is continued to release the inner perichondrium of the thyroid cartilage [9]. The pyriform mucosa is carefully, bluntly dissected and elevated superiorly off the arytenoid [7]. A blunt double skin hook can be used on the thyroid cartilage to better expose the posterolateral cricoid region [8]. The cricoarytenoid joint is located by palpating the arytenoid cartilage. The muscular process is almost on the same level as the vocal folds and can be identified as a minute prominence obliquely upward from the cricothyroid joint [9]. In Isshiki's original description, the joint was opened with a small sharp scissors but was later modified and deemed unnecessary in most cases [7–9]. The arytenoid muscular process is grasped with a fine-toothed forceps, and a 3-0 Prolene suture is passed twice through the muscular process and pulled anteriorly to reproduce the thyroarytenoid, lateral thyroarytenoid muscular pull [7, 8]. The suture is pulled through the paraglottic space, and the suture is tied over either the anterior portion of the implant or the lower border of the thyroid cartilage [7]. This has been described either over a Keith needle or using a 16-gauge angiocath needle placed through a hole in the anteroinferior aspect of the ipsilateral thyroid cartilage and can then be tied over a two-hole microplate as a bolster if needed [8, 24].

If Isshiki's arytenoid adduction recreates the motion of the lateral cricoarytenoid muscle, then Woodson's modification with a posterior suspension suture recreates the lost posterior cricoarytenoid support. The suture originates at the muscular process of the arytenoid and inserts at the inferior cornu of the thyroid lamina to yield a more physiologic and upright position of the arytenoid with less vertical displacement than AA alone [9, 10].

12.10 Adduction Arytenopexy

The adduction arytenopexy was designed to provide a more normal physiological arytenoid closure simulating combined effects of interarytenoid, lateral cricoarytenoid, thyroarytenoid, and posterior cricoarytenoid muscles during normal adduction [12].

The lateral thyroid lamina is exposed to the inferior cornu. The inferior constrictor is separated from the thyroid lamina, and the cricothyroid joint is disarticulated. After the pyriform mucosa is bluntly dissected from the inner aspect of the thyroid lamina and the posterolateral aspect of the cricoid cartilages, the dissection is carried posterosuperiorly along the cricoid. The lateral cricoarytenoid muscle is separated from the muscular process. The posterior cricoarytenoid is also separated from the posterior plate of the cricoid. Next a 4-0 Prolene suture on a cutting needle is placed through the posterior plate of the cricoid medial to the facet, through the joint, through the body of the arytenoid, and finally under the cricoid facet where a slip knot is placed [12].

12.11 Cricothyroid Subluxation

Zeitels as an additional procedure to adduction arytenopexy and/or ML designed the cricothyroid subluxation to increase vocal fold viscoelastic tension and permit aerodynamically efficient oscillation [11]. A double-pronged skin hook is placed lateral to the edge of the thyroid lamina and rotated anteromedially so that the inferior constrictor can be sharply dissected from the lamina. The inferior cornu is identified, and the cricothyroid joint is separated using a Mayo scissors. A 2-0 Prolene suture is placed around the inferior cornu of the thyroid lamina and passed submucosally under the cricoid anteriorly. This increases the distance between the cricoarytenoid joint and attachment of the anterior commissure, thus increasing tension and length of the musculomembranous vocal fold on the paralyzed side simulating cricothyroid muscle contraction [11].

12.12 Tension Altering Procedures

In Isshiki's original work, thyroplasty types 3 and 4 were described in three patients undergoing procedures to alter vocal cord tension. Two were women with androphonia (masculinized voice) undergoing the "cricothyroid approximation" or type 4 laryngoplasty. The third patient had mutational falsetto, undergoing a vocal ligament relaxation or type 3 laryngoplasty. In 1983, Isshiki describes a larger series of 11 patients for pitch elevating procedures with good short-term results [37]. In 1983 LeJeune reported another technique to increase vocal cord tension using an inferiorly based rectangular flap of anterior thyroid cartilage pulled and secured with a tantalum shim. In 1985, Tucker reported a variation of LeJeune's procedure using a superiorly based flap. LeJeune reported another revision in 1987 by creating midline rectangular flap with anterior vocal fold ligament attached and suspended with two tantalum shims. It was later concluded that most patients with mutational falsetto also had "functional problems" and should be referred to a voice therapist and undergo surgical therapy only as a last resort [8, 37].

Likewise, the vocal ligament relaxation or shortening procedures have also not been consistently successful. Originally described by Isshiki in 1976, the technique was utilized in 1985 by Koufman successfully in a woman with a 2 mm strip of cartilage removed bilaterally and unsuccessfully on a man with a 4 mm strip removed; both patients had adductor spastic dysphonia [8]. Tucker described an alternative for relaxation procedure making two vertical incisions on both sides of thyroid alar cartilage anteriorly 3 mm from the midline and displacing the middle portion inward, with the attached anterior vocal fold ligament [38]. Unfortunately, the results are at best 50% success rates [8, 38].

12.13 Lateral Expansion

Type 2 or midline lateralization techniques were described as a possible treatment for adductor spasmodic dysphonia [22]. However, these really are included here only as historical data from Isshiki's original work.

12.14 Arytenoid Abduction (AAb)

Woodson initially described arytenoid abduction for patients with bilateral vocal fold immobility as an alternative to posterior partial cordectomy and arytenoidectomy [20]. The goal of AAb is to enlarge the glottic airway while preserving residual or recovered adductor muscle activity yielding better vocal outcomes [20]. The procedure was designed after 3D motion analysis demonstrated a ball-and-socket joint at the cricoarytenoid complex where laryngeal adductor muscles rotate the arytenoid cartilage in a vertical axis [15, 39].

The dissection is similar to AA surgery as described above. After the muscular process is identified, a permanent stitch is secured and inferior traction placed on the arytenoid cartilage. Direct laryngoscopy is performed to confirm abduction of the paralyzed vocal fold with inferior traction. Next, the stitch is secured at the inferior cornu of the thyroid lamina.

Woodson's initial article described six patients, all of whom subjectively benefited, two of three able to be decannulated, and three of six avoided tracheostomy, with four of the six without decrease in vocal function (much unlike the breathy voice that results from more standard procedures such as cordectomy) [40]. Her follow-up study demonstrated improvement in 7 of 11 undergoing AAb for bilateral vocal fold paralysis and 3 more for neurogenic glottal airway compromise [20]. Her conclusion was that arytenoid abduction can be considered in select patients: those with bilateral vocal fold paralysis duration less than 1 year and who do not show EMG evidence of laryngeal synkinesis (specifically, inspiratory activity in adductor muscles) [20].

12.15 Laryngeal Reinnervation

Laryngeal reinnervation is a general term to describe surgical procedures intended to reestablish lost laryngeal neural connections (more details in Chap. 15). The nerve function may be those of the recurrent laryngeal nerve or the superior laryngeal nerve and may be motor or sensory. The first described reinnervation procedure by Tucker in the canine model was the nerve-muscle pedicle [41]. Other descriptions include muscle-nerve-muscle, direct implantation of a nerve ending into a muscle, and most commonly the end-to-end anastomosis (neurorrhaphy) [42].

Recurrent laryngeal nerve to ansa hypoglossi (cervicalis) was first described by Crumley in 1984 [43]. Ansa hypoglossi provides a physiologic quiet, resting tone to the reinnervated muscle seen clinically as tone, increased bulk, and position stability [1]. While the anastomosis is an unselected laryngeal reinnervation procedure meaning that the thyroarytenoid, lateral cricoarytenoid, *and* posterior cricoarytenoid muscles all receive innervation, giving the PCA tone is actually beneficial by stabilizing the arytenoid posteriorly [1]. Arguments for adductor reinnervation as compared to medialization procedures are that medialization restores geometric symmetry but does not restore viscoelastic symmetry nor muscle tone, which may be improved with reinnervation [44]. The goal of this procedure is not the return of glottal function, but to maintain muscle bulk and provide static tone. If division of RLN has occurred within 2 years and there is no spontaneous regrowth either clinically or based on EMG, then reinnervation should be considered [7].

12.16 Outcomes

There is an abundance of cohort and case control studies but a general paucity of randomized controlled studies comparing framework surgery and injection procedures. Furthermore, there are a number of different outcome measures studied to include: laryngeal stroboscopy, vocal function, aerodynamic, acoustic, clinical assessment of voice quality, and patient self-assessment tools. Since there is a role for both speech therapy and surgical intervention, decision-making is driven by patient symptoms.

The only randomized, prospective study regarding surgical treatment of unilateral vocal fold paralysis compared ML and reinnervation [45]. Both small groups had significant improvement in untrained listener rating and blinded speech language pathologist scales comparing pre- and 12 months posttreatment; however no significance between groups was discovered [45]. However, when separating for age, there was a difference in outcomes. Therefore, laryngeal reinnervation is typically considered for younger patients (less than 52 years old), minimal comorbidities, and those who choose not to have a permanent implant [1, 46].

A meta-analysis comparing injection laryngoplasty (IL) with calcium hydroxylapatite to silicone thyroplasty with primary outcome voice handicap index (VHI) and secondary outcome measures maximum phonation time (MPT) [47]. A total of 24 studies qualified for inclusion, and the result showed comparable outcomes between IL and silicone thyroplasty [47].

Bielamowicz compared pre-/postsurgical conditions between ML and AA; he found no statistical significance in subglottal pressure, glottal resistance, jitter, shimmer, or noise-to-harmonic ratio [24]. Flow rates declined significantly with treatment for both surgical groups [24]. Evaluating pre- versus postoperative subglottic pressure, no statistically significant changes were measured. This is consistent with the notion that the glottis is driven by constant pulmonary pressure and patients adjust airflow to maintain near normal subglottic pressure despite the degree of glottal insufficiency [24].

Several authors have compared medialization laryngoplasty techniques with Montgomery implants (Boston Medical Products, Inc., Westborough, MA) and Gore-Tex (W.L. Gore and Associates, Flagstaff, AZ), most finding comparable results with immediate improvement of phonation after thyroplasty in all patients [48]. Late complications (>1 month) with Gore-Tex include inflammation of the vocal fold and endolaryngeal extrusion as opposed to Montgomery where dislodgement may occur [48].

Using excised human larynges, Hoffman compared injection IL, ML, and ML + AA [49]. Aerodynamic data showed improvement in phonation threshold flow (PTF) for all conditions; however only ML + AA demonstrated significant improvement in phonation threshold pressure (PTP) and phonation threshold power (PTW) [49]. The mucosal wave was also assessed, demonstrating restoration to normal in ML + AA, increased amplitude with ML, and decreased significantly with IL, a detrimental effect compared to the benefits of convenience and minimal invasiveness [49]. Although ML + AA produced the best overall results, the study also demonstrated that hypo- and hyper-adduction may lead to suboptimal vocal outcomes [49].

Maximum flow rate (MFR) and maximum phonation time (MPT) have both been used as a measure of glottal insufficiency [50, 51]. A decrease in MFR and increase in MPT postsurgically reflect an improved glottal competence and efficiency and therefore vocal fatigue [50]. MPT has also been demonstrated to be a useful intraoperative measure. While MPT values increased almost two and a half times from pre- to post-medialization, there is not a critical or absolute value used to predict need for secondary procedure [51]. With improved closure, higher subglottal pressures are attainable thereby generating a stronger cough [50]. Vocal improvements appear stable at 1 month postoperatively with no significant changes beyond 1 year [52].

Probably the most consistent data stems from questionnaires ultimately reflecting patient satisfaction. Quality of life assessments have also proven the benefit of laryngeal framework surgery beyond the objective acoustical data both on voice specific (e.g., voice handicap index or VHI, voice-related quality of life or V-RQOL) and more general medical outcomes (e.g., short form or SF-36) [50, 53, 54].

12.17 Cautions

According to Netterville, in patients suffering cerebrovascular accident, voice results were disappointing. "The projection and volume were reasonable, but oropharyngeal incoordination led to poor articulation that shadowed the voice improvement" [7]. However, aspiration was significantly improved [7].

Two relative contraindications were initially described for ML. First, in patients having undergone vertical hemilaryngectomy, there is an absence of the lateral buttress from the thyroid cartilage to support a silastic implant. Second, previous laryngeal irradiation is a relative contraindication. If the ventricle is violated during the procedure, placement of the implant should be delayed until mucosal healing is complete [7]. Injection augmentation may be a good option in these individuals.

The need for secondary surgical procedures is common up to 33% but usually estimated closer to 10% [29, 55]. This can be subdivided into planned surgical/touchup procedures and laryngoplasty revision [29]. Planned second stages are more likely in professional singers [29]. Laryngoplasty revision may be required for either inadequate medialization (technical) or progression of disease rendering the amount of initial medialization inadequate [29]. Patients with symptomatic glottal incompetence can be offered "fine-tuning" with autologous fat injection laryngoplasty [30]. The only predictive factor for revision surgery was an abnormal noise-to-harmonic ratio on initial objective voice analyses [29]. Maximum phonation time and mean flow rates were not correlated with need for revision surgery; however they may correlate with extent of glottic closure deficit [29].

Based on national survey data regarding framework surgery, 70% of respondents performing ML or AA surgeries are general otolaryngologists, followed by head and neck surgery subspecialists and finally laryngology trained surgeons [55, 56]. Rosen found an overall complication rate for ML/AA procedures between 6% and 8.5%, which is consistent with literature, yielding a high of 9.8% by Cotter and 0% by Netterville [7, 56, 57]. Of the respondents, 13.8% reported having experienced postoperative airway compromise requiring acute interventions (observation, tracheotomy, release of AA suture, removal of implant, or orotracheal intubation) with a suggested increased risk in AA compared to ML [56]. ML implant extrusion may occur in <1% with ML revision rate of 5% [55, 56]. A strong relationship but not significant was identified between major ML complication rate and overall experience of the surgeon, i.e., surgeons performing less than five lifetime ML or less than 2 ml per year [56].

Minor complications are defined as vocal fold hematoma without airway obstruction or prosthesis movement. Major complications are wound hemorrhage, airway obstruction, or prosthesis extrusion. In a 15-year review at a high volume institution, only five patients presented with extruding implants, two Gore-Tex and three Silastic all managed endoscopically with IL augmentation in 4 of 5 extrusions [58]. Especially in Gore-Tex ML, the most common reason for revision is under correction [36]. Minor vocal fold hematomas were relatively frequent, resolved rapidly, and were not associated with airway obstruction [57]. Female patients may be more prone to complication because of smaller laryngeal size [57].

12.18 Future Directions

Orestes is the first to describe the phonatory effects of ML implant depth and medial surface shape [59]. In the canine model, he demonstrated that both depth and shape affect fundamental frequency range and aerodynamic power necessary to reach phonation threshold. The study also demonstrated that ML is less effective in vagal paralysis (lack of TA and CT action) compared to RLN paralysis (lack TA only). The effects of various implants, convergent or divergent, likely resulted from the increased medial edge stiffness. The divergent, long implant yielded the most optimal flow/pressure relationship while maintaining the most favorable glottic stiffness at the vibratory margin [59].

Khosla's recent work describes a novel biomechanical model measuring intraglottal geometry and its effects on acoustic vortices. He has shown adjusting low, medium, and high subglottal pressures can reproduce vortices. He has postulated that the production of vortices may influence the maximum flow declination rate and thereby acoustic intensity [60].

Significant gains have been made in understanding the structural changes performed during framework surgery, but where new research will be beneficial is better understanding the biomechanical model and how it may affect novel theories in speech therapy, ML implant models, and designing new surgeries to improve vocal outcomes.

References

1. Crumley RL, Izdebski K. Voice quality following laryngeal reinnervation by ansa hypoglossi transfer. Laryngoscope. 1986;96(6):611–6.
2. Arnold GE. Paralytic dysphonia. Methods of vocal rehabilitation. Eye Ear Nose Throat Mon. 1964;43:27–36.
3. Arnold GE. Vocal rehabilitation of paralytic dysphonia. III. Present concepts of laryngeal paralysis. AMA Arch Otolaryngol. 1957;65(4):317–36.
4. Isshiki N, Morita H, Okamura H, Hiramoto M. Thyroplasty as a new phonosurgical technique. Acta Otolaryngol. 1974;78(5–6):451–7.
5. Koufman JA, Isaacson G. Laryngoplastic phonosurgery. Otolaryngol Clin N Am. 1991;24(5):1151–77.
6. Isshiki N. Recent advances in phonosurgery. Folia Phoniatr (Basel). 1980;32(2):119–54.
7. Netterville JL, Stone RE, Luken ES, Civantos FJ, Ossoff RH. Silastic medialization and arytenoid adduction: the vanderbilt experience. A review of 116 phonosurgical procedures. Ann Otol Rhinol Laryngol. 1993;102(6):413–24.
8. Koufman JA. Laryngoplasty for vocal cord medialization: an alternative to teflon. Laryngoscope. 1986;96(7):726–31.
9. Isshiki N, Tanabe M, Sawada M. Arytenoid adduction for unilateral vocal cord paralysis. Arch Otolaryngol. 1978;104(10):555–8.
10. Woodson GE, Picerno R, Yeung D, Hengesteg A. Arytenoid adduction: controlling vertical position. Ann Otol Rhinol Laryngol. 2000;109(4):360–4.
11. Zeitels SM, Hillman RE, Desloge RB, Bunting GA. Cricothyroid subluxation: a new innovation for enhancing the voice with laryngoplastic phonosurgery. Ann Otol Rhinol Laryngol. 1999;108(12):1126–31.
12. Zeitels SM, Mauri M, Dailey SH. Adduction arytenopexy for vocal fold paralysis: indications and technique. J Laryngol Otol. 2004;118(7):508–16.
13. Sprinzl GM, Eckel HE, Sittel C, Pototschnig C, Koebke J. Morphometric measurements of the cartilaginous larynx: an anatomic correlate of laryngeal surgery. Head Neck. 1999;21(8):743–50.
14. Armin BB, Head C, Berke GS, Chhetri DK. Useful landmarks in arytenoid adduction and laryngeal reinnervation surgery. Laryngoscope. 2006;116(10):1755–9.

15. Neuman TR, Hengesteg A, Lepage RP, Kaufman KR, Woodson GE. Three-dimensional motion of the arytenoid adduction procedure in cadaver larynges. Ann Otol Rhinol Laryngol. 1994;103(4 Pt 1):265–70.
16. Maranillo E, Leon X, Orus C, Quer M, Sanudo JR. Variability in nerve patterns of the adductor muscle group supplied by the recurrent laryngeal nerve. Laryngoscope. 2005;115(2):358–62.
17. Sanudo JR, Maranillo E, Leon X, Mirapeix RM, Orus C, Quer M. An anatomical study of anastomoses between the laryngeal nerves. Laryngoscope. 1999;109(6):983–7.
18. Masuoka H, Miyauchi A, Yabuta T, Fukushima M, Miya A. Innervation of the cricothyroid muscle by the recurrent laryngeal nerve. Head Neck. 2015;38(Suppl 1):E441–5.
19. Woodson GE. Spontaneous laryngeal reinnervation after recurrent laryngeal or vagus nerve injury. Ann Otol Rhinol Laryngol. 2007;116(1):57–65.
20. Woodson G. Arytenoid abduction: indications and limitations. Ann Otol Rhinol Laryngol. 2010;119(11):742–8.
21. VAN DEN, BERG J, TAN TS. Results of experiments with human larynxes. Pract Otorhinolaryngol (Basel). 1959;21:425–50.
22. Isshiki N. Vocal mechanics as the basis for phonosurgery. Laryngoscope. 1998;108(12):1761–6.
23. Noordzij JP, Perrault DF Jr, Woo P. Biomechanics of arytenoid adduction surgery in an ex vivo canine model. Ann Otol Rhinol Laryngol. 1998;107(6):454–61.
24. Bielamowicz S, Berke GS, Gerratt BR. A comparison of type I thyroplasty and arytenoid adduction. J Voice. 1995;9(4):466–72.
25. Behrman A. Evidence-based treatment of paralytic dysphonia: making sense of outcomes and efficacy data. Otolaryngol Clin N Am. 2004;37(1): 75–104. vi
26. Li AJ, Johns MM, Jackson-Menaldi C, et al. Glottic closure patterns: type I thyroplasty versus type I thyroplasty with arytenoid adduction. J Voice. 2011;25(3):259–64.
27. McNamar J, Montequin DW, Welham NV, Dailey SH. Aerodynamic, acoustic, and vibratory comparison of arytenoid adduction and adduction arytenopexy. Laryngoscope. 2008;118(3):552–8.
28. Fang TJ, Tam YY, Courey MS, Li HY, Chiang HC. Unilateral high vagal paralysis: relationship of the severity of swallowing disturbance and types of injuries. Laryngoscope. 2011;121(2):245–9.
29. Anderson TD, Spiegel JR, Sataloff RT. Thyroplasty revisions: frequency and predictive factors. J Voice. 2003;17(3):442–8.
30. Postma GN, Blalock PD, Koufman JA. Bilateral medialization laryngoplasty. Laryngoscope. 1998;108(10): 1429–34.
31. Zeitels SM, Mauri M, Dailey SH. Medialization laryngoplasty with gore-tex for voice restoration secondary to glottal incompetence: indications and observations. Ann Otol Rhinol Laryngol. 2003;112(2):180–4.
32. Montgomery WW, Blaugrund SM, Varvares MA. Thyroplasty: a new approach. Ann Otol Rhinol Laryngol. 1993;102(8 Pt 1):571–9.
33. Montgomery WW, Montgomery SK. Montgomery thyroplasty implant system. Ann Otol Rhinol Laryngol Suppl. 1997;170:1–16.
34. McCulloch TM, Hoffman HT. Medialization laryngoplasty with expanded polytetrafluoroethylene. Surgical technique and preliminary results. Ann Otol Rhinol Laryngol. 1998;107(5 Pt 1):427–32.
35. Stasney CR, Beaver ME, Rodriguez M. Minifenestration type I thyroplasty using an expanded polytetrafluoroethylene implant. J Voice. 2001;15(1):151–7.
36. Cohen JT, Bates DD, Postma GN. Revision gore-tex medialization laryngoplasty. Otolaryngol Head Neck Surg. 2004;131(3):236–40.
37. Isshiki N, Taira T, Tanabe M. Surgical alteration of the vocal pitch. J Otolaryngol. 1983;12(5):335–40.
38. Tucker HM. Laryngeal framework surgery in the management of spasmodic dysphonia. Preliminary report. Ann Otol Rhinol Laryngol. 1989;98(1 Pt 1):52–4.
39. Bryant NJ, Woodson GE, Kaufman K, et al. Human posterior cricoarytenoid muscle compartments. Anatomy and mechanics. Arch Otolaryngol Head Neck Surg. 1996;122(12):1331–6.
40. Woodson G, Weiss T. Arytenoid abduction for dynamic rehabilitation of bilateral laryngeal paralysis. Ann Otol Rhinol Laryngol. 2007;116(7):483–90.
41. Tucker HM. Human laryngeal reinnervation. Laryngoscope. 1976;86(6):769–79.
42. Paniello RC. Laryngeal reinnervation. Otolaryngol Clin N Am. 2004;37(1):161–81.
43. Crumley RL. Selective reinnervation of vocal cord adductors in unilateral vocal cord paralysis. Ann Otol Rhinol Laryngol. 1984;93(4 Pt 1):351–6.
44. Titze IR. Comments on the myoelastic - aerodynamic theory of phonation. J Speech Hear Res. 1980;23(3):495–510.
45. Paniello RC, Edgar JD, Kallogjeri D, Piccirillo JF. Medialization versus reinnervation for unilateral vocal fold paralysis: a multicenter randomized clinical trial. Laryngoscope. 2011;121(10):2172–9.
46. Blumin JH, Merati AL. Laryngeal reinnervation with nerve-nerve anastomosis versus laryngeal framework surgery alone: a comparison of safety. Otolaryngol Head Neck Surg. 2008;138(2):217–20.
47. Shen T, Damrose EJ, Morzaria S. A meta-analysis of voice outcome comparing calcium hydroxylapatite injection laryngoplasty to silicone thyroplasty. Otolaryngol Head Neck Surg. 2013;148(2):197–208.
48. Nouwen J, Hans S, De Mones E, Brasnu D, Crevier-Buchman L, Laccourreye O. Thyroplasty type I without arytenoid adduction in patients with unilateral laryngeal nerve paralysis: the montgomery implant versus the gore-tex implant. Acta Otolaryngol. 2004;124(6):732–8.
49. Hoffman MR, Witt RE, Chapin WJ, McCulloch TM, Jiang JJ. Multiparameter comparison of injection laryngoplasty, medialization laryngoplasty, and

arytenoid adduction in an excised larynx model. Laryngoscope. 2010;120(4):769–76.
50. Spector BC, Netterville JL, Billante C, Clary J, Reinisch L, Smith TL. Quality-of-life assessment in patients with unilateral vocal cord paralysis. Otolaryngol Head Neck Surg. 2001;125(3):176–82.
51. Lundy DS, Casiano RR, Xue JW. Can maximum phonation time predict voice outcome after thyroplasty type I? Laryngoscope. 2004;114(8):1447–54.
52. Lundy DS, Casiano RR, Xue JW, Lu FL. Thyroplasty type I: short- versus long-term results. Otolaryngol Head Neck Surg. 2000;122(4):533–6.
53. Hogikyan ND, Wodchis WP, Terrell JE, Bradford CR, Esclamado RM. Voice-related quality of life (V-RQOL) following type I thyroplasty for unilateral vocal fold paralysis. J Voice. 2000;14(3):378–86.
54. Jacobson B, Johnson A, Grywalsky C. The voice handicap index (VHI): development and validation. Am J Speech Lang Pathol. 1997;6:66–70.
55. Young VN, Zullo TG, Rosen CA. Analysis of laryngeal framework surgery: 10-year follow-up to a national survey. Laryngoscope. 2010;120(8):1602–8.
56. Rosen CA. Complications of phonosurgery: results of a national survey. Laryngoscope. 1998;108(11 Pt 1):1697–703.
57. Cotter CS, Avidano MA, Crary MA, Cassisi NJ, Gorham MM. Laryngeal complications after type 1 thyroplasty. Otolaryngol Head Neck Surg. 1995;113(6):671–3.
58. Halum SL, Postma GN, Koufman JA. Endoscopic management of extruding medialization laryngoplasty implants. Laryngoscope. 2005;115(6):1051–4.
59. Orestes MI, Neubauer J, Sofer E, Salinas J, Chhetri DK. Phonatory effects of type I thyroplasty implant shape and depth of medialization in unilateral vocal fold paralysis. Laryngoscope. 2014;124(12):2791–6.
60. Khosla S, Oren L, Ying J, Gutmark E. Direct simultaneous measurement of intraglottal geometry and velocity fields in excised larynges. Laryngoscope. 2014;124(Suppl 2):S1–13.

Surgical Treatment of Bilateral Vocal Fold Immobility

13

Vyas M.N. Prasad, Mohammed I. Almohizea, and Marc Remacle

Abstract

Bilateral vocal fold immobility (BVFI) has several aetiologies. Vocal fold paralysis affecting both folds due to recurrent laryngeal nerve (RLN) injury is the commonest cause for bilateral vocal fold immobility syndrome. Other causes include ankylosis resulting in joint arthrodesis.

Patients present paradoxically with a breathy voice that improves with time at the expense of the respiratory function. Management of patients in acute stridor can be medical, surgical or both. Treatment of patients with BVFI is challenging. Tracheotomy has been the historic fail-safe treatment. Modern technology has allowed for the advancement of microsurgical techniques using the operating microscope, endoscopes, lasers and jet ventilation. Laryngeal airway enlargement procedures have gained greater acceptance and are now more commonly undertaken. Surgical techniques to widen the glottic aperture are being performed more commonly. There is a trade-off between the airway aperture, voice and laryngeal competence in limiting aspiration. Nerve reinnervation and pacing techniques are becoming more widely practised.

13.1 Introduction

Bilateral vocal fold immobility (BVFI) is due to several aetiological factors and presents in several different ways [1]. Vocal fold paralysis affecting both folds due to recurrent laryngeal nerve (RLN) injury is the commonest cause for bilateral vocal fold immobility syndrome, but it is important to make the distinction between paralysis (resulting in disruption to neuromuscular innervation) and mechanical fixation.

Many patients present with a breathy voice initially without respiratory compromise and

V.M.N. Prasad (✉)
Department of Otolaryngology-Head and Neck Surgery, Ng Teng Fong General Hospital, National University Health System, 1 Jurong East Street 21, Singapore 609606, Singapore
e-mail: vyasprasad@gmail.com

M.I. Almohizea
Department of Otolaryngology, Head and Neck Surgery, King Abdulaziz University Hospital, King Saud University, Riyadh, Saudi Arabia

M. Remacle
Department of ORL-Head and Neck Surgery, CHL-Eich, Medical Center 3rd Floor, 76 Rue d'Eich, Luxembourg L-1460, Luxembourg

C. Sittel, O. Guntinas-Lichius (eds.), *Neurolaryngology*,
https://doi.org/10.1007/978-3-319-61724-4_13

progress paradoxically to an improved voice over time. They often present with little or no respiratory difficulties in activities of daily life that involve minimal physical exertion. This relative improvement in voice quality can however be exchanged with more emergent symptoms of airway compromise requiring rapid intervention be it medical, surgical or both. Classically, patients initially present with differing levels of dyspnoea and inspiratory stridor, but given the following factors: (1) precarious nature of their airway and the width of the glottic chink, (2) weight of the patient, (3) comorbidities and (4) general health and wellbeing, they can rapidly progress to biphasic stridor, apnoea and respiratory arrest. Approximately 15% of patients tolerate this condition and do not require any surgical intervention unless there are reasons for deterioration resulting in further narrowing of the glottic chink [2–5].

Medical management of patients presenting with acute and progressive stridor secondary to BVFI consists mainly of the administration of intravenous corticosteroids, adrenaline nebulisers, high flow oxygen or helium-oxygen mixture [6] and intubation where possible and when required. These interventions are however usually temporary and definitive surgical management is advocated in almost all cases.

Treatment of patients with BVFI is challenging and no one procedure is risk-free or without compromise. Indeed, no method is yet perfect enough to efficiently treat dyspnoea without affecting phonation and creating a variable degree of laryngeal incompetence [7]. Tracheotomy is still advocated in many instances and has been historically the fail-safe procedure. Up until 1922, tracheotomy was the only surgical solution. Chevalier Jackson described the open ventriculocordectomy technique which provided a widened airway but compromised voice. Woodman suggested open partial arytenoidectomy in 1946, but it was Thornell 2 years thereafter who proposed endoscopic arytenoidectomy [8, 9]. Naturally, the avoidance of an external incision and direct visualisation of the airway made this procedure attractive. The difficulty at that time was that conventional instruments were blunt, ill-suited for fine dissection and caused bleeding and scarring. This is no longer the case with the modern array of diagnostic tools, microscopes, highly specialised surgical instruments [10], lasers and better anaesthetic delivery.

Laryngeal airway enlargement procedures have gained greater acceptance and are now more commonly undertaken. These procedures are either temporary or permanent with respect to glottic enlargement. Broadly speaking, there are four types of interventions: (1) resection of anatomical structures, (2) reorienting and displacing anatomical structures with minimal tissue resection, (3) displacing existing structures without resection of tissue and (4) restoration or rerouting of innervation to the laryngeal musculature. With the exception of the last intervention, all the others are now mainly performed endoscopically.

In this chapter, we will focus on current surgical treatment options for bilateral vocal fold immobility in adults and aim to provide an understanding and awareness of the various options available to treat this challenging condition.

13.2 Anatomy and Physiology

The larynx is primarily designed to prevent aspiration into the lower respiratory tract. It is also involved in speech and, in addition, when the glottis is closed, helps raise intrathoracic pressure which helps in heavy lifting and straining. It consists of three paired and three unpaired cartilages, several intrinsic and extrinsic muscles and their respective nerve and vascular supplies. The level of the true vocal cords corresponds to the narrowest part of the adult airway (cricoid in the child). Any condition that decreases the size of the glottic opening can result in clinically significant airway narrowing usually manifesting as dyspnoea and/or stridor. The lumen in the normal adult trachea is 300–500 mm^2 compared to the subglottis (200–300 mm^2) and glottis (150–200 mm^2). In bilateral vocal fold paralysis, the glottic cross-sectional area is reduced to a mere 30–60 mm^2. This is only 20–30% of the normal area in healthy individuals [11, 12]. By and large, BVFI with glottic cross-sectional areas of greater that 50 mm^2 can compensate without the need for any form of intervention. Unlike fixed airway stenosis, BVFI due to paralysis is characterised by passive abduction of the cords in expiration and adduction through the Bernoulli effect on inspiration [13–15]. This phenomenon contributes to the rapid deterioration of patients when the cross-sectional area of the glottic chink becomes smaller leading to respiratory fatigue, hypo-oxygenation and CO_2 retention.

All the intrinsic muscles of the larynx except for the cricothyroid (external branch of superior laryngeal nerve, SLN) are supplied by the recurrent laryngeal nerves (RLNs) which originate from the vagus nerve. The left nerve has a longer course and passes around the arch of the aorta. For embryological reasons the right passes around the subclavian artery instead. Injury to either the vagus nerve, its nuclei in the brainstem or to the RLNs results in neurogenic paresis or paralysis. The cricoarytenoid joint is a ball-and-socket joint rather than a hinge joint [16]. The arytenoid cartilage rotates and slides on the superior surface of the posterior cricoid lamina. The posterior cricoarytenoid (PCA) muscle is the only true abductor of the glottis; the rest of the muscles attached to the muscular process of the arytenoid are adductors. Disruption to the joint (subluxation, dislocation or fracture) and arthrodesis /ankylosis are also important causes of BVFI.

The glottis can be divided physiologically into two parts, anterior and posterior. The anterior portion extends from the tip of the vocal process of the arytenoid along the vocal ligament to the anterior commissure. This is the vibratory fold and is essentially phonatory. Surgery here usually has an effect on voice. The posterior glottis extends from the medial edge of the arytenoid cartilage anteriorly to the tip of the vocal process and is the 'respiratory' glottis—essentially for ventilation. Hence, BVFI in adduction results in a reduction in the size of the posterior glottis with reduction in airflow but over time much less effect on voice.

13.3 Aetiology

BVFI is most commonly due to injury to both RLNs. Thyroid surgery is still the commonest cause of RLN paralysis although there is a trend towards an increase in BVFI seen as a result of malignancy and nonsurgical trauma (e.g. intubation and blunt or penetrating neck trauma) [1]. Other surgical causes include parathyroid surgery, carotid endarterectomy and cardiothoracic surgery. Rarer causes include lesions of the brain stem, neurological disorders, radiation, infection, autoimmune conditions and degenerative motor unit disorders (e.g. amyotrophic lateral sclerosis) [17].

The most common laryngeal injuries are seen after endotracheal intubation. Most of these are due to the pressure exerted by the tube or cuff on the posterior glottis causing a neurapraxia although subluxation by traumatic intubation can also occur albeit rarely. Medium- to long-term intubation can lead to ulceration of the posterior glottis and interarytenoid region resulting in fibrosis, fixation and posterior glottic stenosis. Demographic data with aetiology from the authors' series between 1985 and 2000 are found in Table 13.1.

Table 13.1 Demographic data

No. of patients	69
Female	34
Male	35
Age (y)	
Mean ± SD	56 ± 16
Minimum	11
Maximum	83
Follow-up (mo)	
Mean ± SD	50 ± 44
Minimum	1
Maximum	181
Paralysis (no. of patients)	49
Thyroidectomy	20
Tumoural compression	9
Cervical or thoracic surgery	7
Other neurogenic causes	
Viral neuritis	5
Neurologic disease	4
Cervical trauma	1
Prolonged intubation	1
Unknown	2
Ankylosis	20
Intubation	11
Radiotherapy	6
Inflammatory process	1
Malformation	1
Trauma	1
Patients already tracheotomised	10

13.4 Diagnostic Assessment

13.4.1 History and Examination

A thorough history is essential but may not be possible in acute situations involving BVFI. In most cases establishing the diagnosis is relatively straightforward as there is usually an obvious cause such as recent thyroidectomy or trauma. Where doubt exists, a comprehensive history followed by examination and diagnostic tests is indicated.

The history should identify any previous surgery to the central nervous system (CNS), head, neck and thorax. Any recent intubation either for medical or surgical reasons should be noted. Examination including fibre-optic laryngoscopy with or without stroboscopy in the clinic setting should be performed and if possible recorded on image-capturing software for future comparison. Thereafter, depending on the history and preliminary examination findings, further imaging studies and specific laboratory tests should be considered [18].

13.4.2 Imaging Studies

A fine cut computer tomogram (CT) scan from the brainstem to the arch of the aorta is essential to rule out any lesion that may either be infiltrating or compressing the vagus nerve or the RLNs. The use of CT in diagnosing BVFI when the diagnosis is uncertain is becoming more common. Magnetic resonance imaging (MRI) of the CNS if such pathology is suspected should be performed as in the case of demyelinating diseases. The use of ultrasound has become more popular in assessing not only the neck but also the vocal folds for complete paralysis but has not been as accurate in diagnosing paresis [19].

13.4.3 Pulmonary Function Tests

Pulmonary function tests are helpful in assessing the extent of airway compromise. Peak inspiratory and expiratory flow (PIF, PEF), airflow resistance and the flow-volume curves are indicated in diagnosing the extent of central airway compromise. PEF has been shown to be more useful (compared to PIF) in comparing post-operative improvement [13, 14, 20, 21].

13.4.4 Laryngeal Electromyography (LEMG)

LEMG is an electrophysiological method of assessing the electrical activity in muscle (details in Chap. 1). Since its introduction by Weddel et al. [22] and its development thereafter by Faaborg-Andersen et al., it has become an increasingly important diagnostic and prognostic tool, although a recent meta-analysis showed that over 40% of patients with findings predictive of recovery did not in fact recover [23]. LEMG has the ability to diagnose neuropathic conditions and distinguish between a neurological cause for BVFI and mechanical immobility. In this regard, visual observation alone may be inadequate, and the use of vocal dynamic studies and videostroboscopy has been shown to be wrong in almost a third of cases after LEMG [24].

13.4.5 Voice Analysis

Where possible, voice analysis should be performed pre- and post-operatively. Phonation can be assessed by measuring maximum phonation time and phonation quotient for aerodynamic parameters. Acoustic evaluation measuring mean vocal intensity and high-resolution frequency analysis allows for the categorisation of intensity according to frequency which can be used to distinguish the spectrum ranging from no sound, noise, harmonics and fundamental frequency [7].

13.4.6 Rigid Microlaryngoscopy

Where the diagnosis of BVFI is uncertain, especially in the case of joint fixation, a rigid microlaryngoscopy and testing the passive mobility of the arytenoids under general anaesthesia are recommended. EMG studies help in this regard although both fixation and paralysis can occur simultaneously or even affect different cords in the same setting.

13.5 Management Options

BVFI as discussed previously can be temporary or permanent, acute or chronic and a result of neurogenic, mechanical or a combination of the two pathological processes. Many patients with chronic BVFI develop some respiratory compensation mechanism (conditioning) which allows them to pursue most activities of daily living comfortably.

Wasserman et al. have shown that inspiratory resistance of more than 2.5 kPa x s/L can be used as an empirical limit above which surgical intervention is necessary [13–15]. Naturally, this measurement is only helpful in the non-acute setting of a centre with facilities to measure such a parameter.

Treatment options should be tailored towards the individual patient and best possible outcome with regards to the airway, voice and swallow. Eventually, surgery can be considered as a definitive indication when compensatory physiological respiratory mechanisms fail to provide adequate oxygenation for the level of physical exertion each individual requires.

13.5.1 Conservative/Medical Treatment

In many cases of acute stridor, patients respond positively to medical treatment. The use of high-dose intravenous steroids and nebulised adrenaline with high flow oxygen or helium-oxygen mixture (heliox) has been shown to be effective. Over time, they compensate well enough to breathe comfortably. Patients should be encouraged to perform, within reason, some physical activity to optimise their respiratory reserve and help overcome the increased inspiratory airway resistance.

The use of antibiotics where a bacterial infection is highly suspected is acceptable, and some practitioners also encourage the use of antireflux agents such as proton pump inhibitors (PPIs) to reduce any laryngopharyngeal reflux (LPR) and its concomitant inflammation to the narrowed glottis.

Short-term intubation either nasotracheally with fibre-optic guidance or orotracheally is helpful in the very short term. The use of adjuncts in managing the acute airway prior to intubation such as a trans-tracheal catheter or cricothyroid needle is well described in the literature. In general, intubated patients should either have a tracheotomy, a reversible lateralisation procedure or a trial of extubation with maximal medical therapy if the acute event precipitating respiratory compromise and life threatening stridor has been effectively treated.

13.5.2 Surgical Treatment

The surgical management of patients with BVFI can be broadly divided into two groups, i.e. tracheotomy and all 'other procedures'. This categorisation may be simplistic but in essence distinguishes the philosophy surrounding surgical management. 'Other procedures' offer a variety of possibilities to treat BVFI—both temporary (reversible) and permanent.

13.5.3 Tracheotomy/Tracheostomy

Despite the many advances in endoscopic microsurgery for BVFI, tracheostomy continues to be the time-tested procedure for both temporary and permanent BVFI. It is understandably much cheaper as it requires no special equipment as is seen with laser microlaryngeal surgery. It provides a safe airway and can be removed if the patient regains cord function in the future. Indeed many of the historical procedures for BVFI were performed with a tracheostomy tube already in place and depending on the level of success—removed accordingly. In the acute setting, there may be little choice but to tracheotomise the patient. However, many patients are loathed to having a tracheotomy and would forsake voice quality over a surgical airway [25]. Tracheotomy is not without risks either both in the early peri-operative period and thereafter and patients should be counselled where possible on the risks and benefits appropriately [26].

13.5.4 'Other Procedures'

Broadly speaking, all other procedures aimed at surgical management of BVFI aim to mainly widen the glottic chink with the exception of procedures that aim to restore the innervation of the intrinsic muscles of the larynx—primarily its only abductor, i.e. the PCA. Theoretically, reinnervation would be the ideal procedure as it does not compromise voice quality over airway size unlike glottis-expansion procedures that have a lesser or greater degree of voice compromise. In some patients who have either had fixation due to radiation or BVFI due to cerebral events, swallow and ensuing aspiration can also be an important factor surrounding decision-making vis-a-vis glottis-expansion surgery.

13.5.5 Indications

Deteriorating respiratory function/exercise tolerance with inspiratory stridor at rest and increase in inspiratory resistance (>2.5 kPa x s/L) are indications for surgical intervention. Some patients are prone to recurrent attacks of upper respiratory tract infections which have a significant effect on the already narrow glottic chink precipitating acute stridor. These patients should be considered for surgical intervention early and pre-emptively. When a diagnosis is made for idiopathic or neurogenic BVFI, it is reasonable to wait up to even a year before performing surgery. LEMG can be used to assess the presence of electrical intramuscular activity although its prognostic success is debatable [27–29]. In cases where bilateral ankylosis (fixation) is suspected initially on the history and confirmed with LEMG and assessment of joint mobility in the operating theatre, treatment options fall broadly into two categories. The first involves surgical procedures attempting mobilisation of the cricoarytenoid (CA) joint. This is performed in cases of joint subluxation or dislocation. The second category consists of the exact same procedures performed in cases of neurogenic pathology requiring glottis-expansion surgery. Posterior glottic stenosis, anterior synechiae and laryngeal, thyroid and pharyngeal malignancy are other causes of BVFI, and their respective treatment options are outside the scope of this chapter.

13.6 Surgical Procedures

Besides tracheotomy, all other surgical procedures for BVFI can be further categorised into four main interventions: (1) resection of anatomical structures, (2) reorienting and displacing anatomical structures with minimal tissue resection, (3) displacing existing structures without resection of tissue and (4) restoration or rerouting of innervation to the laryngeal musculature. These interventions are all permanent except for category 3, i.e. displacing existing structures without resection of tissue. The development of endoscopic techniques and further refinements made to surgical equipment, use of the CO_2 laser and increasing safety and availability of less cumbersome and bulky anaesthetic delivery systems into the larynx have obviated the need for extralaryngeal approaches (requiring thyrofissure, laryngofissure or paralaryngeal approaches) and in the vast majority of cases—the need for a covering tracheotomy.

13.6.1 Temporary Bilateral Vocal Fold Immobility

BVFI may not be permanent. Some surgeons advocate waiting between 6 months and 1 year to see if cord function returns prior to undertaking any procedure that may result in a permanent change to the larynx anatomically or physiologically. Temporary BVFI is most commonly seen from thyroid surgery, and resolution is seen between 40 and 86% [29, 30]. Management options for patients suspected of having temporary BVFI include intubation for acute and short-lived palsies, tracheotomy and reversible lateral fixation suture techniques—category 3. First described by Ejnell, this procedure has been modified by Lichtenberger and involves a specially designed endolaryngeal needle holder which brings two sutures from within the larynx above and below the vocal process out into a small opening in the neck where it is secured over the thyroid cartilage or the extralaryngeal muscles [31–33]. Other modifications on this technique obviating the need for the specially designed needle holder and jet ventilation have been described [34, 35] with equally good results.

13.6.2 Permanent Bilateral Vocal Fold Immobility

Category 1 and 2 procedures include posterior cordotomy, arytenoidectomy, cordectomy (submucosal and posterior) and permanent/definitive lateralisation (with CO_2 ablation of the thyroarytenoid muscles and arytenoid cartilage) as described by Lichternberger.

13.6.3 Transverse/Posterior Cordotomy (Cordectomy)

Dennis and Kashima [36, 37] first described this procedure which involves making a transverse cordotomy anterior to the vocal process using a CO_2 laser. This was combined with division of the conus elasticus (releasing the glottic sphincter) and retraction of the remaining thyroarytenoid muscle anteriorly increasing both the posterior glottic airway and anterior vocal fold (phonatory) mass. Cicatrisation (and granuloma formation) following this procedure has been commonly encountered requiring repetition and/or further resection of either the true cord anteriorly or the vocal process and/or varying extents of the arytenoid posteriorly [36, 38]. Usually a single-sided procedure is sufficient, but occasionally a bilateral procedure is required.

13.6.4 Cordectomy

Modifications of Kashima's technique involving resection rather than purely incising the true and false vocal cords to further increase the laryngeal aperture have been shown in various series to have better results in managing the airway but as stated before may have a detrimental effect on the voice [39, 40]. The cordectomy therefore can be used in a broader sense as a procedure (usually with CO_2 laser) involving resection of greater amounts of the true cord and false cords with or without a degree of resection of the vocal process of the arytenoid as well. Submucosal resection of the phonatory (anterior) part of the true cord with closure of the mucosa with fibrin glue was also shown to be effective not only for respiration but also phonation [41]. Failures of this procedure like cordotomy include cicatrisation, granulation or, in the case of more extensive cordectomy, a resulting scar replacing the cord—the 'pseudocord' which can retract medially [42–46].

13.6.5 Arytenoidectomy

Kleinsasser's introduction of endoscopic techniques and special instruments in the latter half of the last century revolutionised laryngeal surgery and with it the management of BVFI. Initially, arytenoidectomy as described by Thornell was performed under temporary tracheostomy and utilising electrocautery. An obturator was inserted between the cords and removed in the second stage 3–4 weeks later. Things have progressed since with the utilisation of the CO_2 laser by Eskew (in dogs), Lim (in humans) and Ossoff [47–49] to dissect and either resect or ablate the arytenoid. The first description to preserve the mucosal flap overlying the arytenoid and seal the bed using fibrin glue was described by Sato [50]. The main concerns in this technique include frequent transient aspiration along with scarring and granuloma formation as seen in cordectomy and cordotomy. Cricoid chondritis can also occur especially in patients who have had prior radiation treatment to the neck.

13.6.6 Subtotal Arytenoidectomy

A modification of Ossoff's technique has been shown by Remacle et al. to have a stable and lasting effect on airway patency with preservation of laryngeal competence and socially acceptable voice quality [51]. This procedure is a subtotal CO_2 laser arytenoidectomy. It is performed under general anaesthesia with a laser safe orotracheal tube or a tracheostomy tube in an already tracheotomised patent. The use of modern CO_2 laser systems has improved energy delivery, reducing thermal damage and allowing for computerised calculation of power delivery. This scanner software modification to some CO_2 lasers allows the beam to travel across the target in a circle, straight or curved line depending on the shape desired. Various lengths (0.5–3.5 mm) and penetration depths (0.2–2.0 mm) are programmable. The procedure is performed in superpulse mode at a computer adjusted power setting of approximately 10 W using scanner mode with a depth of penetration of two hundred microns and beam length of 2 mm usually. The technique begins at the tip of the vocal process extending laterally to involve sectioning of the ventricular fold up to the rim of the arytenoid and inferiorly to the conus elasticus. A coronal section of the arytenoid body is performed with preservation of the aryepiglottic fold laterally and mucosa of the medial aspect of the arytenoid. A 1–2 mm thin cartilaginous shell of the posterior body of the arytenoid is left in situ along with its remaining mucosa attached behind and medial to it (Fig. 13.1a–d). The muscular process is preserved while the rest of the arytenoid is excised after dislocating the CA joint (Fig. 13.2). Slow-setting fibrin glue (to avoid irritation and post-operative cough) is applied in the resection bed and helps reduce haematoma and granulation post-operatively. Antibiotic prophylaxis is administered perioperatively. Patients are usually discharged on a short course of antibiotics, inhaled steroids and PPIs. Overall, the results from subtotal arytenoidectomy according to Remacle et al. [7] have been very good. All tracheotomised patients were decannulated; voice quality was minimally affected with some reduction in maximum phonation time, but mean conversational vocal intensity was not notably modified over time. Another advantage of subtotal arytenoidectomy is the preservation of the posterior aspect of the arytenoid frame and mucosa. This prevents inward collapse of the mucosa and helps reduce aspiration. Hence, removal of only the intraluminal portion of the arytenoid with resection and cutting through the conus elastics at the level of the tip of the vocal process releases the cricoarytenoid ligament (vocal ligament) allowing for passive glottal opening [52]. Results in a series published by Remacle et al. (Table 13.2) showed significant improvement in the mean ratio of PEF/PIF highlighting sustained respiratory improvement.

13.6.7 Definitive (Permanent) Vocal Cord Lateralisation of Lichternberger

This procedure consists of a partial laser arytenoidectomy with submucosal cordectomy covering the defect with spared mucosa of the arytenoid and vocal cord using the same endoextralaryngeal suture technique employed in the temporary lateralisation technique. A covering tracheostomy is not essential as the procedure can be performed with jet ventilation during surgery. Essentially, an incision is made either with a CO_2 laser or microsurgical instruments a few millimetres in front of the tip of the vocal process of the arytenoid extending posteriorly over the vocal process 1.0–1.5 mm from the edge of the vocal fold on to the superior surface of the arytenoid. It is then connected posteriorly to the muscular process of the arytenoid forming a triangular incisional shape. The arytenoid is dissected and excised. Thereafter, a submucous cordectomy is performed on the thyroarytenoid muscle safeguarding the mucosa. Suture fixation in the neck on the thyroid lamina over the extralaryngeal muscles (as in the temporary procedure) completes the operation [53, 54, 55].

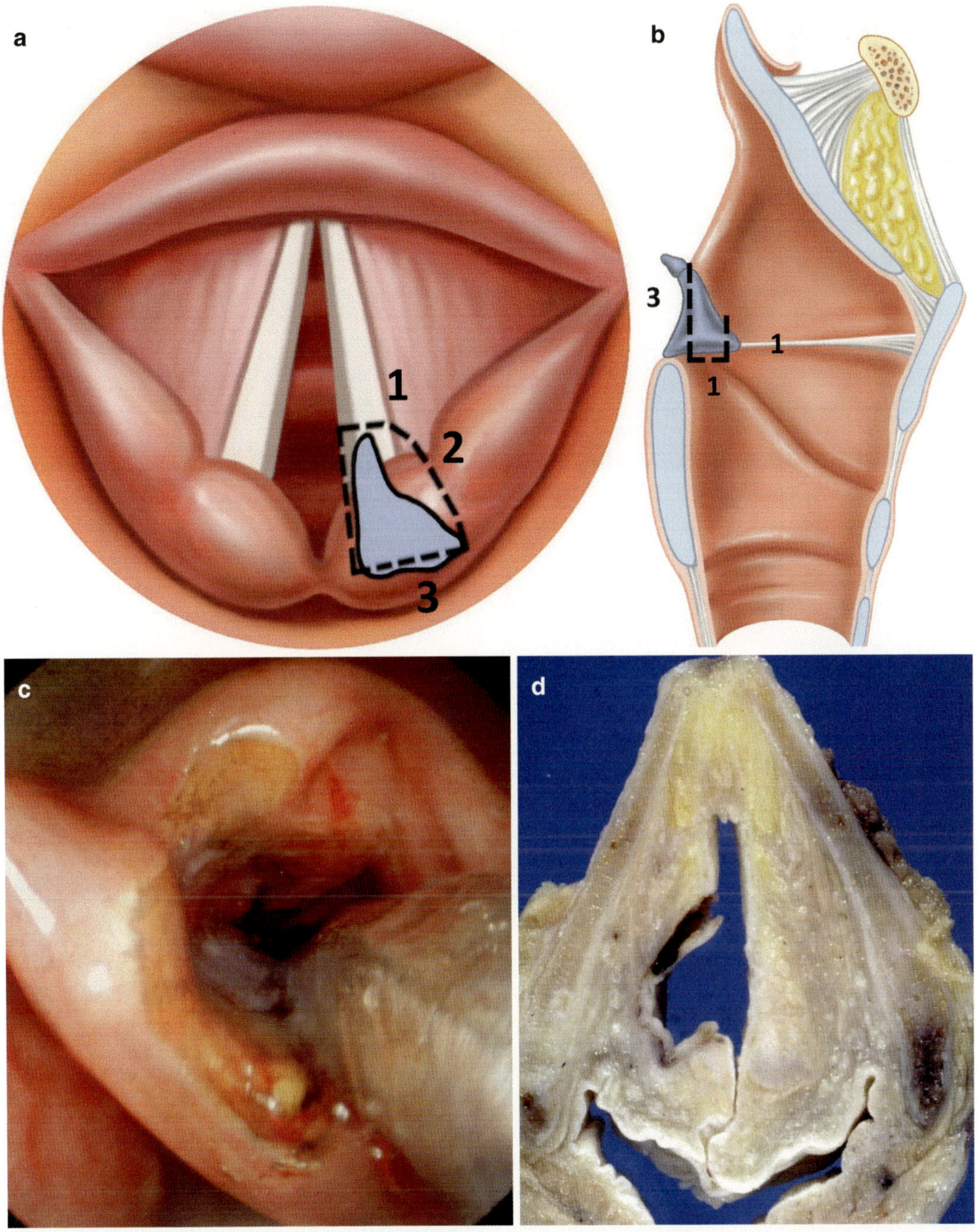

Fig. 13.1 (**a**–**d** clockwise from *top left*). (**a**—superior view, **b**—sagittal view) Limits of subtotal arytenoidectomy. (1) Section of vocal process from membranous part of vocal fold. (2) Section of posterior part of ventricular fold. (3) Section of arytenoid cartilage with preservation of posterior shell. (4) Split between arytenoid and cricoid cartilage. (**c**) Intraoperative view. (**d**) Cadaveric view

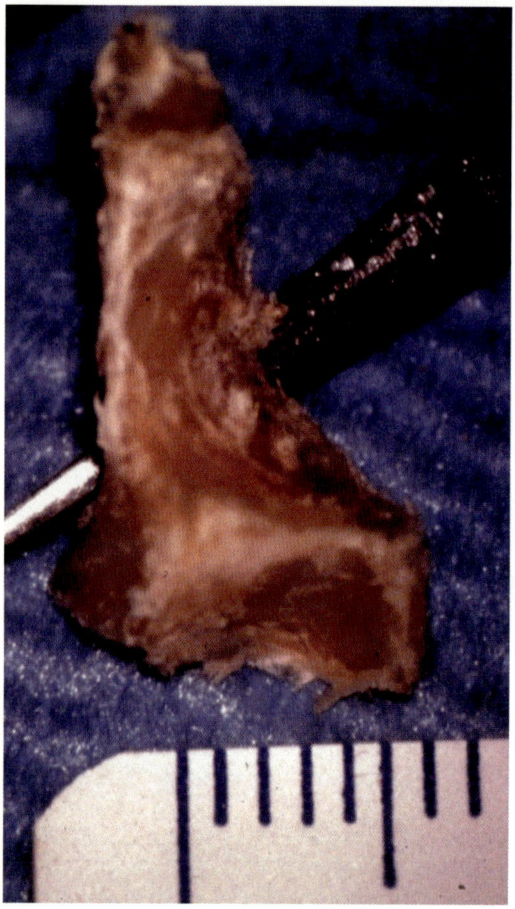

Fig. 13.2 Excised arytenoid from subtotal arytenoidectomy

13.6.8 Reinnervation (for More Details See Chap. 15)

Resection and lateralisation techniques cannot restore activity in the immobile cord which, if possible, could restore complete laryngeal motor function, assuming that the RLNs are involved alone without sensory loss (supplied by the SLN's internal branch). Various procedures have been described in the past including Tucker's nerve muscle pedicle (NMP) technique. In this procedure the branch of the ansa hypoglossi to the anterior belly of the omohyoid (or sternothyroid) is mobilised, and a small block of muscle containing the terminal branches is freed from the muscle proper. Thereafter, the PCA is exposed and the muscle fibres partially cut. The NMP is then sutured to it. Although Tucker and some others did report success with this procedure [56, 57], others have found it to be less than satisfactory [58–61].

Table 13.2 Patients for whom preoperative and post-operative respiratory function values were available

Patient	Preoperative values PEF/PIF ratio	Post-operative values PEF/PIF ratio
1	1.52	1.39
2	1.01	0.77
3	2.22	1.27
4	1.35	1.59
5	1.35	1.23
6	1.00	1.34
7	2.67	1.89
8	1.47	1.45
9	0.54	0.7
10	1.30	1.49
11	2.38	1.89
12	1.14	0.93
13	4.00	1.89
14	5.00	1.00
15	4.76	2.70
16	2.22	1.20

Crumley described a separate procedure involving reinnervation by early anastomosis of the phrenic nerve to the RLN [62]. Others have tried selective anastomosis of the phrenic directly into the PCA muscle or to the nerve to the PCA and so forth. Varying reports of success are described [63, 64].

Laryngeal pacing (cf Chap. 14), introduced by Bergman [65] involving direct electrical stimulation of the PCA muscle using an implantable device in the neck, has shown some success in recent years [66, 67]. Future developments may involve a combination of reinnervation with pacing and further the area of functional laryngeal transplantation (cf Chap. 16) [64].

Conclusion

BVFI remains a challenging condition with a variety of factors to consider prior to making a decision on the appropriate management for each individual patient. A thorough history and clinical examination with the appropriate diagnostic tests should be performed. In cases where a neurogenic cause is unlikely, an EMG and mobilisation of the arytenoid cartilage should be undertaken to confirm the exact nature of the BVFI. Tracheotomy remains a safe and if necessary reversible procedure to safeguard the airway. Lichtenberger's temporary lateral fixation and its variants are an alternative to tracheotomy. Glottis-enlarging surgery such as subtotal arytenoidectomy should be considered in permanent BVFI as a definitive procedure to ameliorate the respiratory issues with minimal effects on voice and laryngeal competence and avoidance of a tracheotomy. Laryngeal nerve reinnervation and pacing are other options with varying degrees of success and should be considered as treatment options for the future.

References

1. Feehery JM, Pribitkin EA, Heffelfinger RN, Lacombe VG, Lee D, Lowry LD, Keane WM, Sataloff RT. The evolving etiology of bilateral vocal fold immobility. J Voice. 2003;17(1):76–81.
2. Benninger MS, Gillen JB, Altaian JS. Changing etiology of vocal fold immobility. Laryngoscope. 1998;108(9):1346–50.
3. Kleinsasser O, Nolte E. Report on the indication, technique and functional results of endolaryngeal arytenoidectomy and submucous partial chordectomy in bilateral paralysis of vocal cord (author's transl). Laryngo-Rhino-Otologie. 1981;60(8):397–401.
4. Leon X, Venegas MP, Orús C, Quer M, Maranillo E, Sañudo JR. Glottic immobility: retrospective study of 229 cases. Acta Otorrinolaringol Esp. 2000;52(6):486–92.
5. Sessions DG, Ogura JH, Heeneman H. Surgical management of bilateral vocal cord paralysis. Laryngoscope. 1976;86(4):559–66.
6. Barach AL. The use of helium in the treatment of asthma and obstructive lesions in the larynx and trachea. Ann Intern Med. 1935;9(6):739–65.
7. Plouin-Gaudon I, Lawson G, Jamart J, Remacle M. Subtotal carbon dioxide laser arytenoidectomy for the treatment of bilateral vocal fold immobility: long-term results. Ann Otol Rhinol Laryngol. 2005;114(2):115–21.
8. Woodman DG. A modification of the extralaryngeal approach to arytenoidectomy for bilateral abductor paralysis. Arch of Otol Head Neck Surg. 1946;43(1):63.
9. Thornell WC. Intralaryngeal approach for arytenoidectomy in bilateral abductor paralysis of the vocal cords: a preliminary report. Arch Otolaryngol. 1948;47(4):505–8.
10. Kleinsasser O. Endolaryngeale Arytenoidektomie und submuköse Hemichordektomie zur Erweiterung der Glottis bei bilateraler Abduktorenparese. Msch Ohr Laryngorhinol. 1968;102:443–6.
11. Eckel HE, Sittel C. Morphometric studies at the level of the glottis as a principle in larynx enlarging microlaryngoscopic surgical procedures in bilateral recurrent nerve paralysis. Laryngo-Rhino-Otologie. 1994;73(8):417–22.
12. Eckel HE, Vössing M. Endolaryngeal surgical procedures in glottis expansion in bilateral recurrent nerve paralysis. Laryngorhinootologie. 1996;75(4):215–22.
13. Wassermann K, Gitt A, Weyde J, Eckel HE. Lung function changes and exercise-induced ventilatory responses to external resistive loads in normal subjects. Respiration. 1995;62(4):177–84.
14. Wassermann K, Koch A, Warschkow A, Mathen F, Müller-Ehmsen J, Eckel HE. Measuring in situ central airway resistance in patients with laryngotracheal stenosis. Laryngoscope. 1999;109(9):1516–20.
15. Wassermann K, Eckel HE. Stenoses of the upper airways. Lung function, local resistance and load compensation. A review. HNO. 1999;47(11):947–56.
16. Woodson G. Arytenoid abduction: indications and limitations. Ann Otol Rhinol Laryngol. 2010;119(11):742–8.
17. Eckel HE, Lichtenberger G. Glottic airway stenosis. In: Surgery of larynx and trachea. Berlin Heidelberg: Springer; 2010. p. 125–35.
18. Eckel HE, Sittel C. Bilateral recurrent laryngeal nerve paralysis. HNO. 2001;49(3):166–79.
19. Carneiro-Pla D, Miller BS, Wilhelm SM, Milas M, Gauger PG, Cohen MS, Solorzano CC. Feasibility of surgeon-performed transcutaneous vocal cord ultrasonography in identifying vocal cord mobility: a multi-institutional experience. Surgery. 2014;156(6):1597–604.
20. Leitersdorfer S, Lichtenberger G, Bihari A, Kovacs I. Evaluation of the lung function test in reversible glottis-dilating operations. Eur Arch Otorhinolaryngol. 2005;262(4):289–93.
21. Leitersdorfer S, Lichtenberger G, Kovacs I. Assessment of the results of glottis-dilating operations using lung function tests. Eur Arch Otorhinolaryngol. 2002;259(2):57–9.
22. Weddell G, Feinstein B, Pattle RE. The electrical activity of voluntary muscle in man under normal and pathological conditions. Brain. 1944;67:178–257.
23. Rickert SM, Childs LF, Carey BT, Murry T, Sulica L. Laryngeal electromyography for prognosis of vocal fold palsy: a meta-analysis. Laryngoscope. 2012;122(1):158–61.
24. Sataloff RT, Praneetvatakul P, Heuer RJ, Hawkshaw MJ, Heman-Ackah YD, Schneider SM, Mandel S. Laryngeal electromyography: clinical application. J Voice. 2010;24(2):228–34.

25. Woodson G, Weiss T. Arytenoid abduction for dynamic rehabilitation of bilateral laryngeal paralysis. Ann Otol Rhinol Laryngol. 2007;116(7):483.
26. Lawson G. Tracheotomy. In: Surgery of larynx and trachea. Berlin Heidelberg: Springer; 2010. p. 159–69.
27. Sittel C, Stennert E, Thumfart WF, Dapunt U, Eckel HE. Prognostic value of laryngeal electromyography in vocal fold paralysis. Arch Otolaryngol Head Neck Surg. 2001;127(2):155–60.
28. Damm M, Eckel HE, Jungehülsing M, Roth B. Management of acute inflammatory childhood stridor. Otolaryngol Head Neck Surg. 1999;121(5):633–8.
29. Lippert BM. Laterofixation der Stimmlippe statt Tracheotomie bei akuter beidseitiger Stimmlippenparese. Dtsch Med Wochenschr. 2002;127:917–22.
30. Jatzko GR, Lisborg PH, Müller MG, Wette VM. Recurrent nerve palsy after thyroid operations--principal nerve identification and a literature review. Surgery. 1994;115(2):139–44.
31. Lichtenberger G. Reversible immediate and definitive lateralization of paralyzed vocal cords. Eur Arch Otorhinolaryngol. 1999;256(8):407–11.
32. Ejnell H, Mansson I, Bake B, Hallén O, Stenborg R, Lindstroum J. A simple operation for bilateral vocal cord paralysis. Laryngoscope. 1984;94(7):954–8.
33. Kirchner FR. Endoscopic lateralization of the vocal cord in abductor paralysis of the larynx. Laryngoscope. 1979;89(11):1779–83.
34. Oysu C, Sahin-Yilmaz A, Uslu C. Emergency endoscopic vocal cord lateralization as an alternative to tracheotomy for patients with bilateral abductor vocal cord paralysis. Eur Arch Otorhinolaryngol. 2012;269(12):2525–9.
35. Ezzat WF, Shehata M, Kamal I, Riad MA. Adjustable laterofixation of the vocal fold in bilateral vocal fold paralysis. Laryngoscope. 2010;120(4):731–3.
36. Dennis DP, Kashima H. Carbon dioxide laser posterior cordectomy for treatment of bilateral vocal cord paralysis. Ann Otol Rhinol Laryngol. 1989;98:930–4.
37. Kashima HK. Bilateral vocal fold motion impairment: pathophysiology and management by transverse cordotomy. Ann Otol Rhinol Laryngol. 1991;100(9 Pt 1):717–21.
38. Wassermann K, Mathen F, Eckel HE. Concurrent glottic and tracheal stenoses: restoration of airway continuity in end-stage malignant disease. Ann Otol Rhinol Laryngol. 2001;110(4):349–55.
39. Pia F, Pisani P, Aluffi P. CO2 laser posterior ventriculocordectomy for the treatment of bilateral vocal cord paralysis. Eur Arch Otorhinolaryngol. 1999;256(8):403–6.
40. Reker U, Rudert H. Die modifizierte posteriore Chordektomie nach Dennis und Kashima bei der Behandlung beidseitiger Rekurrensparesen. Laryngo Rhino Otologie. 1998;77(04):213–8.
41. Eckel HE, Thumfart M, Wassermann K, Vössing M, Thumfart WF. Cordectomy versus arytenoidectomy in the management of bilateral vocal cord paralysis. Ann Otol Rhinol Laryngol. 1994;103(11):852–7.
42. Hoover WB. Bilateral abductor paralysis: operative treatment by sub mucous resection of the vocal cords. Arch Otolaryngol. 1932;15(3):339–5.
43. Jackson C. Ventriculocordectomy: a new operation for the cure of goitrous paralytic laryngeal stenosis. Arch Surg. 1922;4(2):257.
44. Kelly JD. Surgical treatment of bilateral paralysis of the abductor muscles. Arch Otolaryngol. 1941;33(2):293–304.
45. Lore J. Suggested operative procedure for the relief of stenosis in double abductor paralysis: an anatomic study. Ann Otol Rhinol Laryngol. 1936;45(3):679–86.
46. Lore J Jr. An atlas of head and neck surgery. 3rd ed. Philadelphia: WB Saunders; 1988. p. 878–81.
47. Eskew JR, Bailey BJ. Laser arytenoidectomy for bilateral vocal cord paralysis. Otolaryngol Head Neck Surg. 1983;91(3):294–8.
48. Lim RY. Laser arytenoidectomy. Arch Otolaryngol. 1985;111(4):262–3.
49. Ossoff RH, Sisson GA, Moselle HI, Duncavage JA, Andrews PE, McMillan WG. Endoscopic laser arytenoidectomy for the treatment of bilateral vocal cord paralysis. Laryngoscope. 1984;94(10):1293–7.
50. Sato K, Umeno H, Nakashima T. Laser arytenoidectomy for bilateral median vocal fold fixation. Laryngoscope. 2001;111(1):168–71.
51. Remacle M, Lawson G, Mayne A, Jamart J. Subtotal carbon dioxide laser arytenoidectomy by endoscopic approach for treatment of bilateral cord immobility in adduction. Ann Otol Rhinol Laryngol. 1996;105(6):438–45.
52. Reidenbach MM. Anatomical bases of glottic widening surgery related to arytenoidectomy. Clin Anat. 1999;12(2):94–102.
53. Lichtenberger G. Laryngeal microsurgical laterofixation of paralyzed vocal cords using a new suture instrument. Laryngorhinootologie. 1989;68(12):678–82.
54. Lichtenberger G, Toohill RJ. Technique of endo-extralaryngeal suture lateralization for bilateral abductor vocal cord paralysis. Laryngoscope. 1997;107(9):1281–3.
55. Lichtenberger G, Toohill RJ. The endo-extralaryngeal needle carrier. Otolaryngol Head Neck Surg. 1991;105(5):755–6.
56. Tucker HM. Human laryngeal reinnervation. Laryngoscope. 1976;86(6):769–79.
57. Tucker HM. Human laryngeal reinnervation: long-term experience with the nerve-muscle pedicle technique. Laryngoscope. 1978;88(4):598–604.
58. Tucker HM, Harvey J, Ogura JH. Vocal cord remobilization in the canine larynx. Arch Otolaryngol. 1970;92(6):530–3.

59. Maniglia AJ, Dodds B, Sorensen K, Katirji MB, Rosenbaum ML. Newer technique of laryngeal reinnervation: superior laryngeal nerve (motor branch) as a driver of the posterior cricoarytenoid muscle. Ann Otol Rhinol Laryngol. 1989;98(11):907–9.
60. Tóth A, Szócs A, Harasztosi C, Matesz K, Pucsok K, Mikó I, Sziklai I. Intrinsic laryngeal muscle reinnervation with nerve-muscle pedicle. Otolaryngol Head Neck Surg. 2005;132(5):701–6.
61. Crumley RL. Experiments in laryngeal reinnervation. Laryngoscope. 1982;92(S30):1–27.
62. Crumley RL. Phrenic nerve graft for bilateral vocal cord paralysis. Laryngoscope. 1983;93(4):425–8.
63. Zheng H, Zhou S, Li Z, Chen S, Zhang S, Huang Y, Geng L. Reinnervation of the posterior cricoarytenoid muscle by the phrenic nerve for bilateral vocal cord paralysis in humans. Zhonghua Er Bi Yan Hou Ke Za Zhi. 2002;37(3):210–4.
64. Marie JP. Nerve reconstruction. In: Surgery of larynx and trachea. Berlin Heidelberg: Springer; 2010. p. 279–94.
65. Bergmann K, Gerhardt HJ, Warzel H, Eckhardt HU, Hopstock U, Hermann V. Long-term implantation of a system of electrical stimulation of paralyzed laryngeal muscles in dogs. Laryngoscope. 1988;98(4):455–9.
66. Obert PM, Young KA, Tobey DN. Use of direct posterior cricoarytenoid stimulation in laryngeal paralysis. Arch Otolaryngol. 1984;110(2):88–92.
67. Zealear DL, Rainey CL, Herzon GD, Netterville JL, Ossoff RH. Electrical pacing of the paralyzed human larynx. Ann Otol Rhinol Laryngol. 1996;105(9):689–93.

Laryngeal Pacing

14

Andreas H. Mueller

Abstract

Bilateral vocal fold paresis (BVFP) is a rare condition, potentially life-threatening when the associated airway obstruction symptoms are severe. The most frequent etiology is iatrogenic nerve lesion during thyroid gland surgery. Surgical glottic enlargement, even though associated with various degrees of voice impairment, still represents the golden therapeutic standard.

This chapter focuses on neurostimulation as potential alternative treatment strategy. Decades of clinical experience supported by the laryngeal electromyography (EMG) results have provided sound evidence that the majority of peripheral laryngeal nerve lesions do not cause paralysis with atrophy of the intrinsic laryngeal muscles. On the contrary they are generally associated with misdirected, mostly synkinetic reinnervation.

Basic research, including long-term results from animal trials, has shown that a synkinetically reinnervated larynx is the prerequisite for neuromuscular electrical stimulation (NMES). In general, the stimulation of terminal nerve branches near the target muscle can re-establish its original function. In the specific case of BFVP, stimulation of the posterior cricoarytenoid muscle (PCA) restores vocal fold abduction.

The concept of laryngeal pacing (LP) was introduced in the 1970s of the last century. The first proof of principle laryngeal pacing study in human evaluated the use of an implantable pulse generator (IPG) primarily designed for pain therapy. However, due to various technical problems, such as electrode corrosion, this early clinical research was referred back to animal trials after 2003.

A.H. Mueller
Department of Otorhinolaryngology/Plastic Surgery,
SRH Wald-Klinikum Gera, Strasse des Friedens 122,
Gera 07548, Germany
e-mail: andreas.mueller@srh.de

C. Sittel, O. Guntinas-Lichius (eds.), *Neurolaryngology*,
https://doi.org/10.1007/978-3-319-61724-4_14

On account of the technological advancements of the last decade, a new type of medical device for laryngeal pacing has been recently developed. With this device, electrode placement is done in a minimally invasive procedure, thus preventing the occurrence of the technical problems observed in earlier attempts. The first feasibility study in human with this new LP system has been recently published and showed promising results.

14.1 Bilateral Vocal Fold Paresis and Synkinetic Reinnervation

Bilateral recurrent laryngeal nerve (RLN) lesions cause loss of voluntary movement of both vocal folds. The most significant clinical symptom of bilateral vocal fold paresis (BVFP) is airway obstruction. Depending on the severity of the nerve damage, the consequence is either a neurapraxia, an axonotmesis or, in the case of nerve disruption, a neurotmesis. When the RLN has a minor lesion, recovery of the vocal fold mobility can be observed within the first 6–12 months. However, after severe nerve lesions the intrinsic laryngeal muscles may become atrophic and the vocal fold movement is completely inhibited (paralysis). More frequently in RLN lesions a pathological reinnervation of the laryngeal muscles occurs, that preserves a certain amount of muscular volume and tension, but does not lead to recovery of relevant voluntary vocal fold movement (paresis).

Critical clinical symptoms linked to pathologic reinnervation include unexpected voice improvement accompanied with exertion intolerance and stridor, beginning from 4 to 6 months upon BVFP onset. Laryngoscopy reveals a tightening and an almost median position of the fixed vocal folds at this time. Besides, it is possible that fasciculations of the vocal and false vocal folds occur, which negatively affects voice quality. Pathological reinnervation is characterized by axonal sprouting entering the wrong terminal branches of the RLN. These sprouting axons can either be aberrant axons of neighboring nerves (n. laryngeus superior, ansa cervicalis, n. glossopharyngeus) or antagonistic axons of the RLN stem, originally responsible for the opposite movement of the vocal folds (see Fig. 14.1).

This phenomenon, known from facial nerve paresis, causing an autoparalytic reinnervation (synchronous activation of agonist and

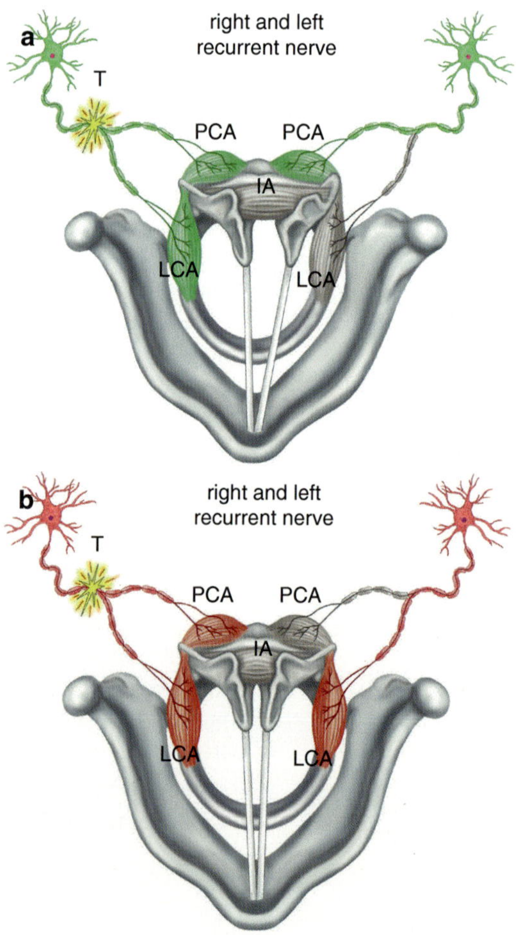

Fig. 14.1 (**a**) Synkinetic Reinnervation right side. Abduction inhibition right side (*green marked RLN*) because of co-stimulation of the PCA and LCA muscles, due to sprouting of abductor axons into adductor RLN fibers after trauma (T). (**b**) Adduction inhibition right side (*red marked RLN*) because of co-stimulation of the LCA and PCA muscles, due to sprouting of adductor axons into abductor RLN fibers after trauma (T)

antagonist muscles), is called "laryngeal synkinesis" and was described for the first time by Crumley in 1982 [1, 2]. Crumley distinguished four types of laryngeal synkinesis [3]. *Type I* does not involve any relevant symptoms concerning the respiration or the voice quality in case of a unilateral paresis (UVFP) because the vocal folds muscles are well preserved, allowing an appropriate closure of the glottal gap during phonation. In the event of bilateral vocal fold paresis (BVFP), voice quality is generally unaffected and due to residual vocal fold mobility, the respiratory function is restricted only during physical exertion, but not at rest. *Type II* synkinesis is characterized by involuntary vocal fold jerks, twitches, or jumps. It is dominated by moderate-to-severe adductor spasmodic-like dysphonia with unpredictable changes in the voice quality. In case of bilateral paralysis, respiration is affected at times. In particular, patients may experience short-term dyspnea caused by minimal saliva aspiration. In *type III* synkinesis, the adductor rather than the abductor reinnervation is predominant, in particular in regards to the m. cricoarytenoideus lateralis (LCA). As a result the vocal fold assumes a tight, almost median position and loses any relevant residual mobility. This can cause respiratory problems even in unilateral paralyses. If there is a BVFP with this type of synkinesis, a tracheotomy or an early glottis enlargement is often necessary. Voice quality is generally only slightly hampered or nearly unaffected. In contrast to type III, *type IV* synkinesis displays a predominance of reinnervated abductor muscles with vocal folds immobilized in a more lateral position. In this case respiration is only slightly affected, but voice quality is strongly impaired.

High-grade nerve lesions accompanied by foreseeable wrong reinnervation may be predicted via larynx-EMG (LEMG), a diagnostic tool that may also offer a suitable assistance for timing of the patient's therapy. Patients with BVFP should also receive speech-language therapy, which should help limit compensatory supraglottic constriction and adapting the breathing technique to that of a stenotic airway [4].

At present, basic research is being undertaken to investigate to what extent the process of reinnervation and the level of synkinesis can be influenced therapeutically. Animal models (rats) have shown that wrapping of RLN-anastomoses with olfactory ensheathing cells, expressing trophic and nerve growth factors, induce an improved synchronization to the respiratory rhythm of the laryngeal muscles after reinnervation [5]. Stem cells derived from bone marrow failed to improve facial nerve reinnervation. Further basic research in animal models is exploring whether continuous electrical stimulation during the reinnervation process could improve the reinnervation of the laryngeal muscles [6, 7]. Hydman first examined the impact of the regeneration-promoting agent nimodipine on reinnervation and neuromuscular function following RLN crush injury [8]. Recent clinical trials showed that through the systemic administration of nimodipine it was possible to achieve a tripled vocal fold motion recovery rate in patients with an acute RLN paresis, in contrast to the untreated reinnervation [9].

14.2 Neurostimulation

In the 1950s and 1960s of the last century researchers made several attempts [10, 11] to inhibit atrophies in denervated muscles by means of therapies based on transcutaneous electrical stimulation. More than 60 years later, there is no clear evidence to confirm that electrostimulation therapy of denervated muscles is truly able to prevent fibrosis and maintain muscle flexibility after peripheral nerve paralysis. This is also the recent status in pareses with a high chance of spontaneous recovery, like in Bell's facial nerve paresis [12]. The possible effects of the electrostimulation therapy are regarded as depending on the frequency range of the electric currents. For instance, frequencies above 100 kHz have no stimulation effects. They are used to warm up the tissue in thermotherapy. In low frequency ranges, up to 1 kHz, a single pulse with sufficient intensity and duration can generate muscle contraction. The current intensities, required to generate a contraction, may cause skin irritations, pain, and an undesired current spreading to other muscles [13]. In the future, optogenetic stimulation could be an alternative to selective muscle stimulation. An experiment with transgenic mice has shown that vocal fold abduction could be induced via optical stimulation [14]. However, in this case, the stimulation is effective only if, along with a direct contact between the optical fibers and the muscle, a specific gene mutation of the muscle fibers is present or induced. These requirements make the clinical application of such a therapy a distant prospect.

For muscles underwent reinnervation during the course of disease, indirect muscle stimulation known as *neuromuscular electrical stimulation (NMES)* may be applied. Since this method is based on nerve rather than muscle stimulation, a 10- to 100-fold lower stimulation intensity is needed than that used for direct muscle stimulation. In otolaryngology, NMES is used for surface stimulation with adhesive electrodes, for example in post-stroke dysphagia and unilateral vocal fold paresis [15]. If NMES is combined with voluntary activity, a strengthening of the weakened muscle tissue seems to be achievable [16]. According to Ptok [17] and Garcia Perez [18], at least in UVFP patients, voice therapy combined with NMES has a higher rate of success than voice therapy alone. Sometimes patients may report that there is a carry-over effect of voice improvement after NMES therapy. However, there is still a lack of knowledge regarding the adaptive mechanisms in cortical connectivity after peripheral nerve stimulation, that enhances the recovery of some amount of voluntary vocal fold movement [19]. In general, neuromuscular stimulation is based on the delivery of peripheral electrical stimuli. Transcranial magnetic stimulation (TMS) may be an alternative, but within a very limited range of indications. To our knowledge TMS is exclusively used for diagnostic purposes [20].

14.3 Early Attempts of Laryngeal Pacing

In 1977 Zealear and Dedo introduced the concept of using electrical stimulation to restore the function of unilaterally paralyzed laryngeal muscles. They used a canine model [21], in which the cricothyroid muscle was electrically stimulated on one side. The stimulation was paced by the activation of the cricothyroid muscle on the other side.

Bergmann et al. implanted electrodes into artificially paralyzed posterior cricoarytenoid muscles (PCA) in guinea pigs, rabbits, and dogs. In all these cases, the stimulation was paced by the respiratory rhythm, detected by means of a chest belt sensor [22]. The stimulation system was chronically implanted and was found stable in 4/6 dogs for a post-implantation follow-up period of 3–11 months. In 2/6 cases over the same follow-up period, the cables broke [23].

Obert et al. showed in a canine model that it is possible to completely restore abduction in bilaterally denervated PCAs by means of unilateral implantation of a bipolar single-stranded Teflon electrode [24]. Otto et al. implanted electrodes into the artificially paralyzed PCA in a canine model and used the EMG signal of the diaphragm muscle in order to use inspiratory diaphragm contraction as stimulation trigger [25].

Zrunek et al. used a sheep model to show that long-term low-frequency direct electrical stimulation of chronically denervated PCA muscles causes a switch of the muscle fibers from type-2 (fast) to type-1 (slow) [26].

Kano and Sasaki developed a canine model in which they used a pair of platinum-tungsten coiled electrodes. The experiment was specifically designed to evaluate the biphasic stimulation of the PCA abduction. They inserted the electrode pair at a distance of 2 mm from each other and delivered biphasic, short pulse duration (2 msec) stimuli to induce PCA abduction. One of the aims of this trial was to determine the effects of the electrode material and of the stimulation parameters on the reduction of electrical charge accumulation on the electrode and consequent risks of corrosion [27].

Sanders systematically evaluated the belly structure of the canine PCA, the abduction effect of different stimulation parameters, and the effects that the electrode insertion site and orientation in respect to the PCA fibers have on the stimulation. He also evaluated the histopathologic changes after long-term stimulation [28].

What we can learn from these animal studies is that residual or recovering reinnervation of the PCA is preferable to a complete denervation in terms of laryngeal pacing. If these results turn out to be reproducible and transferrable into clinical practice, selective neurostimulation of the PCA abductor branches might be considered as the future of laryngeal pacing. The surgical procedure used to place the electrode, the electrode design, the stimulation parameters, and the characteristics of the stimulator shall be carefully adapted to this condition. In the best case, the laryngeal pacing devices should be able to synchronize the PCA stimulation with inspiration.

In 1989 Bergmann received a positive vote from the relevant ethics committee in East Germany for the first clinical trial aiming to evaluate laryngeal pacing in human. However, he did not enroll any patients because he was highly concerned about the long-term stability of the implant and because of the ongoing political changes in Germany at that time [29]. Thus, the first clinical trial was started in 1995 by Zealear in cooperation with an international team, on tracheotomized patients who suffered from BVFP, using a preexisting implantable pulse generator (Itrel II, Medtronic Inc.) with 3- or 4-channel spinal cord electrodes [30]. This proof of principle trial was the first clinical investigation to evaluate the performance of laryngeal pacing in BVFP patients. However, this preliminary study showed issues with the adopted system, e.g. electrode corrosion, and was not followed by further developments of the system or larger cohort studies.

In contrast, innovative technologies are now available that may support a more efficacious implementation of laryngeal pacing. This increases the interest of the scientific and medical community for the potential clinical applications of laryngeal pacing.

14.4 New Laryngeal Pacing Concepts

Three insights from numerous anatomical and clinical studies concerning the innervation patterns of the intrinsic larynx muscles have to be considered.

First, there is a great variability of the natural RLN branching. Between 1 and 6 terminal branches of the RLN innervate the PCA with an asymmetric pattern when the left and the right side are compared. The innervating branches of the RLN enter the PCA with different orientations and through different layers [31].

Second, the anatomic variability and prevalence of intralaryngeal nerve anastomosis (Galen's) between the superior and recurrent laryngeal nerve and their clinical impact are not finally defined. These inconstant neural connection patterns seem to be responsible for the remaining innervation of the laryngeal muscles after RLN lesions, a finding supported by the variability of LEMG results and vocal fold positions [32].

Third, the typical synkinetic reinnervation patterns after RLN lesions have a main impact on newer laryngeal pacing concepts. In cases of BVFP with relevant vocal fold motion impairment, the PCA muscles are mainly reinnervated, but the established reinnervation is generally only partial and misdirected, often synkinetic. Thus, the vocal fold abduction is strongly impaired and asynchronic with respect to the respiration cycle, particularly because of the typical and aberrant reinnervation of abductor axons into adductor muscle fibers. It is important to note, however, that although aberrant, this type of reinnervation still enables the reinnervated muscle fibers to respond to neurostimulation.

Because BVFP is the most suitable indication for such investigational therapy, the stimulation of the terminal abductor branches of the RLN has become one of the most promising targets for laryngeal pacing. In summary, it can be assumed that due to the variability of RLN branching, intralaryngeal neural connection patterns and synkinetic reinnervation status, the position of the spots with the best response to the stimulation may differ in individual PCAs. Accordingly, when Zealear et al. mapped the total surface of chronically denervated/reinnervated canine PCA muscles with plane array multi-electrodes, they were able to identify surface spots located in the lower medial quadrant of the central region of the PCA, that, when electrically stimulated, triggered an effective abduction. The said spots are known as "hot-spots" and their distribution pattern varies from PCA to PCA [33].

In all cases, it is necessary to consider the medical procedure that is used to expose the PCA for electrode implantation. For instance, the use of open surgery may increase the risk of laryngeal immobility following scar formation. Another challenge is the electrode anchoring into the PCA and the mechanical stress on the electrode due to head and neck movement. In this regard, our animal studies showed that there is a risk of electrode dislocation depending on the procedure used to position and anchor the electrode into the PCA. Current research focuses on minimally invasive procedures for the PCA hot-spot detection and consequent electrode placement [34]. In particular, the design of the stimulation electrode should consider the effects of current distribution, electrical charge accumulation, and potential electrode corrosion in order to avoid the occurrence of the same problems observed by Zealear [30]. Furthermore, the design of the stimulator should consider the need of delivering biphasic stimulation with amplitudes, pulse length, and frequencies that support the most efficient nerve stimulation in a pathologically reinnervated PCA, potentially showing a high rate of synkinesis. Ideally, the stimulator should permit the modulation of the stimulation parameters based on the individual needs of each patient and synchronization with the respiratory cycle.

14.5 Candidates for Laryngeal Pacing

The perspective clinical use of laryngeal pacing should preferably be considered when the target PCA reinnervation, particularly favorable synkinetic reinnervation, is established and no vocal fold movement recovery occurred [35]. However, in principle, laryngeal pacing can also be used in patients who have been suffering from BVFP for more than a decade. BVFP patients who underwent a previous surgical glottis enlargement but nonetheless are unable to sustain their physical activities are potentially suitable candidates for laryngeal pacing as long as at least one vocal fold isn't impaired in its mobility. The selection of potential candidates for laryngeal pacing in BVFP shall require the documented evidence that at least one PCA is able to respond to selective neuromuscular stimulation with vocal fold abduction. The application of laryngeal pacing should not be considered in patients suffering from pathologies that impair larynx functionality not related to the BVFP onset, such as ankylosis of the cricoarytenoid joint, tumor infiltration of the vocal fold or extensive scar formations. In the same way, laryngeal pacing is not considered suitable for the therapy of subjects suffering from respiratory problems caused by pharyngeal obstruction, laryngotracheal stenosis, asthma, pulmonary or heart failure or underlying neurologic diseases.

Future applications of a laryngeal pacemaker systems may include the implantation of such a system early upon onset of BVFP, after microsurgical selective reinnervation [36] of the larynx in BVFP or after larynx transplantation (please see Chap. 15) [37]. The aim of such an early implantation could be the transient relief from respiratory symptoms, avoiding the otherwise necessary tracheostomy, until either the spontaneous recovery of at least one vocal fold occurs or a definitive treatment can be performed. In these cases, it is important to remember that BVFP onset correlates with a gradual denervation that, in the first weeks following the paresis, is associated with a shift of the current threshold required to efficaciously stimulate the PCA towards the range used for muscle rather than nerve stimulation. This may increase the risks related to current spreading. In this indication the laryngeal pacing device would be a life support system like a heart pacemaker in complete A-V block with all the associated device failure risks.

The hypothesis that continuous electric stimulation of the PCA during reinnervation may enhance selective reinnervation [6] would support an early application of laryngeal pacing, but there is still no clear evidence from the basic research results.

Even considering the costs and the patient's dependence of an active medical implant in laryngeal pacing, such technology should still be preferred to other destructive therapies because of its reversibility and its expected lack of negative effects locally on the functionality of the intrinsic laryngeal muscles, the cricoarytenoid joint (CAJ), and in general on the overall laryngeal nerve and muscle network. However such aims can be achieved only by the implementation of minimally invasive electrode insertion technology.

Another potential target for laryngeal pacing is evoked vocal fold adduction. This application of laryngeal pacing may be a valid alternative to the current treatment options for selected unilateral vocal fold paresis (UVFP) patients, such as voice professionals [38]. This application would be of particular interest in treating UVFP with type IV synkinesis (lateral vocal fold position), for which the type I thyroplasty is not a valid solution and the arytenoid-adduction is associated with vocal fold muscle atrophy, due to potential RLN dissection.

14.6 Neurolaryngologic Diagnostics

Laryngo(strobo)scopy is today considered the gold standard of diagnostics for laryngological diseases. Nonetheless, electrophysiological examinations have become more and more important whenever the extent of laryngeal muscle denervation/reinnervation is expected to affect the therapeutic decision. In this context, laryngeal EMG (LEMG) is the most common tool to determine if the impairment of the vocal fold movements observed via laryngoscopy is caused by a paresis and, if so, whether the paresis involves either the RLN or the whole vagal nerve.

In short, the number of motor unit action potentials during volitional activity, the so-called recruitment pattern, reflects the denervation or reinnervation status of the relevant laryngeal muscles. Strongly decreased or single fiber recruitment patterns are associated with reduced strength of voluntary muscle contraction.

While the predictive value of LEMG in prognosticating the regeneration of the abductor fibers is low (60%), its predictive value for poor prognosis of nerve regeneration is close to 100% (97%), particularly when it is based on the results of multiple examinations [39]. The predictive value of LEMG for poor prognosis may help the surgeon make the best therapeutic decisions for the patients in the early stages of the BVFP.

The LEMG is able to discriminate between synkinetic reinnervation of abductors and adductors muscles. For instance, increased EMG recruitment patterns of the LCA during sniffing or of the PCA during phonation are typical signs of synkinetic reinnervation.

Unlike LEMG, electrical PCA test stimulation is a relatively new type of neurolaryngologic diagnostic method. This type of diagnosis is performed in TIVA in absence of muscle relaxants and by means of standard neuromonitoring devices with stimulation channels, similar to those used for RLN or facial nerve stimulation during thyroid or parotid gland surgery. The stimulation can be delivered into the PCA either with surface or with needle electrodes. In the former case, transmucosal surface stimulation of the PCA is applied and monitored via laryngoscopy. In short, a standard diagnostic catheter, similar to those used for intracardiac sensing or heart stimulation, is connected to the stimulation channel of the external neuromonitoring device, which delivers the current, until clear vocal fold abduction is seen. In the latter case, a bipolar electrode is positioned in the PCA in the same way as for LEMG (see Fig. 14.2). Compared

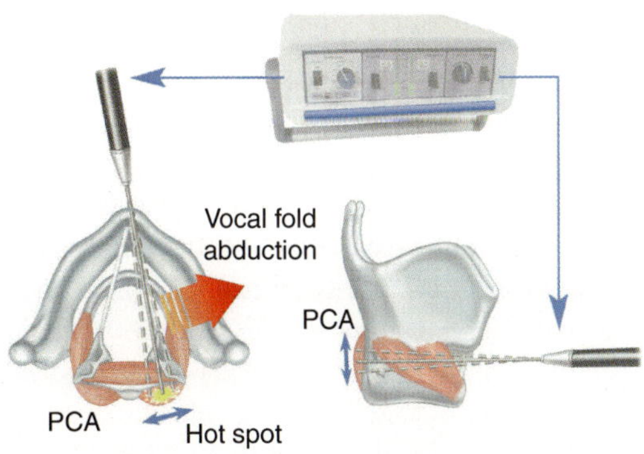

Fig. 14.2 Electrical Needle PCA Test Stimulation

with surface stimulation, the use of needle electrodes requires lower amplitudes to induce clear vocal fold abduction, because of the closer contact between the electrode tip and the nerve branches. The transluminal approach via the cricothyroid ligament eases the change of the needle tip position during the searching for a hot-spot (point with best abduction). The use of needle electrodes can also be performed in awake patients or in local anesthesia, but in this case the results are of lower quality than those performed in TIVA and often accompanied by drawbacks such as discomfort and repeated cough urge, especially when the needle electrode is moved in order to find the hot-spot. The use of needle electrode stimulation of the PCA in TIVA gives particularly good results when the anesthesia is administered via a larynx mask. Laryngoscopic monitoring performed during PCA test stimulation helps to identify the relevant hot-spots on the PCA for later electrode insertion and to decide whether their stimulation induces a selective abduction or rather unwished combined responses such as anterior adduction of the vocal fold with posterior abduction of the vocal process.

Positive stimulation results would make the subject a potentially promising candidate for laryngeal pacing.

An interesting spin-off of this kind of laryngeal surface or needle test stimulation is that the induced vocal fold motion is a good indicator of the cricoarytenoid joint (CAJ) mobility. In this context, this type of diagnosis is more sensitive than standard palpation methods during suspension laryngoscopy.

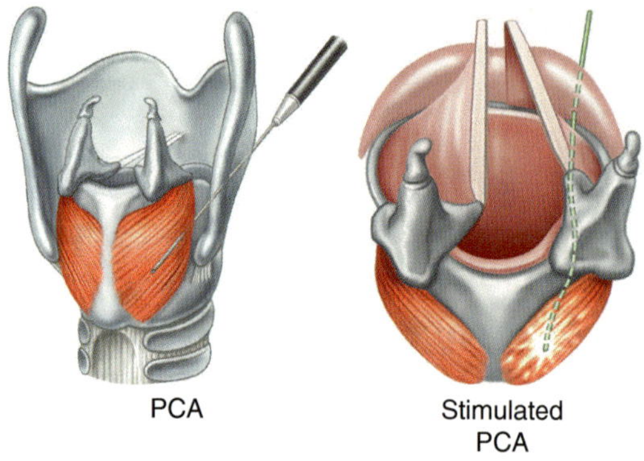

Fig. 14.3 Minimal invasive PCA-stimulation electrode insertion

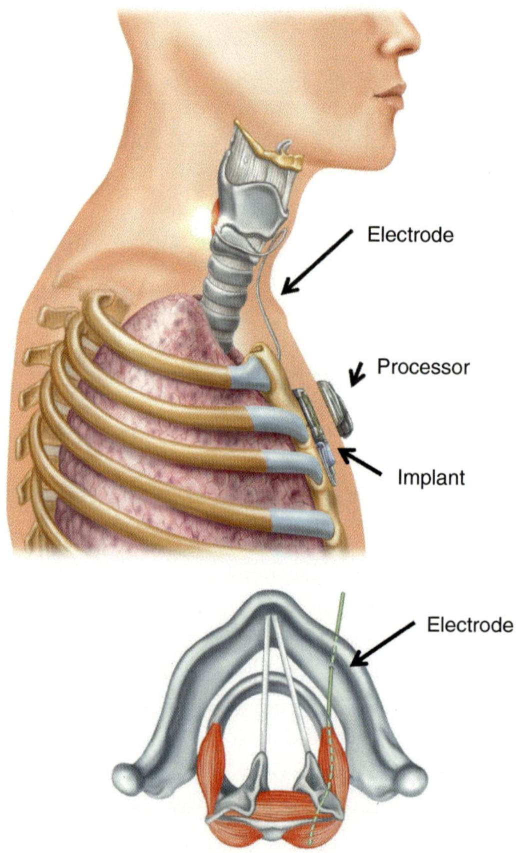

Fig. 14.4 Laryngeal pacemaker system (MED-EL)

14.7 Clinical Studies and Potential Benefits for Patients

In the context of laryngeal pacing, our group has been involved in the development of a new Laryngeal Pacemaker (LP) System for the treatment of BVFP (see Fig. 14.3). Pre-clinical research was completed in cooperation with a center in Germany and one in Austria. Medical Electronics (MED-EL), Innsbruck, Austria, sponsored the research. The medical procedure has been designed to ensure that no irreversible tissue damage is done, contrarily to what happens in the most cases of surgical glottis enlargement (see Fig. 14.4). Thus the stimulation electrode of this LP System can be implanted and removed in a minimally invasive procedure [34, 40]. The reversibility of the LP System implantation ensures that, in case of lack of benefit, the patient can be explanted and treated with an alternative therapy without conflict.

The LP System was evaluated for the first time in human in a feasibility study conducted between 2012 and 2014, which included the above mentioned three centers. The study was approved by the relevant Ethics Committees and National Competent Authorities and involved nine subjects.

The study included a post-implantation follow-up of 6 months. 8/9 subjects were unilaterally implanted with the LP System. In one subject it was not possible to implant the LP electrode in a sufficiently stable way. 7/9 subjects completed the follow-up period of the study. One subject became pregnant and thus was withdrawn from the study.

The study evaluated the effects of the LP System in terms of safety and patient's quality of life, in addition to the impact of the LP System on the respiratory function, voice quality, and capability to sustain physical activity. The results of the study have been recently published [41]. In short, the LP System implantation and its therapeutic effect was very positively received by all the subjects enrolled in the study, including those with long-term BVFP of iatrogenic origin, who had refused any other surgical treatment. Accordingly, the adherence of the subjects to the study provisions and the instruction for the handling of the LP System at home was excellent.

In 2/9 subjects who were tracheotomized before, it was possible to close it within 6 months after the LP implantation.

In terms of respiratory function, the values of both the peak expiratory and inspiratory flow increased significantly within 14 days after the implantation of the LP System, reaching values comparable to those observed in cases of surgical glottis enlargement [42]. In addition, it is important to note that unlike the results with the LP System, the results of the glottis enlargement are expected to show an improvement starting at least 3 months after the surgery, with intended scar formation. In the same way, results with the selective reinnervation with initial complete RLN transection showed that an improvement could be seen starting from 6–9 months post-treatment (please see Chap. 15).

The subjects enrolled in the LP System study did not show any post-implantation swallowing problems at all and, according to the SF-36, they showed an improvement of the mental component and no worsening in the other SF-36 domains or in the patient's benefit, as measured with the Glasgow Benefit Inventory (GBI). However, due to the minimal sample size, the results are not yet confirmatory.

A potentially significant advantage of the LP System to the standard surgical glottis enlargement is the preservation of the voice quality. Indeed, it is well known that in standard surgical glottis enlargement a balance has to be found between improved respiratory function and loss of voice quality. In our modern world, where communication is of paramount importance, the loss in voice quality may have a severe impact on patient's social and working life [43]. Thus, generally the attempt to achieve minimal voice quality loss in surgical glottis enlargement necessitates a series of revision surgeries due to the minimal gain in the respiratory voice obtained with the first surgery [44].

In this context, the LP System may become a promising alternative. As shown in the study described above, the LP System is able to stimulate the abduction of the vocal fold at the implanted side, without disturbing the work of the adductor muscles that were shown to be able to override the stimulated PCA abduction during phonation and swallowing. The analysis of the voice handicap index (VHI-12) in the aforementioned study showed that at baseline (pre-implantation situation) subjects suffered from a moderately disturbed voice quality. Such situation is explained by the fact that 4/7 subjects of this study had undergone unilateral glottis enlargement before LP System implantation. The study confirmed that voice quality was preserved for the entire duration of the follow-up [44, 45].

References

1. Crumley RL, McCabe BF. Regeneration of the recurrent laryngeal nerve. Otolaryngol Head Neck Surg. 1982;90:442–7.
2. Crumley RL. Laryngeal synkinesis: its significance to the laryngologist. Ann Otol Rhinol Laryngol. 1989;98:87–92.

3. Crumley RL. Laryngeal synkinesis revisited. Ann Otol Rhinol Laryngol. 2000;109:365–71.
4. Baker SE, Sapienza CM, Martin D, Davenport S, Hoffman-Ruddy B, Woodson G. Inspiratory pressure threshold training for upper airway limitation: a case of bilateral abductor vocal fold paralysis. J Voice. 2003;17:384–94.
5. de Corgnol AC, Guerout N, Duclos C, Verin E, Marie JP. Olfactory ensheathing cells in a rat model of laryngeal reinnervation. Ann Otol Rhinol Laryngol. 2011;120:273–80.
6. Zealear DL, Mainthia R, Li Y, et al. Stimulation of denervated muscle promotes selective reinnervation, prevents synkinesis, and restores function. Laryngoscope. 2014;124:E180–7.
7. Cheetham J, Perkins JD, Jarvis JC, et al. Effects of functional electrical stimulation on denervated laryngeal muscle in a large animal model. Artif Organs. 2015;39:876–85.
8. Hydman J, Remahl S, Bjorck G, Svensson M, Mattsson P. Nimodipine improves reinnervation and neuromuscular function after injury to the recurrent laryngeal nerve in the rat. Ann Otol Rhinol Laryngol. 2007;116:623–30.
9. Rosen CA, Smith L, Young V, Krishna P, Muldoon MF, Munin MC. Prospective investigation of nimodipine for acute vocal fold paralysis. Muscle Nerve. 2014;50:114–8.
10. Iakovleva I, Iliutovich GM, Iuvalova ND. On the use of sinusoidal low-frequency modulated currents in vocal disorders in patients with paralysis and paresis of the laryngeal muscles. Vestn Otorinolaringol. 1965;27:93–8.
11. Scarabicchi S. Isolated left diaphragmatic paresis; improvement after galvanic stimulation. Minerva Pediatr. 1952;4:1026–7.
12. Guntinas-Lichius O. Rehabilitation options for lesions of the facial nerve. HNO. 2007;55:605–12.
13. Kim Y, Zieber HG, Wang FE. Uniformity of current density under stimulating electrodes. Crit Rev. Biomed Eng. 1990;17:585–619.
14. Bruegmann T, van Bremen T, Vogt CC, Send T, Fleischmann BK, Sasse P. Optogenetic control of contractile function in skeletal muscle. Nat Commun. 2015;6:7153.
15. Miller S, Kuhn D, Jungheim M, Schwemmle C, Ptok M. Neuromuscular electric stimulation therapy in otorhinolaryngology. HNO. 2014;62:131–8. quiz 139-140
16. Low J, Reed A. Electrical stimulation of nerve and muscle. In: Low J, Reed A, editors. Electrotherapy explained: principles and practice. Oxford: Elsevier LTD; 2000. p. 53–140.
17. Ptok M, Strack D. Electrical stimulation-supported voice exercises are superior to voice exercise therapy alone in patients with unilateral recurrent laryngeal nerve paresis: results from a prospective, randomized clinical trial. Muscle Nerve. 2008;38:1005–11.
18. Garcia Perez A, Hernandez Lopez X, Valadez Jimenez VM, Minor Martinez A, Ysunza PA. Synchronous electrical stimulation of laryngeal muscles: an alternative for enhancing recovery of unilateral recurrent laryngeal nerve paralysis. J Voice. 2014;28:524 e521–7.
19. Rushton DN. Functional electrical stimulation and rehabilitation—an hypothesis. Med Eng Phys. 2003;25:75–8.
20. Urban PP. Transcranial magnetic stimulation in brainstem lesions and lesions of the cranial nerves. Suppl Clin Neurophysiol. 2003;56:341–57.
21. Zealear DL, Dedo HH. Control of paralysed axial muscles by electrical stimulation. Acta Otolaryngol. 1977;83:514–27.
22. Bergmann K, Warzel H, Eckhardt HU, Gerhardt HJ. Respiratory rhythmically regulated electrical stimulation of paralyzed laryngeal muscles. Laryngoscope. 1984;94:1376–80.
23. Bergmann K, Warzel H, Eckhardt HU, Hopstock U, Hermann V, Gerhardt HJ. Long-term implantation of a system of electrical stimulation of paralyzed laryngeal muscles in dogs. Laryngoscope. 1988;98:455–9.
24. Obert PM, Young KA, Tobey DN. Use of direct posterior cricoarytenoid stimulation in laryngeal paralysis. Arch Otolaryngol. 1984;110:88–92.
25. Otto RA, Templer J, Davis W, Homeyer D, Stroble M. Coordinated electrical pacing of vocal cord abductors in recurrent laryngeal nerve paralysis. Otolaryngol Head Neck Surg. 1985;93:634–8.
26. Zrunek M, Carraro U, Catani C, et al. Functional electrostimulation of the denervated posticus muscle in an animal experiment: histo- and biochemical results. Laryngo-Rhino-Otologie. 1986;65:621–7.
27. Kano S, Sasaki CT. Pacing parameters of the canine posterior cricoarytenoid muscle. Ann Otol Rhinol Laryngol. 1991;100:584–8.
28. Sanders I. Electrical stimulation of laryngeal muscle. Otolaryngol Clin N Am. 1991;24:1253–74.
29. Bergmann K. History of the laryngeal pacing in the GDR in the 80th. FSU Jena: Jena/Gera; 2015.
30. Zealear DL, Billante CR, Courey MS, et al. Reanimation of the paralyzed human larynx with an implantable electrical stimulation device. Laryngoscope. 2003;113:1149–56.
31. Maranillo E, Leon X, Ibanez M, Orus C, Quer M, Sanudo JR. Variability of the nerve supply patterns of the human posterior cricoarytenoid muscle. Laryngoscope. 2003;113:602–6.
32. Martin-Oviedo C, Maranillo E, Lowy-Benoliel A, et al. Functional role of human laryngeal nerve connections. Laryngoscope. 2011;121:2338–43.
33. Zealear DL, Rainey CL, Jerles ML, Tanabe T, Herzon GD. Technical approach for reanimation of the chronically denervated larynx by means of functional electrical stimulation. Ann Otol Rhinol Laryngol. 1994;103:705–12.

34. Foerster G, Arnold D, Bischoff SJ, Schubert H, Scholle HC, Mueller AH. Laryngeal pacing in minipigs: in vivo test of a new minimal invasive transcricoidal electrode insertion method for functional electrical stimulation of the PCA. Eur Arch Otorhinolaryngol. 2013;270:225–31.
35. Mueller AH, Blechschmidt K. Laryngeal pacing in RLNP. In: ELS, ed. 5th ELS Congress, 10. Lisboa, Portugal: ELS; 13 Jul 2004.
36. Marina MB, Marie JP, Birchall MA. Laryngeal reinnervation for bilateral vocal fold paralysis. Curr Opin Otolaryngol Head Neck Surg. 2011;19:434–8.
37. Farwell DG, Birchall MA, Macchiarini P, et al. Laryngotracheal transplantation: technical modifications and functional outcomes. Laryngoscope. 2013;123:2502–8.
38. Mueller AH, Foerster G. Who are suitable candidates for laryngeal pacing? In: 7th Congress of the European Laryngological Society. Barcelona, Spain: Eur Arch Otorhinolaryngol (2009), Springer; 2008. p. 586.
39. Grosheva M, Wittekindt C, Pototschnig C, Lindenthaler W, Guntinas-Lichius O. Evaluation of peripheral vocal cord paralysis by electromyography. Laryngoscope. 2008;118:987–90.
40. Foerster G, Arnold D, Bischoff S, Boltze K, Scholle HC, Schubert H, Mueller AH. Pre-clinical evaluation of a minimally invasive laryngeal pacemaker system in mini-pig. Eur Arch Otorhinolaryngol. 2016;273:151–8.
41. Mueller AH, Hagen R, Foerster G, Grossmann W, Baumbusch K, Pototschnig C. Laryngeal pacing via an implantable stimulator for the rehabilitation of subjects suffering from bilateral vocal fold paralysis: a prospective first-in-human study. Laryngoscope. 2016;126:1810–6.
42. Nawka T, Sittel C, Gugatschka M, Arens C, Lang-Roth R, Wittekindt C, Hagen R, Mueller AH, Volk GF, Guntinas-Lichius O. Permanent transoral surgery of bilateral vocal fold paralysis: a prospective multicenter trial. Laryngoscope. 2015;125:1401–8.
43. Nawka T, Sittel C, Arens C, Lang-Roth R, Wittekindt C, Hagen R, Nasr AI, Guntinas-Lichius O, Friedrich G, Gugatschka M. Voice and respiratory outcomes after permanent transoral surgery of bilateral vocal fold paralysis. Laryngoscope. 2015;125:2749–55.
44. Djugai S, Boeger D, Buentzel J, Esser D, Hoffmann K, Jecker P, Mueller AH, Radtke G, Bohne S, Finkensieper M, Volk GF, Guntinas-Lichius O. Chronic vocal cord palsy in Thuringia, Germany: a population-based study on epidemiology and outcome. Eur Arch Otorhinolaryngol. 2014;271:329–35.
45. Mueller AH, Hagen R, Pototschnig C et al. Laryngeal pacing for bilateral vocal fold paralysis: Voice and respiratory aspects. Laryngoscope. 2017;127:1838–1844.

Surgical Reinnervation

15

Jean-Paul Marie and Kate Heathcote

Abstract

Laryngeal reinnervation can be performed in the treatment of both unilateral and bilateral vocal cord palsy. Here we discuss the development, technical steps and clinical outcomes of these procedures.

In unilateral palsy, the aim of reinnervation is to increase tonicity of the hemilarynx. This is achieved by a straight-forward anastomosis of the recurrent laryngeal nerve to a branch of the ansa hypoglossi. This non-selective reinnervation acts to rebalance the laryngeal muscles, preventing muscular atrophy, and giving good long-term voice results.

In bilateral paralysis, the vocal cords are usually in a paramedian position. This results in inspiratory dyspnea. However, phonation is satisfactorily preserved in most cases.

Classical modes of treatment for bilateral vocal fold paralysis are aimed at enlarging the glottis which can result in variable hoarseness and inadequate protective closure. Laryngeal reinnervation can theoretically solve these problems. The posterior cricoarytenoid muscles are responsible for abduction of the vocal folds and thus are the main target of selective reinnervation.

The initial technique using a nerve muscle pedicle of a branch of the hypoglossal was disappointing with poor visible abduction. This has now been superseded by new techniques using phrenic nerve roots, anastomosed to the posterior cricoarytenoid branches of the recurrent laryngeal nerves, or moreover, implanted into both posterior cricoarytenoid muscles to

J.-P. Marie (✉)
Otorhinolaryngology, Head and Neck Surgery, University Hospital of Rouen, 1 rue de Germont, Rouen, Normandy 76000, France
e-mail: jean-paul.marie@chu-rouen.fr

K. Heathcote
Otolaryngology, Poole Hospital NHS Trust, Longfleet Road, Poole, Dorset BH15 2 JB, UK

C. Sittel, O. Guntinas-Lichius (eds.), *Neurolaryngology*, https://doi.org/10.1007/978-3-319-61724-4_15

induce neurotisation. Adductor muscle reinnervation can also be performed to improve closure of the larynx and avoid inappropriate synkinetic reinnervation.

Using these techniques, dyspnea is relieved in three out of four cases, without degradation of the voice. Bilateral active abduction on inspiration is observed in approximately one half of cases where there is no previous intralaryngeal scar.

15.1 Introduction

Vocal fold immobility of neurological origin is a common problem that may present in different manifestations depending on the site of the lesion, whether it is unilateral or bilateral and the degree of natural reinnervation at the time of presentation. It must also be considered that the clinical outcome will evolve over time with increasing muscle atrophy and prolapse of the arytenoid cartilages.

Consequently, the approach to treating this condition is far from straight-forward. To achieve the best outcome for the patient it is vital that a thorough assessment of the neurological, structural and functional state of the larynx is made as well as that of the patient in general.

The aim of surgical reinnervation is to improve laryngeal performance for the patient. In the case of unilateral palsy the issues are poor voice, weak cough and sometimes aspiration. In bilateral palsy the voice and cough are often preserved, but the airway is compromised.

Traditional approaches to unilateral palsy aim to reposition the paralysed vocal cord with a surgically inserted implant with or without arytenoid adduction or to increase its bulk with an injectable substance. With reinnervation the position and bulk of the vocal cord is improved by increasing the muscle tone of the hemilarynx.

In bilateral palsy the vocal cords are usually in the paramedian position. The aim of reinnervation is to achieve abduction of the vocal cords on inspiration whilst preserving voice. This restoration of mobility and tonicity is in contrast with traditional techniques, which prioritise the airway and enlarge the glottis at the expense of voice and cough.

There is a long history of reinnervation research in animal models but limited experience in humans. In this chapter we present the current state of clinical applications and outcomes. However, it must be noted that some of the techniques have not been used extensively and require comparison with passive techniques.

The neuroanatomy of the larynx has been extensively covered in other chapters but it is important to note that the intralaryngeal branch of the recurrent laryngeal nerve (RLN) to the posterior cricoarytenoid muscle (PCA) may be single or multiple, originating from the common branch to the adductor muscles. There is no topographical separation between the motor fibres to the adductors and those to the abductors in the main trunk of the RLN. The plexiform organisation of axons in the trunk explains the failure of direct nerve anastomosis to restore normal function as regenerating axons misdirected to antagonistic muscles (synkinesis).

As with other nerves, the RLN has a strong propensity to recover. Fully functional recovery may be expected in crush injuries where there is no disruption of the axons, but regrowth following interruption of the axons is likely to have a poorer outcome with synkinesis. Either of these situations may arise with iatrogenic lesions and careful clinical evaluation is required before making a decision on invasive procedures. Temporary techniques may be used for symptomatic improvement whilst observing the evolution of the lesion.

RLN nerve malfunction may be due to damage at any point from the emergence of the vagal nerve at the brainstem to the insertion of the RLN branches in the larynx. It may be unilateral or bilateral, solitary or combined with superior laryngeal nerve (SLN) or other cranial nerve pathologies. This will be reflected in the resting position of the paralysed vocal cord. For example, if the SLN is preserved the cord is likely to be held in the paramedian position, possibly due to unopposed activity of the cricothyroid muscle or reinnervation of the hemilarynx from the SLN. Effectively, the greater the residual or recovered nerve supply, the more trophic the hemilarynx and the more favourable the position of a unilateral, paralysed vocal cord allowing closure of the glottis on phonation [1]. This preservation (or recovery) of the viscoelasticity is required for optimum voice outcomes and is a strong justification for laryngeal reinnervation. In addition, reinnervation avoids disruption and scarring in the larynx, which is inevitable with traditional techniques and destroys the viscoelasticity.

The motor units of the adductor muscles are small with only 2–20 muscle fibres per motor unit and mainly fast contraction times. In contrast, the abductor muscle (PCA) has 200 to 250 fibres per unit and these have mainly slower contraction times. These characteristics are determined by the axonal supply and thus may change if the nerve supplying the muscle is changed. This is relevant in the choice of donor nerves for reinnervation.

Another feature that is important to appreciate in reinnervation surgery is that a muscle will only accept the donor nerve axons if it is not already adequately innervated. Thus, irrespective of axonal sprouting at the end of the donor nerve, these axons will not be utilised by the target muscle unless that muscle is denervated to some degree. This may require removal of the spontaneous, recovered innervation.

However, it is this natural, spontaneous reinnervation that is vital in preserving the muscle as the atrophy that occurs with denervation thwarts surgical reinnervation. This preservation of the muscle, even if synkinetic, should conserve the conditions for surgical reinnervation for many years after the original injury. The other issue on these delayed cases is the condition of the cricoarytenoid joint which must be mobile to allow favourable repositioning/movement of the arytenoid with surgical reinnervation. In our experience, ankylosis of the joint is rare, even many years later. In fact, successful reinnervation has been claimed 50 years after the onset of the palsy.

Surgical reinnervation of the larynx has evolved over many years from animal models to applications in humans. Over this course, different techniques have been used although not many have been widely adopted.

In general terms, reinnervation can be categorised as selective or non-selective and as unilateral or bilateral.

Selective reinnervation is the technique of reinnervating the abductors and adductors separately with the aim of restoring vocal cord mobility. Thus, inspiratory glottic opening may be achieved as well as improved laryngeal tonicity with adduction as required for good voice production. This is required in bilateral palsy.

Non-selective reinnervation involves anastomosis to the main stump of the RLN and thus, indiscriminate reinnervation of adductors and abductors. The aim is to increase tonicity and stabilise the arytenoids much as the springs on a trampoline suspend and work to neutralise the position of the canvas. This is effective in unilateral paralysis.

What has become apparent is that the properties of the donor nerve have to be very similar to those of the original nerve, particularly in selective reinnervation, if function is to be restored. This has to be considered in the context of the clinical impact of disruption of the donor nerve. With recent developments, we have now reached a point where the phrenic nerve can be safely utilised in humans [2–8].

15.2 Unilateral Vocal Cord Palsy: Non-Selective Reinnervation

A unilateral palsy may present in many ways and have many underlying causes. The lesion may be at any point from the origin of the vagal nerve to the point at which the RLN enters the larynx. In fact, a length of only a few millimetres of residual RLN nerve is adequate to perform reinnervation. The residual stump of the nerve can be identified by intralaryngeal retrograde dissection.

Important Factors in Consideration of Non-selective Reinnervation:

Quality of voice: If the patient scores well on the voice handicap index and quality of life scores, the potential gains to be made from reinnervation should be carefully considered (even if objective voice analysis is not as good).

Presence or absence of aspiration: If the patient reports coughing on drinking and/or has had lower respiratory tract infections, this must be dealt with urgently. The patient should be instructed on swallowing techniques and temporary medialisation performed before or at the time of reinnervation.

Life expectancy and comorbidity of the patient: The procedure requires a general anaesthetic of up to 2 h duration and has no benefit for approximately 4 months.

Mobility of the cricoarytenoid joint: If the joint is fixed, correction of the arytenoid malposition with reinnervation will not occur, although there may be improvement in voice due to increasve muscle tone of the cord alone.

Vagal trunk lesion; RLN and SLN palsy with sensory deficit: consider SLN and sensory reinnervation.

Severe muscle atrophy: The muscle will have irreversible fibrosis and will not gain tone or bulk with reinnervation.

Previous surgery and potential donor nerves: In the case of extensive neck surgery, the ansa may have been resected. In these cases it is possible to utilise the contralateral ansa if that is preserved.

Vocal cord scars: Previous vocal cord or framework surgery will result in scarring and fibrosis of the muscle reducing its potential increase in trophicity.

Previous Radiotherapy: This causes generalised fibrosis and may cause joint fixation and nerve lesions.

Other cranial nerve lesions: The outcome of the surgery must be in the context of other functional issues.

Factors Indicative of Muscle Atrophy:

Longstanding palsy
EMG findings:
- *Electric silence, lack of fibrillation potential*
- *Absence of muscle contraction on neurostimulation*

Nasal endoscopy findings: *thin, bowed vocal cord, wide-open piriform fossa. Arytenoid prolapse.*

Direct laryngoscopy: retrocricoid palpation with direct cartilage contact.

CT/MRI findings [9, 10]

- *Coronal view demonstrates loss of vertical height*
- *Axial view shows gaping of the piriform sinus aperture and reduced volume of the PCA and TA.*

Laryngeal echography: thin laryngeal muscles.

Non-selective reinnervation should bring about adequate tonicity of the hemilarynx to produce optimum voice after 4–6 months. If there is aspiration, inadequate cough or a pressing need to return to work/voicing activities, then injection medialisation should be considered at the time of reinnervation surgery. A short acting substance such as fat, Gelfoam or collagen is appropriate and it may be that this also improves the outcome from the reinnervation by facilitating normal voicing and stimulating the muscles. This seems to be the case for early injection following nerve injury [11].

15.2.1 Acute Nerve Lesion

If transection of the nerve is expected or is seen to occur at the time of neck surgery, an immediate repair should be attempted. The options are: to reanastomose the cut ends of the nerve, with or without a free nerve graft to bridge any gap between the ends; or to utilise a neighbouring nerve such as the ansa hypoglossi as described by Crumley [12].

If the nerve is damaged in the thorax, direct reanastomosis at this level should be attempted [13]. If this is not possible, there is not the option to use the Ansa and so immediate injection medialisation is recommended. This does not preclude secondary reinnervation.

Transection of the vagal trunk above the origin of the RLN and SLN may be treated by direct anastomosis of the cut ends, with or without a free nerve graft. If a graft is required, as in vagal paraganglioma resection, it is unlikely that results will be observed much before 12 months. The alternative is to perform Ansa to RLN anastomosis, which can achieve results within 4 months. With these high vagal lesions, the vocal cord usually lies in a lateral position and when combined with the sensory deficit, ineffective pharyngeal contraction and additional relaxation problems of the upper oesophageal sphincter there is a very high risk of aspiration. Immediate injection medialisation—or thyroplasty in some cases—is advised. Reinnervation may be performed at the same time, or at a later date if medialisation has not been satisfactory.

15.2.2 Longstanding Nerve Lesion

Relatively recent lesions (less than 36 months) are preferable to older lesions as muscle atrophy is less marked. However, even fairly minimal residual innervation will preserve trophicity that is adequate for successful reinnervation. Benefit is also seen even if there is ankylosis of the joint, so long as the arytenoid is not prolapsed and blocking posterior glottic closure.

Factors as noted above must be considered and Laryngeal EMG (LEMG) should be performed to ensure that there is denervation but not complete atrophy. A severe neurogenic pattern or fibrillation potentials are the most suitable traces. If there is big enrichment on phonation, this would indicate good residual innervation and thus it is unlikely to bring about any improvement with reinnervation.

15.2.3 Technique

Several techniques have been developed over the years. The most widely adopted is Ansa Cervicalis to RLN Anastomosis which was pioneered by Crumley et al. [14–16] from the 1980s. Tucker [17, 18] championed nerve-muscle pedicle implantation into the adductor muscles and had some long-term success.

15.2.3.1 Ansa Cervicalis to RLN Anastomosis (Fig. 15.1)

A horizontal skin crease incision is made at the level of the lower border of the cricoid cartilage. It may be possible to approach through a previous scar in cases such as post thyroid surgery palsy. The platysma is incised and then the superficial fascia, taking care to preserve the branches of the ansa. Passing medial to the sternocleidomastoid muscle, the Internal Jugular Vein (IJV) is identified by blunt dissection. The superior root of the ansa is the descendens hypoglossi and this lies anterior to the IJV and turns posteriorly to join the inferior root (descendens cervicalis) to form a loop overlying the IJV. This loop is easily identified lying on the IJV just superior to the omohyoid muscle. The nerves to the strap muscles branch off at various points along this loop and can be identified using a nerve stimulator. The descendens hypoglossi is released from the surrounding fascia and followed proximally. A rubber sling is placed around the nerve but the nerve is not transected at this stage.

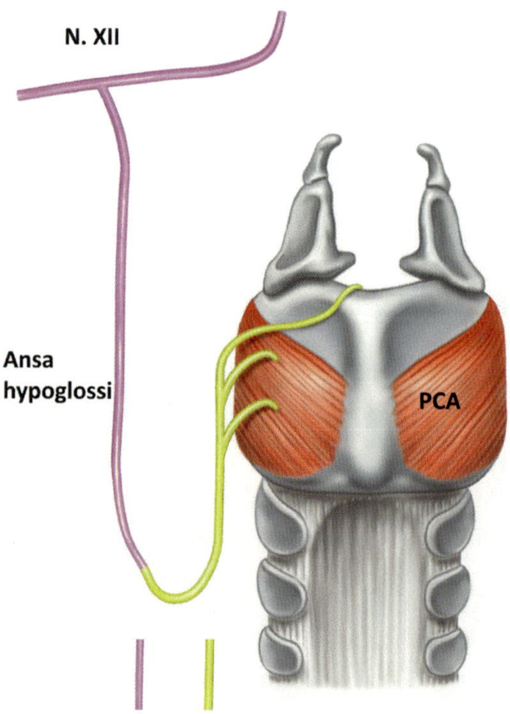

Fig. 15.1 Ansa-recurrent nerve anastomosis [14–16, 24]. Schematic posterior view of the procedure. *Left side*. XII: Hypoglossal nerve. *PCA* posterior cricoarytenoid muscle

The next step is to identify the RLN. In cases where there has been previous neck surgery, the nerve is most reliably found adjacent to the cricothyroid joint. The larynx must be rotated by applying upward traction on a skin hook carefully placed on the posterior border of the thyroid cartilage. The constrictor muscles are dissected off the cartilage and the nerve revealed lying just deep to them. The nerve is then followed in a retrograde direction and a sling is passed around the nerve.

Once the nerves have been identified it is possible to judge the lengths required to form a tension free anastomosis between them. The ascending movement of the larynx on swallowing must also be taken into account.

The nerves are then transected and the axons that subsequently protrude beyond the epineurium are trimmed so that they are flush to the epineurium. A 9/0 suture is used to perform an end-to-end anastomosis of the epi/perineurium and a small amount of tissue glue applied to support it. Haemostasis is secured and the wound closed in layers. It is usually not necessary to insert a drain and the procedure can be carried out as a day case.

It is unlikely that there will be any improvement before 4 months and so a short-acting injection augmentation with fat, collagen or hyaluronic acid should be considered, particularly if there is an immediate aspiration risk.

In a series of 20 patients reinnervated with this technique, Crumley et al. [12, 15, 17, 19] report excellent to normal phonatory quality with excellent medialisation of the cord and correction of the arytenoid malposition. Other authors have achieved similar results [20, 21].

Paniello et al. [22] performed a comparative trial of ansa-RLN reinnervation versus thyroplasty with 12 patients in each arm. They showed an improved outcome with reinnervation in those patients less than 52 years of age.

Wang et al. [23] reported a series of 237 patients receiving ansa-RLN reinnervation with a mean follow-up of 5.2 years. They found no significant difference in the voice outcome compared to that of the healthy control group.

Jean-Paul Marie [24, 25] has a 10-year experience with this technique. He has found that with appropriate selection of patients, including LEMG, the short-term and long-term results are excellent with normal voice. He has not experienced a worse outcome in the over 52 age group.

15.2.3.2 Combination Technique

In cases where there is incomplete closure of the posterior glottis, some authors advocate performing a simultaneous arytenoid adduction procedure at the time of reinnervation [26]. Tucker [27, 28] demonstrated poor long-term results following thyroplasty due to muscle atrophy and proposed performing reinnervation at the time of thyroplasty to augment and preserve results. Equally, we have seen good results from reinnervation in cases with inadequate improvement following thyroplasty where the implant is left in situ but also following extrusion of the implant.

15.2.3.3 Unilateral Reinnervation in Children

In the paediatric population, reinnervation offers several advantages over the alternatives of injection medialisation or framework surgery. It provides a permanent result without disruption of the growing larynx. It is well recognised that the patient should be awake and able to vocalise on command to achieve the best voice outcome with thyroplasty. As this is not possible in children, reinnervation under general anaesthetic is favourable.

Smith et al. [29, 30] have developed this technique in children and report significant success.

15.2.3.4 Superior Laryngeal Nerve Injury

Paralysis of the cricothyroid muscle may occur due to damage of the main trunk of the vagus or SLN or due to damage of the external branch of the SLN only as this branch supplies the muscle. The clinical consequence is mild dysphonia, poor pitch control and loss of the higher register. Before considering surgery, it is important to await the results of speech therapy and spontaneous recovery. The traditional surgical approach is a cricothyroid approximation but this increases the tension in the vocal cords at all times and risks feminisation of a male voice and loss of the low register. Reinnervation is a viable alternative that has been used with some success. El Kashlan et al. [31] used a muscle-nerve-muscle technique, also described in cats by Hogikyan et al. [32]. It involves a nerve implanted at one end in the donor muscle and at the other in the recipient denervated muscle. An alternative is reinnervation with the ansa to distal stump of the external branch of the SLN if it can be identified.

When there is transection of the vagus, there is a high risk of aspiration. Sensory rehabilitation by reinnervation of the SLN may be considered. Based on our animal experiments, we have developed a new approach to this problem by anastomosing the SLN to a branch of the superficial cervical plexus [33].

15.3 Conclusion

Unilateral non-selective reinnervation has been shown to be a highly successful alternative to type 1 thyroplasty. Insertion of an implant in thyroplasty carries a risk of infection and extrusion, has cost implications and must be taken into consideration in future intubations due to its position in the airway. Overall, reinnervation seems to have better long-term results by preventing muscle atrophy, avoids glottic scarring and does not require an implant. It is suitable for paediatric patients in whom the larynx is still growing and if not successful a thyroplasty can always be performed.

However, laryngeal reinnervation has not been widely adopted. This is possibly due to a lack of surgical confidence with microsurgical techniques.

15.4 Bilateral Vocal Cord Palsy: Selective Reinnervation

The ultimate aim of selective reinnervation is the restoration of vocal cord trophicity and mobility coordinate with respiration and phonation.

It is observed that in bilateral palsy the vocal cords usually lie in the paramedian position resulting in dyspnea but good voice quality. The main issue therefore is the recovery of abduction on inspiration.

The key is to apply an inspiratory trigger to the sole abductor muscles, the posterior cricoarytenoids (PCA). To this end, after decades of animal experiments, two techniques went into trial in humans. The nerve-muscle pedicle with ansa hypoglossi technique pioneered by Tucker [34–38] and the phrenic nerve reinnervation of the PCA as championed by Crumley, van Lith-Bijl et al. and Marie et al.

Tucker used the ansa hypoglossi with an island of strap muscle attached distally and swung this across to be imbedded into the PCA. He reported 214 patients with bilateral palsy of which 202 had at least 2 years follow-up with 74% success [38]. He reports deterioration in 17% of these 2–5 years later, which he attributes to cricoarytenoid ankylosis. However, other surgeons failed to achieve similar results with this technique and it is not performed today. In conclusion it was felt that any improvement of the glottic airway was static and due to contractile scarring of the PCAs. No active arytenoid abduction was achieved. On closer consideration of the ansa it is apparent that whilst it is active on deep inspiration, this is not the case in quiet breathing. This limits it usefulness as a donor nerve in this clinical scenario. The other possible drawback of this technique is that the RLNs are not actively cut at the time of the procedure and so there is no re-denervation and thus the muscles are not in a state of actively seeking innervation, although some double innervation may be possible.

15.4.1 Selective Reinnervation Using the Phrenic Nerve

We demonstrated in animal models that the phrenic nerve, unlike the ansa, is active in quiet breathing [39]. This makes it a far more physiologically appropriate donor nerve if the goal is inspiratory activity of the recipient abductor muscles. However, unlike the ansa, the phrenic nerve serves a central role in respiration. The challenge was to utilise the phrenic without negatively impacting on respiratory function. Thus techniques were developed to preserve adequate nerve supply to the diaphragm.

1. Crumley et al. [40–42] used a split phrenic graft, first in animals and then in humans (Fig. 15.2). The main trunk of the RLN was transected to remove the residual innervation of the larynx and to stimulate the muscles to

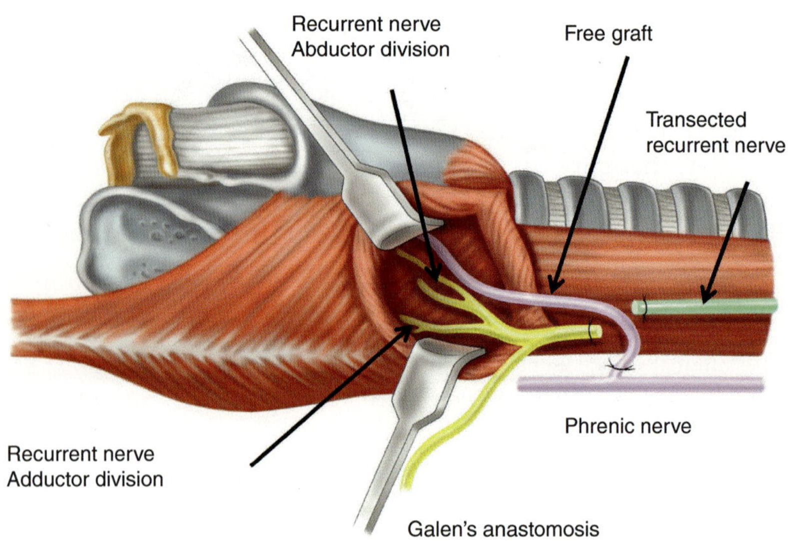

Fig. 15.2 Split-phrenic nerve graft procedure. Inspiratory phrenic nerve fibres are connected to the abductor branch of the RLN (for the PCA), through a free nerve graft [40–42]

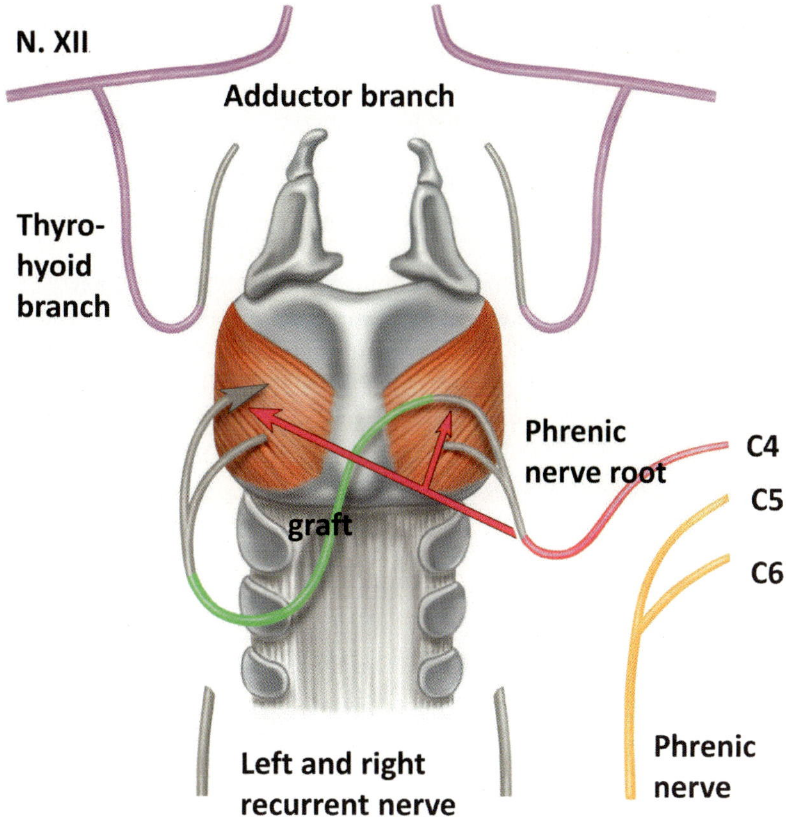

Fig. 15.3 Schematic view of total motor reinnervation of the larynx: both PCA reinnervation by the upper root of one phrenic nerve; both adductors muscles reinnervation by thyrohyoid branches of both hypoglossal nerves [2, 49, 53–62]. The free interposition nerve graft (*green*) is now replaced by a Y shaped lengthening nerve graft (*red*), implanted in both PCA

accept the new innervation. The phrenic nerve graft was anastomosed onto the diminutive abductor branch of the RLN inside the larynx.

Good results were obtained in animals but the first human results [42], presented in 1983, showed some improvement in glottis diameter but no active arytenoid abduction.

2. Variations of this technique have been described by Rice [43], Mahieu et al. [44] and van Lith Bijl [45, 46]. They performed an extra-laryngeal anastomosis onto the more robust, main trunk of the RLN. They then sectioned the adductor branch inside the larynx and implanted its proximal stump also into the RLN to direct all the donor fibres to the PCAs.

Crumley [47], van Lith-Bijl et al. [48] and Marie et al. [49] refined this technique by simultaneously reinnervating the adductors using the ansa. They achieved some success in animals.

3. Zheng et al. [50] performed a hybrid technique on humans using the phrenic nerve, as above, to reinnervate one side and the ansa nerve-muscle pedicle technique on the other side. Inspiratory abduction of the arytenoids was only noted on the side reinnervated by the phrenic.

Li et al. [51, 52] subsequently performed and presented a series of bilateral PCA reinnervation in humans using the left phrenic and reported some success.

4. Bilateral Selective Motor Reinnervation of adductor and abductor muscles of the larynx (Fig. 15.3).

Having obtained successful results in dogs with unilateral reinnervation of both the adductor and abductor muscles using the ansa and phrenic nerves, respectively [2, 3, 49], we endeavored to develop these techniques for use in humans.

We studied the effects of partial phrenic nerve resection on the respiration of dogs and rabbits, observing that the resection of the upper phrenic nerve root had only a slight and temporary impact on respiration [3, 7, 8, 39].

In order to optimise glottic opening it was clearly desirable to achieve bilateral inspiratory abduction of the arytenoids. However utilising the phrenic nerve on both sides carried the risk of significant respiratory morbidity. In exploring these possibilities it became apparent that the arytenoid abduction achieved was in fact better if the PCA received fewer axons from the donor phrenic nerve [2]. This awakened us to the potential of using one phrenic root to supply both PCAs.

For the simultaneous reinnervation of the adductors, the nerve to the thyrohyoid (a branch of the hypoglossal) emerged as the best candidate [53]. This nerve is the only nerve to the strap muscles that fires during phonation and swallowing. As such it can provide appropriate supply to the adductors in phonation and protection of the airway on swallowing [54].

As this technique involves re-denervation of the larynx (by transecting the RLNs), it can be done at any stage after the initial injury as any established synkinesis is removed and so cannot work against the donor nerve supply.

Having formulated and trialed this technique in animals, we obtained approval for a prospective trial in humans. Today, more than 50 patients have undergone the procedure [55–59]. Here we describe the technique and present the results (Fig. 15.3). We are confident that this procedure can offer these patients a significant improvement in quality of life. It is a single surgical procedure requiring no expensive implants or on-going medical involvement. It can free a patient of their uncomfortable, unsightly, time-consuming, and expensive tracheostomy whilst preserving voice.

On the basis of these positive results we have extended the remit of the procedure to include those patients with previous cordotomy. This is on the condition that the cricoarytenoid joints are mobile and that the patient appreciates that there may be the need for secondary medialisation to improve voice.

15.4.2 Technique (Fig. 15.3)

1. *Tracheostomy*: This is performed if the patient does not already have a tracheostomy. It should be low in the neck to avoid the unsterile tracheostomy site becoming in continuity with the operative site.
2. *Surgical Incision*: A skin crease incision is made at the level of the cricothyroid membrane.
3. *Harvesting the free graft from the Great Auricular Nerve*: This is a convenient stage to harvest a section of the right great auricular nerve. This may be done by extension of the original incision or through a small additional skin crease incision overlying the upper third of the sternocleidomastoid. A Y shaped graft of about 10 cm in length is acquired by following the nerve superiorly into the parotid gland where it branches.
4. *Phrenic nerve exploration*: For the right-handed surgeon it is convenient to utilise the right phrenic nerve. Having identified the main trunk, it is followed in a retrograde direct to its roots as they emerge from the spinal foramina. The upper nerve root is isolated and a vascular sling passed around it for ease of identification later in the procedure. It is important to remember that this root may be only 2 cm in length. The root is tested with a nerve stimulator (with prior warning to the anaesthetist) and a hand place on the patient's abdomen to feel for contractions of the diaphragm. The other roots and accessory phrenic (if present) are also tested to ensure that the diaphragm will receive adequate innervation once the upper root is transected.
5. *Identification of the Nerve to thyrohyoid*: This is performed bilaterally. It is a small branch of the hypoglossal nerve that comes off anterior to the descendens hypoglossi, crossing the hyoid bone to lie on the superficial aspect

thyrohyoid muscle, which it enters in the superior part of the muscle. Vascular slings are placed around the nerves, which are not at this stage transected.

6. *Intralaryngeal dissection of the RLNs*: The larynx is rotated to the contralateral side by applying traction to a skin hook placed behind the posterior border of the thyroid cartilage. The inferior constrictors are dissected off the cartilage and the RLN is seen lying between the just posterior to the cricothyroid joint. Sometimes it is possible to identify and the small branch to the PCA. This is performed bilaterally and vascular slings placed for ease of location of the nerves.
7. *Retrolaryngeal dissection*: A tunnel is created posterior to the cricoid cartilage, superficial to the PCAs. This dissection must be minimised to avoid significant disruption to the retropharyngeal plexus.
8. *Reinnervation of the adductors*: The adductors are reinnervated by transecting the main trunks of the RLNs as low as the previous nerve lesions allow. The distal stumps of the RLNs are swung upwards and a free nerve graft is interposed between the stump and ipsilateral nerve to thyrohyoid on each side.
9. *Reinnervation of the PCAS with the phrenic nerve*: The y-shaped, free nerve graft is passed from left to right (single end first) through the retrocricoid tunnel such that the single end is ready to be attached to the previously identified root of the right phrenic. The double ends of the y then come to lie each one adjacent to its ipsilateral PCA. The double ends of the y graft are then implanted one into each PCA. This is done by inserting the end of the graft into a small pocket, which is created in the muscle. A 9/0 suture is used to secure the nerve in place and some tissue glue applied. The single end of the graft is anastomosed onto the root of the phrenic using a 9/0 epi-perineural suture and tissue glue. It is essential to ensure there is no tension on these anastomoses and it may be prudent to pass the graft through a tunnel between the jugular vein and the carotid artery to shorten the distance.

In the situation where the PCA branch of the RLN has been identified, it is possible to make the anastomosis of the phrenic root, via a graft, to the main trunk of the RLN. The adductor branch is then transected and the proximal stump anastomosed to another free cable graft (harvested from the ansa), which is passed through the retrocricoid tunnel to reach the contralateral side where it is anastomosed onto the PCA branch of the RLN. The distal stump of the adductor branch is then anastomosed via a free nerve graft to the nerve to thyrohyoid on both sides.

15.4.3 Post-Operative Instructions

In fact, the act of severing both RLNs removes the paradoxical adduction during phonation and usually reduces laryngeal resistance with improvement of the airway. However, it is strongly advisable to leave the tracheostomy in situ for 5 days. Aspiration can occur in the immediate post-operative period and so the patient is initially fed by nasogastric tube, which is also removed at 5 days.

Post-Operative Investigations

Voice analysis: questionnaire, perceptual and computer analysis to assess vocal impact.

Lung flow volume loops and transdiaphragmatic manometry: to assess the laryngeal resistances and impact of phrenic nerve root transection.

Chest X-Rayand MRI: to assess the position of the diaphragm and trophicity.

Flexible laryngoscopy: to assess active arytenoid mobility.

LEMG: to objectively analyse muscle condition and innervation.

15.5 Results

To date we have performed 49 cases and the technique has been adopted by other centres with success (Paniello and Birchall, personal reports). Here we present the summarised evaluation of 40 cases who have a follow-up of at least 1 year. Publication of results is in preparation. The most common etiology was iatrogenic damage to the nerves during thyroid surgery. There were three children with congenital paralysis and ten patients had had previous glottic enlargement procedures.

Voice: Preservation or improvement of the voice was observed in almost all cases.

Airway: 35 out of 40 cases were decannulated. 30 out of 40 cases showed improvement in ventilation parameters although three required additional arytenoidectomy or posterior cricoid enlargement.

Arytenoid abduction: 27 out of 40 patients had endoscopically observed arytenoid abduction on inspiration on at least one side. Of these, 16 had bilateral abduction although this figure is improved to 14 out of 30 patients if those with previous endolaryngeal scarring are excluded (Figs. 15.4 and 15.5a, b). In one case with previ-

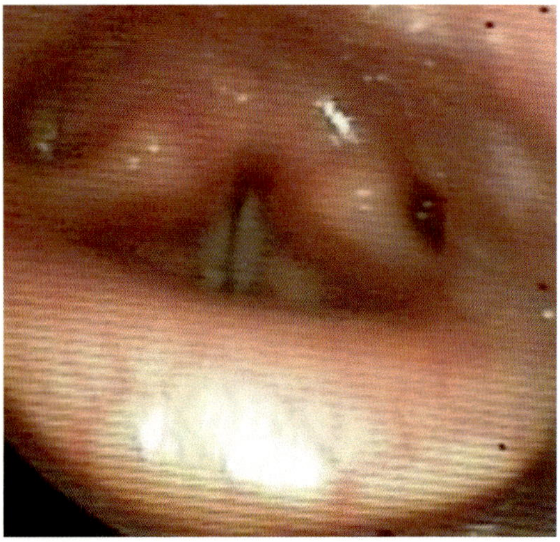

Fig. 15.4 Direct laryngoscopy of bilateral vocal fold paralysis during deep inspiration: no abduction, very narrow glottis

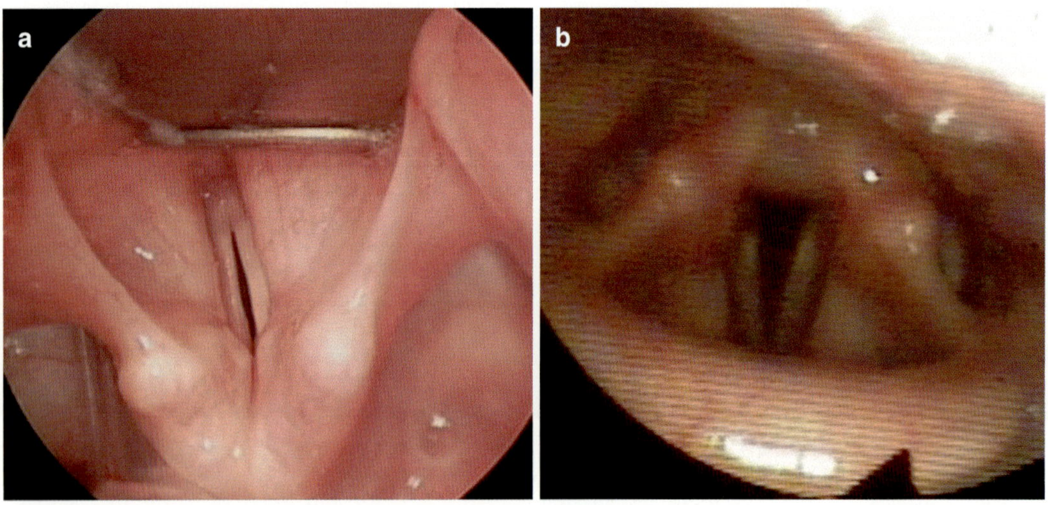

Fig. 15.5 (**a**) Same patient (as Fig. 15.4). Nasofibroscopic view 3 years after bilateral selective reinnervation with the total selective reinnervation technique [2, 56, 58]. Phonation. (**b**) Same patient, nasofibroscopic view 3 years after bilateral selective reinnervation with the total selective reinnervation technique [2, 56, 58]. Inspiration

ous, unsuccessful endolaryngeal enlargement and scarring, the reinnervation result good enough to allow secondary medialisation of the scarred hemilarynx to improve voice.

Phrenic nerve function: recovery was observed in most cases.

Paediatric cases: Using the above technique, we have performed three cases in children under 3 years of age. Two of them were of congenital origin, with some preserved PCA trophicity and passive arytenoid mobility. The third case was secondary to cervicothoracic removal of a lymphangioma, with bilateral RLN and left phrenic nerve paralysis [60]. The first two to be operated on have been decannulated and one has greatly improved with only slight stridor on rigorous exercise. We are waiting to evaluate the second and third patients.

We have also performed the procedure on a 17 years old who recovered inspiratory abduction bilaterally and 3 years later is playing rugby [61].

15.5.1 Additional Points of Interest and Research

There are rare cases of bilateral palsy where the vocal cords are in an open position, probably due to severe denervation with negligible natural, spontaneous reinnervation. Our impression is that good results can also be achieved with reinnervation surgery. We have a short experience of two cases.

We have received ethical approval for a new trial into reinnervation in cases with previous endolaryngeal scarring where the arytenoids are still mobile.

There is ongoing research into how to optimise nerve regeneration and target nerves to specific muscles to prevent synkinesis.

Hydman et al. [63, 64] showed enhanced neuromuscular function, an increased number of regenerated motor neurons and preservation of the somatotopic arrangement in the nucleus ambiguus following nerve transection in rats that were treated with nimodipine.

We are currently investigating the use of olfactory ensheathing cells to enhance regeneration of the RLN in a rat model [65–67].

Rubin et al. [68] have demonstrated a neurotrophic effect of injecting a viral vector into a crushed RLN.

Kanemaru et al. [69] have found polyglycolic acid tubes coated in collagen to make effective conduits for RLN regeneration in dogs. Thus mitigating the need to harvest autologous donor nerves. Suppress many other synthetic materials are also under investigation for use in peripheral nerve injury as well the possibility of these materials delivering growth factors to enhance recovery.

Toll et al. [70] observed a beneficial effect of low-dose tacrolimus on RLN regeneration in minipigs.

Laryngeal pacing (as described in another chapter) has had some success and may be a good adjunct to reinnervation by stimulating the PCA muscles during the months of recovery. There is evidence that suggests mechanical stimulation of a muscle promotes reinnervation [71].

Selective reinnervation is also key to achieving functionality in laryngeal transplantation [72, 73].

Conclusion

Bilateral selective laryngeal reinnervation has the potential to transform the life of someone with bilateral vocal fold palsy. It involves a single procedure and requires no expensive hardware or ongoing management. It avoids destructive procedures to the larynx and has good voice and airway outcomes.

Enhanced results may be possible in the future with developments in tissue engineering.

References

1. Blitzer A, Jahn AF, Keidar A. Semon's law revisited: an electromyographic analysis of laryngeal synkinesis. Ann Otol Rhinol Laryngol. 1996;105:764–9.
2. Marie JP. Contribution à l'étude de la réinnervation laryngée expérimentale; intérêt du nerf phrénique [Laryngeal reinnervation: special interest with the phrenic nerve]. PhD Thesis. University of Rouen, Normandy, France.1999:p300.
3. Marie JP, Lacoume Y, Laquerriere A, et al. Diaphragmatic effects of selective resection of the upper phrenic nerve root in dogs. Respir Physiol Neurobiol. 2006;154:419–30.

4. Verin E, Marie JP, Tardif C, Denis P. Spontaneous recovery of diaphragmatic strength in unilateral diaphragmatic paralysis. Respir Med. 2006;100:1944–51.
5. Verin E, Marie JP, Similowski T. Cartography of human diaphragmatic innervation: preliminary data. Respir Physiol Neurobiol. 2011;176:68–71.
6. Marie J-P, Bon Mardion N, Paviot A, Brami P, Dehesdin D, Verin E. Bilateral functional reinnervation in bilateral vocal fold paralysis: new indications. Seoul: IFOS Congress; 2013.
7. Marie JP, Tardif C, Lerosey Y, et al. Selective resection of the phrenic nerve roots in rabbits. Part II: respiratory effects. Respir Physiol. 1997;109:139–48.
8. Marie JP, Laquerriere A, Lerosey Y, et al. Selective resection of the phrenic nerve roots in rabbits. Part I: cartography of the residual innervation. Respir Physiol. 1997;109:127–38.
9. Mat Baki M, Punwani S, Birchall M, Menys A, Atkinson D, Beale T, Naduvilethil G, Stevens N, Kumar U, Rubin J. Quantitative measure of vocal fold motion—a feasibility study. radiological society of North America 2012. In: Scientific Assembly and Annual Meeting, 25–30 Nov 2012, Chicago, IL.
10. Chin S-C, Edelstein S, Chen C-Y, Som PM. Using CT to localize side and level of vocal cord paralysis. AJR Am J Roentgenol. 2003;180(4):1165–70.
11. Alghonaim Y, Roskies M, Kost K, Young J. Evaluating the timing of injection laryngoplasty for vocal fold paralysis in an attempt to avoid future type 1 thyroplasty. J Otol-HNS. 2013;42:24.
12. Crumley RL. Update: ansa cervicalis to recurrent laryngeal nerve anastomosis for unilateral laryngeal paralysis. Laryngoscope. 1991;101:384–8.
13. Yumoto E, Sanuki T, Kumai Y. Immediate recurrent-laryngeal nerve reconstruction and vocal outcome. Laryngoscope. 2006;116:1657–61.
14. Crumley RL, Izdebski K. Voice quality following laryngeal reinnervation by ansa hypoglossi transfer. Laryngoscope. 1986;96:611–6.
15. Crumley RL. Muscle transfer for laryngeal paralysis: restoration of inspiratory vocal cord abduction by phrenic-omohyoid transfer. Arch Otolaryngol Head Neck Surg. 1991;117:1113–7. Reinnervation: New Frontiers 867
16. Crumley RL. Unilateral recurrent laryngeal nerve paralysis. J Voice. 1994;8:79–83.
17. Tucker HM. Reinnervation of the unilaterally paralyzed larynx. Ann Otol Rhinol Laryngol. 1977;86:789–94.
18. Tucker HM, Rusnov M. Laryngeal reinnervation for unilateral vocal cord paralysis: long-term results. Ann Otol Rhinol Laryngol. 1981;90:457–9.
19. Crumley RL. Teflon versus thyroplasty versus nerve transfer: a comparison. Ann Otol Rhinol Laryngol. 1990;99:759–63.
20. Olson DE, Goding GS, Michael DD. Acoustic and perceptual evaluation of laryngeal reinnervation by ansa cervicalis transfer. Laryngoscope. 1998;108: 1767–72.
21. Lorenz RR, Esclamado RM, Teker AM, et al. Ansa cervicalis-to-recurrent laryngeal nerve anastomosis for unilateral vocal fold paralysis: experience of a single institution. Ann Otol Rhinol Laryngol. 2008;117:40–5.
22. Paniello RC, Edgar JD, Kallogjeri D, Piccirillo JF. Medialization versus reinnervation for unilateral vocal fold paralysis: a multicenter randomized clinical trial. Laryngoscope. 2011;121:2172–9.
23. Wang W, Chen D, Chen S, et al. Laryngeal reinnervation using ansa cervicalis for thyroid surgery-related unilateral vocal fold paralysis: a long-term outcome analysis of 237 cases. PLoS One. 2011;6:e19128.
24. Marie J-P, Bon Mardion N, Mayeur A, Brami P, Magnier P, Verin E. Unilateral vocal fold paralysis: which place for the reinnervation? Seoul: IFOS Congress; 2013.
25. Marie JP, Navarre I, Brami P, Magnier P, Dehesdin D. Réinnervation non sélective des paralysies larynges unilatérales. Une solution optimale pour les cas difficiles. Société de Laryngologie des Hôpitaux de Paris: Paris; 2007.
26. Chhetri DK, Gerratt BR, Kreiman J, Berke GS. Combined arytenoid adduction and laryngeal reinnervation in the treatment of vocal fold paralysis. Laryngoscope. 1999;109:1928–36.
27. Tucker HM. Long-term preservation of voice improvement following surgical medialization and reinnervation for unilateral vocal fold paralysis. J Voice. 1999;13:251–6.
28. Tucker HM. Combined surgical medialization and nerve-muscle pedicle reinnervation for unilateral vocal fold paralysis: improved functional results and prevention of long-term deterioration of voice. J Voice. 1997;11:474–8.
29. Smith ME, Roy N, Houtz D. Laryngeal reinnervation for paralytic dysphonia in children younger than 10 years. Arch Otolaryngol Head Neck Surg. 2012;138:1161–6.
30. Smith ME. Pediatric ansa cervicalis to recurrent laryngeal nerve anastomosis. Adv Otorhinolaryngol. 2012;73:80–5.
31. El-Kashlan HK, Carroll WR, Hogikyan ND, Chepeha DB, Kileny PR, Esclamado RM. Selective cricothyroid muscle reinnervation by muscle-nerve-muscle neurotization. Arch Otolaryngol Head Neck Surg. 2001;127:1211–5.
32. Hogikyan ND, Johns MM, Kileny PR, Urbanchek M, Carroll WR, Kuzon WM Jr. Motion-specific laryngeal reinnervation using muscle-nerve-muscle neurotization. Ann Otol Rhinol Laryngol. 2001;110:801–10.
33. Bouchetemble P, Marcolla A, Lacoume Y, Verin E, Dehesdin D, Marie JP. Laryngeal sensation recovery by reinnervation in rabbits. Laryngoscope. 2007;117:897–902.
34. Tucker HM, Harvey J, Ogura JH. Vocal cord remobilization in the canine larynx. Arch Otolaryngol. 1970;92:530–3.
35. Tucker HM. Laryngeal transplantation: current status 1974. Laryngoscope. 1975;85:787–96.
36. Tucker HM. Human laryngeal reinnervation: long-term experience with the nerve-muscle pedicle technique. Laryngoscope. 1978;88:598–604.

37. Tucker HM. Nerve-muscle pedicle reinnervation of the larynx: avoiding pitfalls and complications. Ann Otol Rhinol Laryngol. 1982;91:440–4.
38. Tucker HM. Long-term results of nerve-muscle pedicle reinnervation for laryngeal paralysis. Ann Otol Rhinol Laryngol. 1989;98:674–6.
39. Marie JP, Lerosey Y, Dehesdin D, Jin O, Tadie M, Andrieu-Guitrancourt J. Experimental reinnervation of a strap muscle with a few roots of the phrenic nerve in rabbits. Ann Otol Rhinol Laryngol. 1999;108:1004–11.
40. Crumley RL, Horn K, Clendenning D. Laryngeal reinnervation using the split-phrenic nerve-graft procedure. Otolaryngol Head Neck Surg. 1980;88:159–64.
41. Crumley RL. Experiments in laryngeal reinnervation. Laryngoscope. 1982;92:1–27.
42. Crumley RL. Phrenic nerve graft for bilateral vocal cord paralysis. Laryngoscope. 1983;93:425–8.
43. Rice DH. Laryngeal reinnervation. Laryngoscope. 1982;92:1049–59.
44. Mahieu HF, van Lith-Bijl JT, Groenhout C, Tonnaer JA, de Wilde P. Selective laryngeal abductor reinnervation 868 diagnosis and treatment of voice disorders in cats using a phrenic nerve transfer and ORG 2766. Arch Otolaryngol Head Neck Surg. 1993;119:772–6.
45. van Lith-Bijl JT, Mahieu HF, Stolk RJ, Tonnaer JA, Groenhout C, Konings PN. Laryngeal abductor function after recurrent laryngeal nerve injury in cats. Arch Otolaryngol Head Neck Surg. 1996;122:393–6.
46. van Lith-Bijl JT, Stolk RJ, Tonnaer JA, Groenhout C, Konings PN, Mahieu HF. Laryngeal abductor reinnervation with a phrenic nerve transfer after a 9-month delay. Arch Otolaryngol Head Neck Surg. 1998;124:393–8.
47. Crumley RL. Selective reinnervation of vocal cord adductors in unilateral vocal cord paralysis. Ann Otol Rhinol Laryngol. 1984;93:351–6.
48. van Lith-Bijl JT, Stolk RJ, Tonnaer JA, Groenhout C, Konings PN, Mahieu HF. Selective laryngeal reinnervation with separate phrenic and ansa cervicalis nerve transfers. Arch Otolaryngol Head Neck Surg. 1997;123:406–11.
49. Marie JP, Dehesdin D, Ducastelle T, Senant J. Selective reinnervation of the abductor and adductor muscles of the canine larynx after recurrent nerve paralysis. Ann Otol Rhinol Laryngol. 1989;98: 530–6.
50. Zheng H, Zhou S, Li Z, et al. Reinnervation of the posterior cricoarytenoid muscle by the phrenic nerve for bilateral vocal cord paralysis in humans. Zhonghua Er Bi Yan Hou Ke Za Zhi. 2002;37:210–4.
51. Li M, Zheng H. Reinnervation of the bilateral posterior cricoarytenoid muscle using left phrenic nerve in patients with bilateral vocal cord paralysis. Seoul: IFOS Congress; 2013.
52. Li M, Chen S, Zheng H, Chen D, Zhu M, et al. Reinnervation of bilateral posterior cricoarytenoid muscles using the left phrenic nerve in patients with bilateral vocal fold paralysis. PLoS One. 2013;8(10):e77233. doi:10.1371/journal.pone.0077233.
53. Marie J-P, Lacoume Y, Magnier P, Dehesdin D, Andrieu-Guitrancourt J. Selective bilateral motor reinnervation of the canine larynx. Laryngo-Rhino-Otologie. 2000;79:S188–9.
54. Marie J-P, Laquerriere A, Choussy O, Lacoume Y, Dehesdin D, Andrieu-Guitrancourt J. Thyrohyoid branch of the hypoglossal nerve in the canine: perspectives for larynx reinnervation. Eur Arch Otorhinolaryngol. 2000;257:S1–S11.
55. Marie J-P, Bon Mardion N, Paviot A, et al. Bilateral functional reinnervation in bilateral vocal fold paralysis: new indications. In: IFOS Congress. Seoul, South Korea; 2013.
56. Marie J-P. Human bilateral laryngeal réinnervation: implications for transplantation. In: American Laryngological Association (ALA) Combined Otolaryngology Spring Meetings. Phoenix, AZ, USA; 2009.
57. Marina MB, Marie JP, Birchall MA. Laryngeal reinnervation for bilateral vocal fold paralysis. Curr Opin Otolaryngol Head Neck Surg. 2011;19(6):434–8.
58. Marie J-P. Nerve reconstruction. In: Remacle M, Eckel HE, editors. Surgery of larynx and trachea. Berlin: Springer-Verlag; 2009.
59. Marie J-P. Ten years'experience in selective bilateral reinnervation of the larynx in humans. In: American Laryngological Association. Neurolaryngology Study Group, 14–15 May 2014; Las Vegas, NV, USA; 2014.
60. Marie J-P. Laryngeal reinnervation in bilateral vocal fold paralysis in children. In: American Association of Pediatric Otorhinolaryngology, COSM, 16–18 May 2014; Las Vegas, Nevada, USA; 2014.
61. Marie JP, Vérin E, Woisard V, et al. Successful reinnervation of congenital bilateral vocal cord paralysis. In: IX Congress of European Society of Pediatric Otorhinolaryngology; 18–21 Jun 2006. Paris; 2006.
62. Marie JP, Vérin E, Woisard V, et al. Réinnervation sélective des paralysies laryngées bilatérales en fermeture. Premiers résultats. In: Société de Laryngologie des Hôpitaux de Paris; 24 Nov 2007. Paris; 2007.
63. Mattsson P, Bjorck G, Remahl S, et al. Nimodipine and microsurgery induced recovery of the vocal cord after recurrent laryngeal nerve resection. Laryngoscope. 2005;115:1863–5.
64. Hydman J, Remahl S, Bjorck G, Svensson M, Mattsson P. Nimodipine improves reinnervation and neuromuscular function after injury to the recurrent laryngeal nerve in the rat. Ann Otol Rhinol Laryngol. 2007;116:623–30.
65. de Corgnol AC, Guerout N, Duclos C, Verin E, Marie JP. Olfactory ensheathing cells in a rat model of laryngeal reinnervation. Ann Otol Rhinol Laryngol. 2011;120:273–80.
66. Paviot A, Guerout N, Bon-Mardion N, et al. Efficiency of laryngeal motor nerve repair is greater with bulbar than with mucosal olfactory ensheathing cells. Neurobiol Dis. 2011;41:688–94.
67. Guerout N, Paviot A, Bon-Mardion N, et al. Co-transplantation of olfactory ensheathing cells from mucosa and bulb origin enhances functional recovery after peripheral nerve lesion. PLoS One. 2011;6:e22816.

68. Rubin AD, Hogikyan ND, Oh A, Feldman EL. Potential for promoting recurrent laryngeal nerve regeneration by remote delivery of viral gene therapy. Laryngoscope. 2012;122(2):349–55.
69. Kanemaru S, Nakamura T, Omori K, Kojima H, Magrufov A, Hiratsuka Y, Ito J, Shimizu Y. Recurrent laryngeal nerve regeneration by tissue engineering. Ann Otol Rhinol Laryngol. 2003;112(6):492–8.
70. Toll EC, Murison PJ, Jones A, Kingham PJ, Sedaghati T, Seifalian AM, Birchall MA. The effect of low-dose tacrolimus on recurrent laryngeal nerve regeneration in pigs: a pilot study. Arch Clin Exp Surg. 2014;3(2):78–86.
71. Zealear DL, Rodriguez RJ, Kenny T, Billante MJ, Cho Y, Billante CR, Garren KC. Electrical stimulation of a denervated muscle promotes selective reinnervation by native over foreign motoneurons. J Neurophysiol. 2002;87:2195–9.
72. Knott PD, Hicks D, Braun W, Strome M. A 12-year perspective on the world's first total laryngeal transplant. Transplantation. 2011;91:804–5.
73. Farwell DG, Birchall MA, Macchiarini P, et al. Laryngotracheal transplantation: technical modifications and functional outcomes. Laryngoscope. 2013;123:2502–8.

16 Laryngeal Transplantation

David G. Lott and Robert R. Lorenz

Abstract

Laryngeal transplantation has the potential to restore voice, breathing, and swallowing in patients with severe laryngeal dysfunction. Following the first successful human laryngeal transplant in 1998, significant research has been performed and advancements have been made in an effort to expand the applicability of laryngeal transplantation to a larger cohort of patients. The main areas of focus have included efforts to reduce or bypass the need for immunosuppression and to establish volitional control of the laryngeal musculature through reinnervation or pacing techniques. This chapter details the world's first human total laryngeal transplantation and describes the lessons learned until its explantation almost 15 years later. We also summarize many of the major studies and findings that have furthered the science and have contributed to the goal of one day transplanting a fully functional larynx in any patient in need.

16.1 Introduction

Human laryngeal transplantation was first studied in the 1960s in animal models by Boles [1], Ogura [2], and Silver [3]. Kluyskens and Ringoir [4] first performed a subtotal laryngeal transplant in 1969 in the setting of reconstruction after cancer extirpation. There were no neuronal or microvascular anastamoses performed, and the recipient perichondrium was preserved as the blood supply to the transplanted cartilage. Unfortunately, the tumor quickly recurred while on immunosuppression and interest in laryngeal transplantation waned for the next two decades.

Electronic Supplementary Material The online version of this chapter (doi:10.1007/978-3-319-61724-4_16) contains supplementary material, which is available to authorized users.

D.G. Lott (✉)
Department of Otolaryngology Head and Neck Surgery, Mayo Clinic Arizona,
5777 E. Mayo Blvd, Phoenix, AZ 85054, USA
e-mail: lott.david@mayo.edu

R.R. Lorenz
Head and Neck Institute, Cleveland Clinic,
9500 Euclid Avenue, A-71, Cleveland,
OH 44195, USA

C. Sittel, O. Guntinas-Lichius (eds.), *Neurolaryngology*,
https://doi.org/10.1007/978-3-319-61724-4_16

There are barriers to overcome for laryngeal transplantation to become a viable option for a large patient cohort. First, the larynx is considered a non-vital organ since it is possible to survive following its removal. The ethics of subjecting patients to the potential complications of transplantation for a non-vital organ are of primary concern. This topic is discussed thoroughly in a publication by Genden and Urken [5]. Second, transplantation requires lifelong immunosuppression which is accompanied by many known adverse side effects. Most notably, the relative risk of developing a malignancy while on immunosuppression has been estimated to be up to 400 times that of the general population [6]. This increase in risk currently prohibits transplantation in cancer patients. Despite this risk, 75% of surveyed laryngectomy patients said they would accept a larynx transplant if offered [7]. The patient desire for larynx functionality puts into question the "non-vital" classification. Lastly, restoring vocal fold motion is in its infancy with some successes reported to date.

In 1987, Marshall Strome began to investigate the potential of laryngeal transplantation, focusing on reinnervation, revascularization, immunosuppression, and the ethics of laryngeal transplantation. A rat laryngeal transplantation model was developed to investigate the maximum tolerated total ischemia time [8], preservative solutions, stages of histologic rejection [9], and immunosuppressive regimens [10]. Once the research supported the feasibility, the first human total laryngeal transplantation was performed on January 4, 1998 by a team of surgeons at the Cleveland Clinic led by Strome, the details of which were later reported in a New England Journal publication [11].

16.2 The First Total Human Composite Laryngeal Transplant

Following extensive interviews, counseling, and testing, a 40-year-old man with a dysfunctional larynx secondary to trauma was chosen. He had suffered a crush injury to his larynx and pharynx during a motorcycle accident 20 years earlier. Despite multiple attempts at another institution to reconstruct his larynx, he remained aphonic and tracheotomy dependent.

The donor was a 40-year-old brain dead man from a ruptured cerebral aneurysm who met all the predetermined criteria for acceptance in regard to HLA matching (4 of 5) and serum virology. The donor organ harvest included the entire pharyngolaryngeal complex, including six tracheal rings and the thyroid and parathyroid glands (Fig. 16.1).

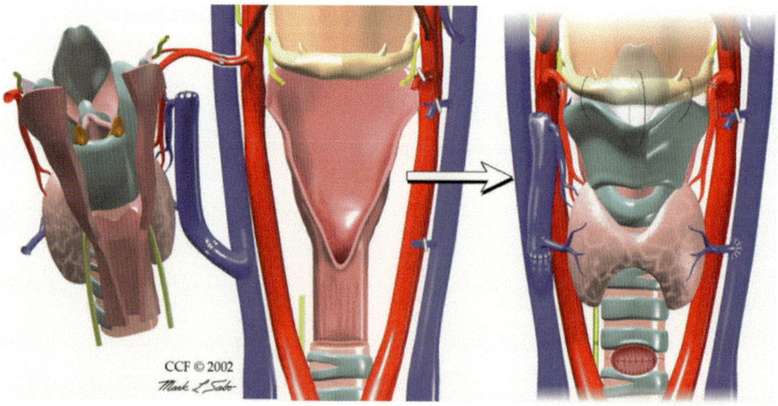

Fig. 16.1 Surgical technique of the first successful composite total laryngeal transplant. Vascular anastomoses included the donor right internal jugular vein to the recipient right facial vein, donor left middle thyroid vein to recipient left internal jugular vein, donor superior thyroid arteries to the recipient superior thyroid arteries. Nerve anastomoses included both superior laryngeal nerves and the only the right recurrent laryngeal nerve. [Reprinted with permission, Cleveland Clinic Center for Medical Art & Photography© 2015. All Rights Reserved.]

The organ complex was stored in solution during transport until revascularization 10 h later.

The recipient received cyclosporine, azathioprine, and methylprednisolone prior to surgery. Perfusion was re-established to the donor organ as the first step of the transplant via the donor's right superior thyroid artery anastomosed to the same artery of the recipient. The proximal end of the donor's right internal jugular vein was anastomosed to the patient's right common facial vein. Blood flow through the transplanted thyroid gland, six tracheal rings, larynx, and pharynx was observed within 30 min of clamp release.

Once perfusion was established, a narrow field laryngectomy was performed on the recipient. His thyroid lobes were kept in situ but lateralized and the hyoid bone was left in place. A majority of the donor's pharynx was utilized to widen the patient's stenotic pharyngoesophageal complex. The donor laryngeal cartilage was sutured to the hyoid bone to create fixed, laryngeal elevation. Five of the donor's tracheal rings were sutured to the recipient tracheostoma. The stoma was left open given that bilateral vocal fold paralysis in the cadaveric position was anticipated.

The left-sided vascular anastomoses were then completed, including the donor's superior thyroid artery to the recipient's superior thyroid artery and the donor middle thyroid vein to the recipient internal jugular vein. Both superior laryngeal nerves were located and reanastomosed. Only the recipient's right recurrent laryngeal nerve could be located for reinnervation to the donor's right recurrent laryngeal nerve. The donor's left recurrent laryngeal nerve was allowed to remain free within the soft tissues of the neck, and not connected to a recipient nerve. A gastrostomy tube was placed for perioperative nutrition.

Postoperatively, the patient was maintained on muromonab-CD3, cyclosporine, methylprednisolone, and mycophenolate mofetil. Initial aspiration was controlled with glycopyrrolate and atropine, which were later discontinued. After observation in the hospital for 1 month, the patient's transplanted trachea was noted to be slightly edematous on endoscopy but showed no signs of rejection on biopsy. Three months post-transplant, the supraglottis and vocal folds became sensitive to touch. Purposeful swallowing, taste, and smell returned. Subsequent barium swallows revealed no aspiration. To evaluate thyroid function, a 4 h uptake of iodine-123 demonstrated 83% activity in the transplanted thyroid lobes, as well as 17% in the patient's native thyroid.

The first post-transplant voicing occurred on the third postoperative day. Endoscopy at 1 month revealed that both true vocal folds were in a lateral (cadaveric) position, creating a breathy voice. The right fold (the side of the recurrent nerve anastomosis) was midline at the 4 month endoscopy. By 6 months post-transplant, the left had medialized. Neither vocal fold demonstrated abduction, but rather appeared to be synkinetic. Electromyographic (EMG) measurements confirmed reinnervation of both thyroarytenoid muscles and bilateral volitional cricothyroid function [12] (Figs. 16.2a,b). It was postulated that the innervation on the left was likely due to "field-reinnervation," in which the left thyroarytenoid muscle is supplied by surrounding motor nerves. Subjective and objective measures of phonation including pitch, jitter, intensity, and maximal phonation time were within the normal range at 36 months post-transplant. As a vocation, the patient became a motivational speaker and stated his quality of life improved "immeasurably" subsequent to the transplantation.

Postoperative complications included three early episodes of tracheobronchitis which were successfully treated with oral amoxicillin clavulanate. At 16 weeks post-transplant, the patient inadvertently stopped his trimethoprim sulfamethoxazole and developed Pneumocystis carinii pneumonia, which cleared rapidly with intravenous antibiotics. Fifteen months post-transplant, the patient presented with a decrease in voice quality. He was noted to have an episode of acute rejection. After three daily doses of methylprednisolone 1gm/day, his larynx and voice returned to normal. A second episode of rejection occurred about 5 years later due to laboratory error in tacrolimus values measuring levels falsely high. As a result the patient's medication became below therapeutic levels. Laryngeal edema was

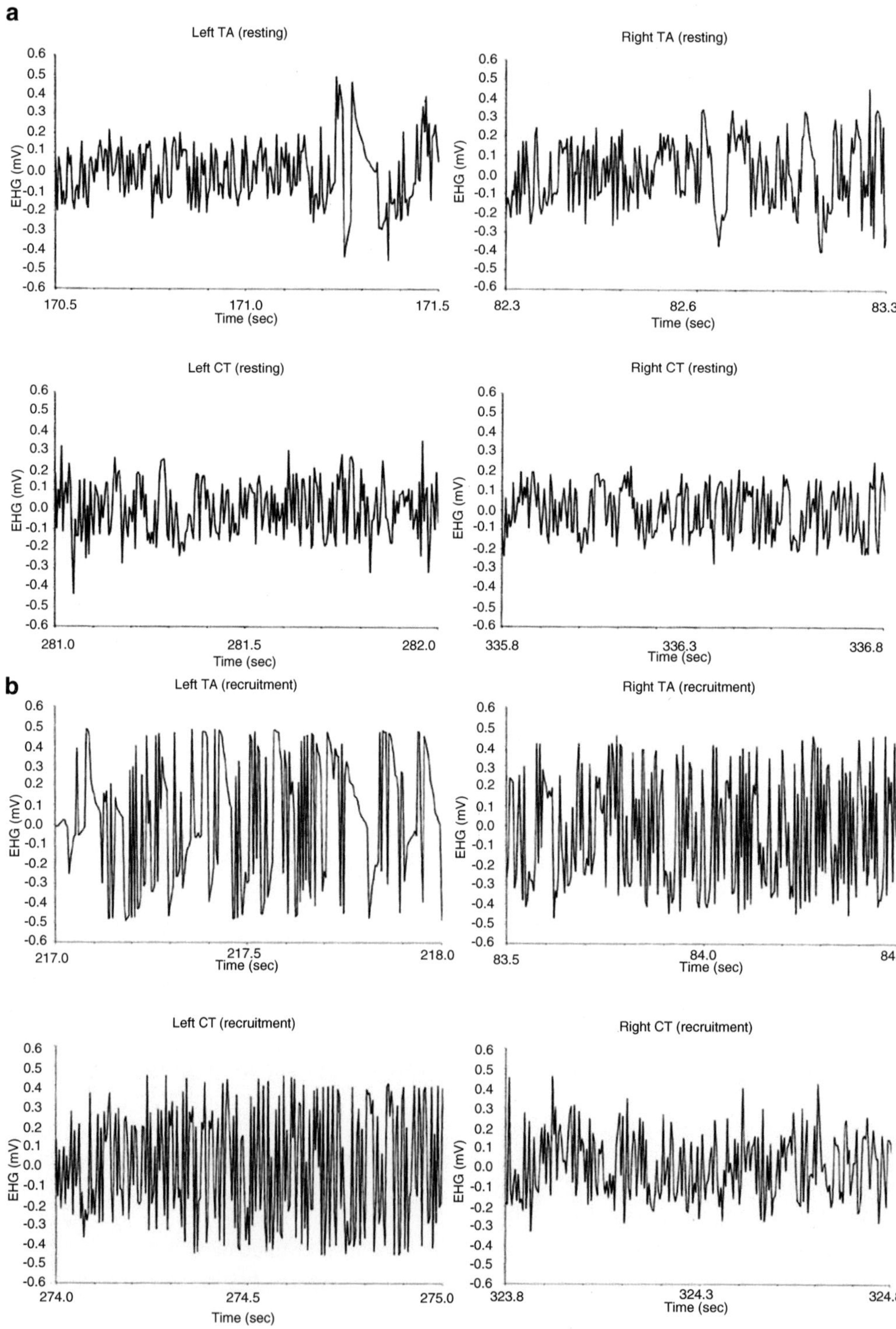

Fig. 16.2 EMG results in laryngeal transplant patient at 3 years. (**a**) EMG findings at rest, including bilateral thyroarytenoid muscles (TA) and cricothyroid (CT) muscles. (**b**) EMG findings during sustained/ee/phonation (TA) and raising and lowering of pitch (CT). Upon volitional movement, the left TA and CT muscles demonstrated moderately reduced recruitment patterns, whereas the right muscle groups showed mild reductions in recruitment. All 4 muscles demonstrated increased numbers of polyphasic motor unit potentials of mildly increased duration and normal amplitude, firing at moderate to rapid rates

observed during the acute rejection episode, but returned to normal once medication levels returned to the therapeutic range.

16.3 Immunosuppression Reduction

As previously discussed, the primary limitation to laryngeal transplantation, and transplantation in general, is immunosuppression. Our lab and others have investigated possible ways to reduce the amount of immunosuppression given to a patient while still preventing rejection.

A variety of animal models have been developed to lessen the necessary immunosuppression for laryngeal transplantation including dog [1–3], mouse [13, 14], and pig [15]. All offer complementary information forming the basis on which to build further understanding into laryngeal transplantation. The two authors' work focused on the rat and mouse models since they are well-established transplant models, significant information is known about their immune systems, and are relatively inexpensive. This model places the transplanted organ in tandem with the native larynx (Fig. 16.3a–c). In 2002, the rat model's revisions were published, as well as a revised grading scale of rejection [16]. The mouse model [14] and a mouse rejection grading scale [17] were published later. Over time and more than 3000 transplants, these models have shown overall nearly 100% survivability, and a greater than 90% graft evaluability. Furthermore, it was demonstrated that performing a total parathyroidectomy on the recipient during transplantation can utilize the production of parathormone from the rat transplanted larynx as a marker of graft viability rather than having to sacrifice the animal for histologic evaluation [18]. This has allowed for a new generation of studies examining the ability to "pulse" immunosuppressives and "salvage" the organ if parathormone levels drop.

In early studies on immunosuppression for laryngeal transplantation, Haug et al. [19] have correlated the laryngeal rejection grade, cyclosporine A (CSA) concentration, and CSA intramuscular dosing. They found that significant

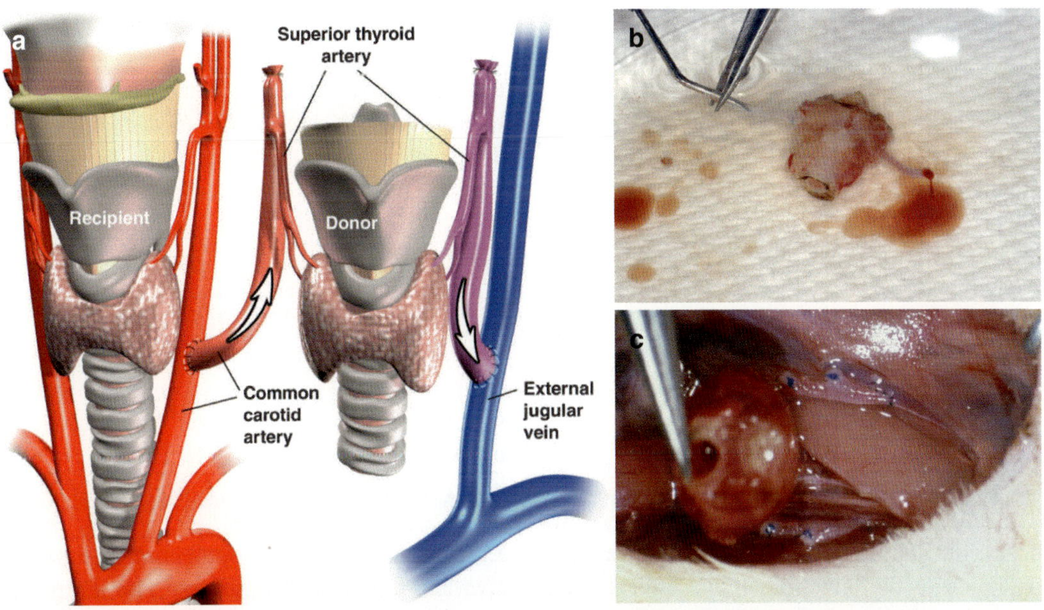

Fig. 16.3 (**a–c**) Mouse and rat laryngeal transplantation diagram. Arterial inflow is achieved through the donor common carotid artery anastomosed to recipient common carotid artery. Direct graft inflow and outflow is based on superior thyroid artery pedicled via the external carotid artery. Venous outflow continues through the donor contralateral common carotid artery anastomosed to recipient internal jugular vein. (**a**) [Reprinted with permission, Cleveland Clinic Center for Medical Art & Photography© 2015. All Rights Reserved]

pathologic allograft rejection correlated with CSA concentrations below 250 ng/cc. This study helped to develop the minimum level of CSA required to obtain optimum graft survival when used as the sole agent for immunosuppression.

Lorenz et al. [20] studied in rats the ability to decrease the amount of CSA by adding prednisone to cyclosporine. In a multiarm study containing 220 transplantations, multiple doses of both cyclosporine and prednisone were administered. The transplanted organs were evaluated at both 15 days and 30 days post-transplantation. It was demonstrated that the addition of 1.0 mg/kg/day of prednisone allowed CSA doses to be reduced to 2.0 mg/kg and still demonstrate no significant rejection at 30 days post-transplantation. Although the combination of low-dose CSA and prednisone significantly improved graft survival when compared to CSA alone at the equivalent dose, prednisone monotherapy demonstrated rates of rejection similar to no immunosuppression at all.

Additional studies further demonstrated that combination therapy of other immunosuppressives would also allow for decreased levels while maintaining graft viability [21, 22]. Akst et al. [22] treated transplanted rats with tacrolimus and mouse anti-rat alpha beta T-cell receptor monoclonal antibodies (αβ-TCR) for only 7 days following the transplant. All grafts demonstrated viability at 100 days. Skin grafting, mixed lymphocyte reaction, and flow cytometry revealed that tolerance was neither donor specific nor related to prolonged depletion of T-cell populations.

16.4 Immunosuppression in the Cancer Patient

The ability to induce tolerance with very low doses of immunosuppression and subsequent reduction of the undesirable side effects facilitates the ability to transplant more patients. However, that degree of immunosuppression is still prohibitive in cancer patients, which represents the vast majority of laryngeal transplantation candidates. It may be allowable to transplant patients with large benign or low-grade malignant laryngeal tumors or those with laryngeal cancer who are already on a post-transplant immunosuppression regimen. A patient with a combination of laryngotracheal stenosis who was post kidney-pancreas transplant underwent laryngeal transplantation under such circumstances in 2010 [23], but these patients are relatively rare.

The recipient pool may be further expanded by transplanting patients who have already undergone laryngectomy for cancer and there is no sign of recurrent cancer after 5 years. Ultimately, the largest group of patients who stand to benefit are those presenting with locally advanced laryngeal cancer. There are approximately 7000 new cases of advanced laryngeal cancer per year in the United States [24]. To date, two transplants have been performed for locally advanced head and neck cancer reconstruction—the non-revascularized partial laryngeal transplant in 1969[4] and a tongue transplant in 2003. Unfortunately, both patients rapidly succumbed to recurrent disease. There are at least three areas of investigation that are promising for possible transplantation in malignancy. The first is to add an antineoplastic agent to the immunosuppression regimen. The second is to directly modify immune cells to maintain immunocompetence while accepting the transplant. Lastly, bioengineering of an organ with the patients own cells should bypass the need for immunosuppression altogether. The second and third areas will be discussed later in the chapter.

Everolimus (SDZ-RAD) is an intriguing immunosuppressive option for transplantation in cancer patients [25]. It is a derivative of rapamycin and belongs to the mTOR (mammalian target of rapamycin) class of immunosuppressants. It blocks the translation of mRNA in critical cell cycle regulatory proteins, thereby inhibiting proliferation of intimal cells, lymphocytes, and tumor cells. Everolimus has shown both immunosuppressive and antitumor properties. The antitumor properties have been demonstrated in several animal and human tumor cell lines, including squamous cell carcinoma [26–28], which is the predominant laryngeal cancer type. In addition, it has been shown to inhibit the development of post transplant lymphoproliferative disorders [29].

Data from our laryngeal transplant models have provided support for the use of everolimus as an effective immunosuppressive and antineoplastic agent in laryngeal transplantation [30, 31]. A mouse squamous cell carcinoma cell-line was used to determine the effect of everolimus on the growth of both intradermal tumors and pulmonary metastases [28]. Tumor inhibition occurred in both the intradermal primary tumors and pulmonary metastasis models studied (Figures 16.4a–d). The authors concluded that everolimus provides potent tumor inhibition in animals inoculated with squamous cell cancer cells by decreasing local spread of disease as well as distant metastases. Everolimus was then studied as a single agent immunosuppressive in the mouse transplantation model [31]. The study showed that everolimus monotherapy successfully prevented laryngeal allograft rejection up to the study endpoint (60 days post-transplantation).

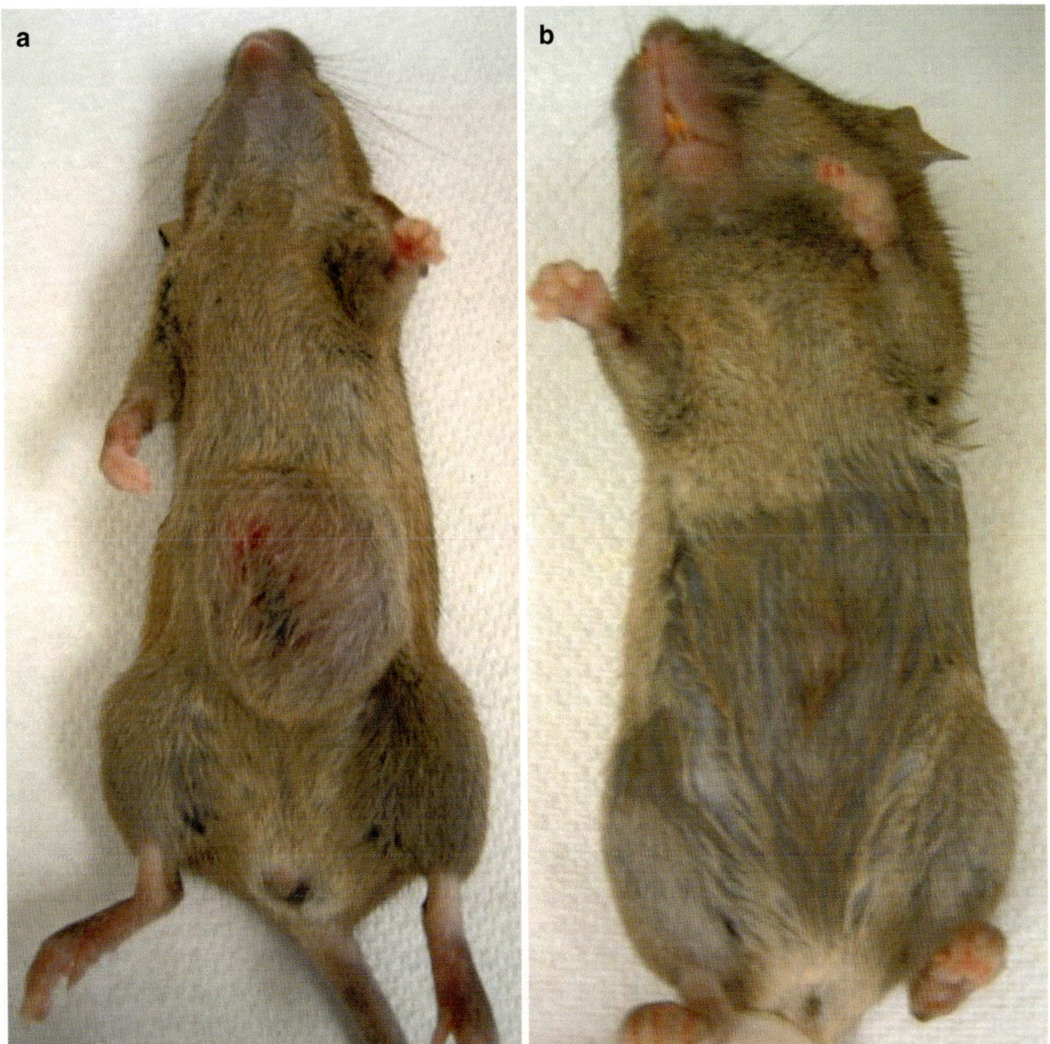

Fig. 16.4 Results of everolimus therapy in mouse squamous cell carcinoma. (**a**) Intradermal tumor in untreated animal. (**b**) Intradermal tumor in treated animal. (**c**) Pulmonary metastasis in untreated animal. (**d**) Pulmonary metastasis in treated animal

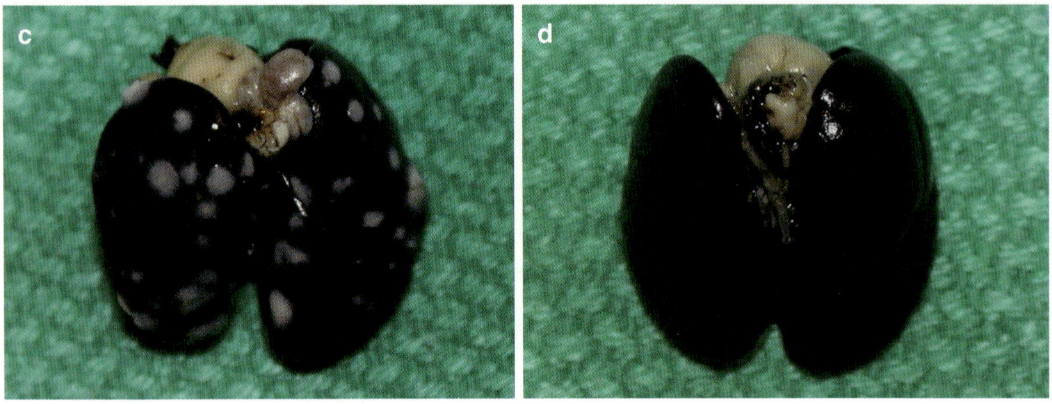

Fig. 16.4 (continued)

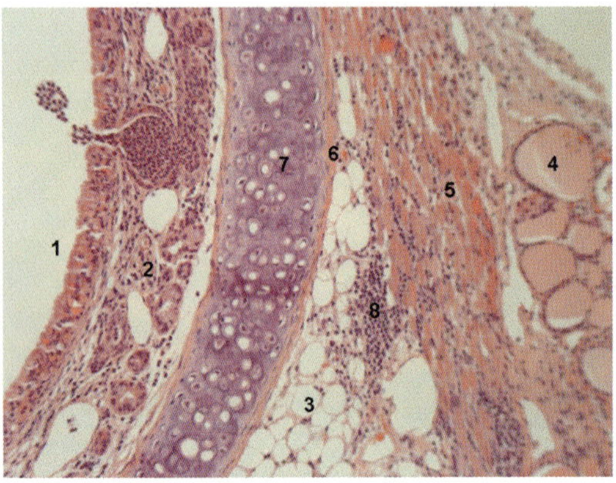

Fig. 16.5 Preservation of transplanted larynx with everolimus monotherapy. Hematoxylin-eosinophil analysis of laryngeal allograft at 60 days post-transplant. Note moderate lymphocytic infiltration with normal structures including ciliated epithelium. (1) epithelium; (2) minor salivary glands; (3) fat; (4) thyroid gland; (5) muscle; (6) perichondrium; (7) cartilage; (8) lymphocytic infiltration

(Fig. 16.5) It appeared to increase the production of regulatory T-cells while decreasing the cytotoxic T-cell and dendritic cell response. This is a favorable environment for transplantation.

Once everolimus demonstrated efficacy for both immunosuppression and antineoplastic activity in our mouse transplantation model, our lab investigated the feasibility of using it as a combination therapy (everolimus and αβ-TCR) in a pulsed-dose regimen to reduce the total amount of immunosuppression and induce tolerance [32]. This study had the remarkable finding that tolerance can be achieved via a pulsed-dose combination therapy for 10 months with just a total of 15 days of immunosuppression. The promising immunosuppressive and antitumor profile of everolimus continues to suggest a prominent role for this agent in the future of laryngeal transplantation, and may 1 day serve to enable transplantation in the setting of malignancy.

16.5 Immunomodulation

An ideal immunosuppression regimen would be metabolically inert and induce donor-specific tolerance while leaving the remainder of the recipient's immune system functional. One way to achieve this would be to directly alter immune cells. This concept was supported by Genden et al. [33] when they demonstrated that a single injection of UV-B irradiated donor splenocytes was sufficient to prevent rejection in a rat tracheal graft model.

To further investigate immunomodulation as a viable immunosuppressive regimen for laryngeal transplantation, several studies were undertaken to better understand the immunological environment of the larynx and trachea. A dense, organized network of immunologically active cells has been identified in both pig and human laryngeal mucosa [34, 35]. The morphology of the cells in these early studies was suggestive of dendritic cells. These dendritic cells were more closely analyzed by Friedman et al. [36] in the rat model. In that study, rat larynges were stained for dendritic cells and enumerated by a combination of immunofluorescence, confocal microscopy, and imaging software. They found that the vast majority of dendritic cells were located in epithelium and subepithelium when compared to other laryngeal subsites. The epithelium was 11 times more highly populated than the subepithelium. Interestingly, Govindaraj et al. [37] studied the role of tracheal epithelium in the rejection process. Their studies of mouse tracheal grafts showed that replacement of the epithelium by host epithelial cells prevents rejection after withdrawal of immunosuppression.

The vastly increased density of dendritic cells in the epithelium coupled with the knowledge of the important role the epithelium has in graft rejection suggested an important role of dendritic cells in transplant tolerance. Dendritic cells are the primary antigen presenting cells in the body and have a large role in determining graft rejection or survival. In the immature state (lack of a T-cell costimulatory molecule), they work to induce tolerance through T-cell anergy and apoptosis. Once maturation occurs through the presentation of a T-cell costimulatory molecule, dendritic cells facilitate rejection.

Lott et al. [38] were able to modify dendritic cells to become maturation resistant through the addition of nuclear factor kappa B (NF-κB) decoy oligodeoxyribonucleotides. This results in the suppression of costimulatory molecule expression causing resistance to maturation even after contact with activated allogenic T-cells, lipopolysaccharide [39], and antigen [40]. In their study, a single injection of immature dendritic cells (iDC) were injected into mice 7 days before transplantation. iDC treated mice had significantly less rejection at all time points compared to non-immunosuppressed mice. Flow cytometry showed inhibition of cytotoxic T-cell infiltration and expansion of regulatory T-cells at the allograft site. The authors postulated that iDC immunotherapy may facilitate graft tolerance as a monotherapy or favorably affect concurrent immunosuppressive dose sequencing.

16.6 Laryngotracheal Regeneration

The ability to regenerate a structure from one's own cells obviates the need for immunosuppression since no immune response is elicited. Tissue regeneration requires the combination of a biologic scaffold, cells with regenerative capacity, and growth factors. Over time, many studies have focused on different aspects of regeneration but none were able to get to the point where human transplantation was feasible. An exciting paradigm shift occurred when a diseased human trachea was successfully replaced with an engineered tracheal graft in 2008 [41]. The tissue-engineered graft replaced a 5 cm section of the trachea and left bronchus. Follow-up biopsies demonstrated revascularization and incorporation of the graft with no evidence of rejection at 4 months after surgery.

Restoration of laryngeal anatomy and function is significantly more difficult than the trachea given the complex nature of this organ. Promising examples of bioengineered laryngeal structures have been reported. The successful use of a porcine-derived xenogeneic extracellular matrix for reconstruction of the larynx in adult dogs has been demonstrated [42]. Histologic examination of the reconstructed tissue 3 months after surgery showed the presence of a simple squamous epithelial lining, organized glandular structures deep to the epithelial layer, reconstructed thyroid cartilage, vasculature, and bundles of skeletal muscle.

Decellularized tissue scaffolds are a good option for airway tissue engineering due to their ease of manufacturing and good replication of native architecture. A major benefit of acellular grafts is the ability to elicit a natural tissue remodeling response. A recent study reported successful enzymatic decellularization of whole human larynges [43]. In this study, larynges were treated by a detergent-enzymatic method for decellularization. Histological analysis demonstrated a near-complete decellularized human larynx matrix. The authors reported that the decellularization process also maintained the presence of both bFGF and vascular endothelial growth factor, which is important to the angiogenesis and neovascularization of the graft. The mechanical response and tensile strength of the cartilaginous laryngeal structures was similar to native tissues and reflected their different compositions (elastic cartilage in the epiglottis and hyaline cartilage in cricoid and thyroid cartilages).

This study represents a significant step toward successful laryngeal superstructure bioengineering. Once refined, this procedure might provide a functional partial laryngectomy reconstruction option or allow for a scaffold for total laryngeal regeneration. Although it won't allow for vocal fold motion, proper positioning and architecture might enable improved voicing and airway protection.

16.7 Reinnervation Research in Laryngeal Transplantation

The donor and recipient superior and recurrent laryngeal nerves are anastamosed together during transplantation. However, mass reinnervation of both the abductor and adductor muscle groups by the recurrent laryngeal nerve prevents net movement of the vocal folds. This process, called synkinesis, prevents complete glottic functionality. Similar to bilateral vocal fold paralysis, the patient is left with the option of having a permanent tracheostomy or a breathy voice following a laser cordotomy. In our transplanted patient, he rated his voice quality as "excellent," and was reluctant to undergo either lateralization of the true vocal cord or cordotomy in order to achieve closure of his tracheostomy, in the fear that such procedures would lessen his voice quality. In their 2010 transplant experience, Farwell et al. attempted to achieve some volitional movement on their recipient's left side, anastomosing the adductor branch of the RLN to the ansa cervicalis system, and the RLN truck end-to-side into the recipient's phrenic nerve [23]. By 18 months post-operatively, the authors described the glottis opening as limited, and the patient continued to be tracheotomy tube dependent.

Return of volitional movement of the vocal folds is critical to the wide acceptance of laryngeal transplantation. Part of this difficulty is the complex anatomy of the recurrent laryngeal nerve. Stavroulaki and Birchall [44] reviewed the anatomy of the laryngeal nerves in humans, dogs, cats, and pigs. In their review, the authors demonstrate that nerve specification is more complicated than the dogma suggests. The anterior recurrent laryngeal nerve is responsible for adductor function and the posterior recurrent laryngeal nerve controls abductor function. However there are many branches of the anterior and posterior nerves and areas of cross-innervation that make reinnervation much less straightforward.

Perhaps the most promising techniques described to date include those of Marie et al. [45–47] who have developed a bilateral selective reinnervation schema. Both PCA muscles are reinnervated with one right upper phrenic nerve root using an interposition free nerve graft. The adductors are reinnervated with the thyrohyoid branches of the hypoglossal nerve. In a preliminary report of the first 12 patients [48], four of six evaluable patients had decreased dyspnea. Three of six patients achieved active arytenoid abduction. All patients were decannulated. One of them did require an arytenoidectomy.

Ultimately what is requisite for laryngeal innervation in the context of transplantation is to consistently achieve a glottic aperture on abduction of 14–16 mm. The two episodes of rejection experienced by our patient were associated with a sudden alteration in voice quality followed shortly thereafter by the onset of significant edema. Without attaining the aforementioned aperture, the airway could be seriously compromised during an episode of acute rejection.

Sensory function of the transplanted larynx is also important to the success of the transplant. Blumin et al. [49] studied reinnervation of the transplanted dog larynx. In a randomized, controlled study, ten dogs had their superior laryngeal nerves transected. Five of the dogs had the nerves reanastomosed. All dogs were tested for laryngospasm in response to hydrochloric acid stimulation both preoperatively and 6 months postoperatively. None of the dogs regained normal laryngospastic responses but the reanastomosed dogs exhibited protective EMG activity and coughing. The control group exhibited no response. In our human laryngeal transplant patient, the supraglottis and vocal folds were sensitive to touch at 3 months postoperatively, initiating a severe cough. Stimulation through the stoma on the right side of the upper trachea elicited a sensation of touch without cough. Stimulation of the left side was not sensed.

16.8 Explantation

At fourteen and a half years after the first composite head and neck transplant, that included the larynx, explantation was necessary [50] (Fig. 16.6). Over the prior 5 years, a subtle but progressive contracture of the larynx could be noted in retrospect on sequential videos, suggesting chronic rejection. Clinically, over the last year prior to explantation, our patient experienced increased aspiration with fluids, a decrease in voice quality, and persistent pain. Sensory testing revealed a dramatic reduction in sensation compared to prior testing. The thyroid function, which for 3 years post-transplant was found to be 80% donor derivation and 20% recipient, reverted to 100% recipient just prior to explant. Fibrosis seen histologically in our chronic rejection animal model was undoubtedly the reason for this. The patient, on his own, decreased his steroid dose to help with the aspiration. The subsequent increased laryngeal swelling initially helped decrease the aspiration but was insufficient in the long-term. Attempted vocal fold augmentation by injection was unsuccessful. The decision was made to explant the larynx. Following extirpation, the pharyngeal remnant was augmented with a free flap. The histology of the excised larynx showed ulceration, acute and chronic inflammation, and dense fibrosis.

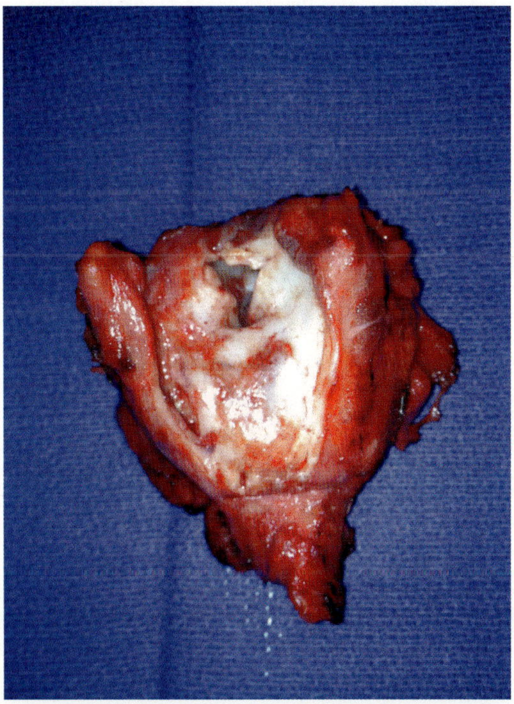

Fig. 16.6 Explanted larynx. 14 years after his transplant, the recipient and the senior author determined that the day had come for explantation. A fibrotic and shrunken organ was removed, with free-flap reconstruction of the pharyngeal defect and voice restoration with TEP speech (see post-explantation video)

On post-explant follow-up, a small 3–4 mm HPV-associated oropharyngeal squamous cell carcinoma was identified and treated with endoscopic resection alone. The relationship of HPV and immunosuppression in the context of the etiology of his cancer remains an open question. After 2 years, the patient continues to be free of recurrence, and did not undergo adjuvant treatment after the resection. Our patient considers his experience worthwhile for multiple reasons (see Video 16.1). Some of which include the ability to have a human voice with pitch control, sense of smell, and an overall feeling of well-being. Today he communicates via TEP speech. He has recently stated that, if given the opportunity, he would opt for another transplant.

Conclusion

Total laryngeal transplantation is now a reality. With it, comes the potential of restored laryngeal function for many patients who have had to suffer the hardships and embarrassment of life without human voicing capability. There is still much to be learned and improved upon from the first transplant and the few that have followed.

With all of the research currently underway in transplantation medicine, the day is likely not too far away when many of the questions highlighted in this chapter will be answered. The immune system will be modified to allow for donor-specific tolerance while keeping immunosurveillance intact; or immunosuppression may be completely bypassed through regenerative techniques. Glottic function might be restored through selective reinnervation or laryngeal pacing. Once these are a reality, laryngeal transplantation will be able to benefit the many people who have undergone a laryngectomy for malignancy. At that time, thousands of people will regain their voices, and their identities.

References

1. Boles R. Surgical replantation of the larynx in dogs: a progress report. Laryngoscope. 1966;76:1057–67.
2. Ogura JH, Kawasald M, Takenouchi S, et al. Replantation and transplantation of the canine larynx. Ann Otol. 1966;75:295–312.
3. Silver CE, Liebert PS, Som ML. Autologous transplantation of the canine larynx. Arch Otolaryngol. 1967;86:95–102.
4. Kluyskens P, Ringoir S. Follow-up of a human larynx transplantation. Laryngoscope. 1970;80:1244–50.
5. Genden EM, Urken ML. Laryngeal and tracheal transplantation: ethical limitations. Mt Sinai J Med. 2003;70:163–5.
6. Lott DG, Manz R, Koch C, Lorenz RR. Aggressive behavior of non-melanotic skin cancers in solid organ transplant recipients. Transplantation. 2010;90: 683–7.
7. Potter CP, Birchall MA. Laryngectomees' views of laryngeal transplantation. Transpl Int. 1998;11:433–8.
8. Strome M, Wu J, Strome S, et al. A comparison of preservation techniques in a vascularized rat laryngeal transplant model. Laryngoscope. 1994;104:666–8.
9. Strome S, Brodsky G, Darrell J, et al. Histopathologic correlates of acute laryngeal allograft rejection in a rat model. Ann Otol Rhino/Laryngol. 1992;101:156–60.
10. Strome M, Strome S, Darrell J, Wu J, Brodsky G. The effects of cyclosporin a on transplanted rat allografts. Laryngoscope. 1993;103:394–8.
11. Strome M, Stein J, Esclamado R, et al. Laryngeal transplantation: a case report and 40-month follow-up. N Engl J Med. 2001;344:1676–9.
12. Lorenz RR, Hicks DM, Shields RW Jr, et al. Laryngeal nerve function after total laryngeal transplantation. Otolaryngol Head Neck Surg. 2004;131:1016–8.
13. Genden EM, Iskander A, Bromberg JS, Mayer L. The kinetics and pattern of tracheal allograft reepithelialization. Am J Respir Cell Mol Bioi. 2003;28:673–83.
14. Shipchandler TZ, Lott DG, Lorenz RR, et al. New mouse model for studying laryngeal transplantation. Ann Otol Rhinol Laryngol. 2009;118:465–8.
15. Birchall MA, Bailey M, Barker EY, Rothkotter HJ, Otto K, Macchiarini P. Model for experimental revascularized laryngeal allotransplantation. Br J Surg. 2002;89:1470–5.
16. Lorenz RR, Dan O, Fritz MA, Strome M. Rat laryngeal transplant model: technical advancements and a redefined rejection grading system. Ann Otol Rhinol Laryngol. 2002;111:1120–7.
17. Lott DG, Shipchandler TZ, Dan O, et al. A new mouse laryngeal transplantation rejection grading system. Laryngoscope. 2010;120(1):39–43.
18. Nelson M, Dan O, Strome M. Evaluation of parathyroid hormone as a functional biological marker of rat laryngeal transplant rejection. Laryngoscope. 2003;113:1483–6.
19. Haug M III, Dan O, Wimberley S, et al. Cyclosporine dose, serum trough levels, and allograft preservation in a rat model of laryngeal transplantation. Ann Otol Rhinol Laryngol. 2003;112:506–10.
20. Lorenz RR, Dan O, Fritz MA, et al. Immunosuppressive effect of irradiation in the murine laryngeal transplantation model: a controlled trial. Ann Otol Rhinol Laryngol. 2003;112:712–5.
21. Nelson M, Fritz M, Dan O, et al. Tacrolimus and mycophenolate mofetil provide effective immunosuppression in rat laryngeal transplantation. Laryngoscope. 2003;113:1308–13.
22. Akst LM, Siemionow M, Dan O, et al. Induction of tolerance in a rat model of laryngeal transplantation. Transplantation. 2003;76:1763–70.
23. Farwell DG, Birchall MA, Macchiarini P, et al. Laryngotracheal transplantation: technical modifications and functional outcomes. Laryngoscope. 2013;123:2502–8.
24. Birchall MA, Lorenz RR, Berke GS, et al. Laryngeal transplantation in 2005: a review. Am J Transplant. 2006;6:20–6.
25. Sedrani R, Cottens S, Kallen J, Schuler W. Chemical modification of rapamycin: the discovery of SDZ RAD. Transplant Proc. 1998;30:2192–4.
26. Mabuchi S, Altomare DA, Cheung M, et al. RAD001 inhibits human ovarian cancer cell proliferation, enhances cisplatin-induced apoptosis, and prolongs survival in an ovarian cancer model. Clin Cancer Res. 2007;13:4261–70.
27. Fernandez A, Marcen R, Pascual J, et al. Conversion from calcineurin inhibitors to everolimus in kidney transplant recipients with malignant neoplasia. Transplant Proc. 2006;38:2453–5.
28. Khariwala SS, Kjaergaard J, Lorenz R, et al. Everolimus (RAD) inhibits in vivo growth of murine squamous cell carcinoma (SCC VII). Laryngoscope. 2006;116:814–20.
29. Boulay A, Zumstein-Meeker S, Stephan C, et al. Antitumor efficacy of intermittent treatment schedules with the rapamycin derivative RADOO 1 correlates with prolonged inactivation of ribosomal protein

S6 kinase 1 in peripheral blood mononuclear cells. Cancer Res. 2004;64:252–61.
30. Khariwala SS, Knott PD, Dan O, Klimczak A, Siemionow M, Strome M. Pulsed immunosuppression with everolimus and anti-αβ TCR: laryngeal allograft preservation at six months. Ann Otol Rhinol Laryngol. 2006;115:74–80.
31. Lott DG, Dan O, Lu L, et al. Long-term laryngeal allograft survival using low-dose everolimus. Oto-HNS. 2010;142:72–8.
32. Lott DG, Khariwala S, Dan O, et al. Ten-month laryngeal allograft survival using pulsed everolimus and anti-αβ TCR antibody immunosuppression. Ann Otol Rhinol Laryngol. 2011;120:131–6.
33. Genden EM, Mackinnon SE, Yu S, et al. Portal venous ultraviolet B-irradiated donor alloantigen prevents rejection in circumferential rat tracheal allografts. Otolaryngol Head Neck Surg. 2001;124:481–8.
34. Gorti GK, Birchall MA, Haverson K, et al. A preclinical model for laryngeal transplantation: anatomy and mucosal immunology of the porcine larynx. Transplantation. 1999;68:1638–42.
35. Rees LE, Ayoub O, Haverson K, et al. Differential major histocompatibility complex class II locus expression on human laryngeal epithelium. Clin Exp Immunol. 2003;134:497–502.
36. Friedman AD, Dan O, Drazba JA, et al. Quantitative analysis of OX62-positive dendritic cell distribution in the rat laryngeal complex. Ann Otol Rhinol Laryngol. 2007;116(6):449–56.
37. Govindaraj S, Gordon R, Genden EM. Effect of fibrin matrix and vascular endothelial growth factor on reepithelialization of orthotopic murine tracheal transplants. Ann Otol Rhinal Laryngol. 2004;113:797–804.
38. Lott DG, Dan O, Lu L, et al. Decoy NF-kB fortified immature dendritic cells maintain laryngeal allograft integrity and provide enhancement of regulatory T-cells. Laryngoscope. 2010;120(1):44–52.
39. Xu MQ, Suo YP, Gong JP, et al. Prolongation of liver allograft survival by dendritic cells modified with NF-kB decoy oligodeoxynucleotides. World J Gastroenterol. 2004;10:2361–8.
40. Tiao MM, Lu L, Tao R, Wang L, Fung JJ, Qian S. Prolongation of cardiac allograft survival by systemic administration of immature recipient dendritic cells deficient in NFkB activity. Ann Surg. 2005;241:497–505.
41. Macchiarini P, Jungebluth P, Go T, et al. Clinical transplantation of a tissue-engineered airway. Lancet. 2008;372(9655):2023–30.
42. Huber JE, Spievack A, Simmons-Byrd A, et al. Extracellular matrix as a scaffold for laryngeal reconstruction. Ann Otol Rhinol Laryngol. 2003;112(5):428–33.
43. Baiguera S, Gonfiotti A, Jaus M, et al. Development of bioengineered human larynx. Biomaterials. 2011;32(19):4433–42.
44. Stavroulaki P, Birchall M. Comparative study of the laryngeal innervation in hwnans and animal employed in laryngeal transplantation research. J Laryngol Otol. 2001;115:257–66.
45. Marie JP, Tardif C, Lerosey Y, et al. Selective resection of the phrenic nerve roots in rabbits: part II: respiratory effects. Respir Physiol. 1997;109:139–48.
46. Marie J-P, Lacoume Y, Laquerrie're A, et al. Diaphragmatic effects of selective resection of the upper phrenic nerve root in dogs. Respir Physiol Neurobiol. 2006;154:419–30.
47. Marie J, Lacoume Y, Magnier P, et al. Selective bilateral motor reinnervation of the canine larynx. Laryngo-Rhino-Otologie. 2000;79:S188–9.
48. Marie JP. Nerve reconstruction. In: Remacle M, Eckel HE, editors. Surgery of larynx and trachea. Heidelberg: Springer; 2010. p. 279–94.
49. Blumin JH, Ye M, Berke GS, et al. Recovery of laryngeal sensation after superior laryngeal nerve anastomosis. Laryngoscope. 1999;109:1637–41.
50. Lorenz RR, Strome M. Total laryngeal transplant explanted: 14 years of lessons learned. Otolaryngol Head Neck Surg. 2014;150:509–11.

17 Neurolaryngological Disorders and Deglutition

Carmen Górriz Gil and Gauthier Desuter

Abstract

Dysphagia and dysphonia are commonly associated with neuromuscular disorders. The symptoms and complications arise from the sensorimotor dysfunction of the oral and pharyngeal phases of swallowing. These symptoms may be unapparent due to compensation strategies, absent sensory cough reflex, or altered cognition. The risks of dysphagia are malnutrition, dehydration, and aspiration. Finding patients at risk is key to avoiding unnecessary complications. Dysphagia could be the first sign of a neuromuscular disease. Videoendoscopy, videofluoroscopy, manometric and electrophysiological studies are complementary tests and should be selected according to patient complaints and availability. In general, neuromuscular diseases tend to affect most phases of deglutition with variable expression and progression among patients. The association with old age of many degenerative conditions further impairs swallowing. Knowledge and awareness of neuromuscular diseases, the signs and symptoms that could affect speech and swallowing, along with familiarity performing a detailed neurological pharyngolaryngeal examination, is essential in understanding the mechanisms altering swallowing and in planning the best treatment. This chapter gives an overview of the physiopathology, the signs and symptoms, the evaluation, and the medical and surgical treatments of the most common neuromuscular conditions.

C.G. Gil (✉)
Otolaryngology Head and Neck Surgery, Hospital Puerta de Hierro Majadahonda, Manuel de Falla 1, Majadahonda 28222, Madrid, Spain
e-mail: carmengorriz@yahoo.co.uk

G. Desuter
ENT Head & Neck Surgery, Cliniques Universitaires Saint-Luc, Université Catholique de Louvain, Voice and Swallowing Clinic, Suite 407, 10 Avenue Hippocrate, Brussels 1200, Belgium

C. Sittel, O. Guntinas-Lichius (eds.), *Neurolaryngology*,
https://doi.org/10.1007/978-3-319-61724-4_17

17.1 Introduction

Prevalence of dysphagia in neuromuscular (NM) disorders is very high especially if we consider that many patients will not recognize the problem due to cognitive impairment, absence of cough or compensating habits. Swallowing problems could also be the first sign of a NM disease. The symptoms could be very subtle such as necessity of double swallow or throat clearing after meals or could accompany others if the patient has a known NM condition. NM diseases tend to affect all phases of deglutition in varying degrees and can start earlier or later in the disease changing over time. Feeding strategies could imply modifications in the volume and viscosity of the food or change from oral to nonoral diet. The patient's ability to cooperate will be essential in the rehabilitation.

Oropharyngeal dysphagia (OPD) arises from the sensorimotor dysfunction of the oral and pharyngeal phases of deglutition and represents a potentially life-threatening condition that leads to malnutrition, dehydration, and aspiration pneumonia. Its prevalence ranges from 30 to 100% depending on the population scrutinized and the definition of OPD that is used.

Approximately one third of one-month post-stroke patients will present some degree of aspiration observed during videofluoroscopy and 100% of amyotrophic lateral sclerosis (ALS) patients will present some degree of OPD at the moment of their death. Likewise, it is true to say that all individuals above the age of 75 will present some degree of OPD affecting one or more stages of the swallowing physiology [1].

A proper swallow will consist in propelling a bolus, whatever its consistency, from the oral cavity to the esophagus keeping the airway clear of any aspiration and the pharynx clear of any residue.

To achieve this result, the oral cavity musculature, the larynx, the pharynx, and the esophagus will have to interdependently act under the NM control of medullary, supramedullary, and cortical centers.

This chapter will cover basic OPD anatomy and physiology knowledge. A pathophysiological model will be proposed and linked with various etiologies. Eventually, adapted multidisciplinary treatment approaches will be exposed.

17.2 Physiology and Functional Modelization of Swallowing

Normal deglutition is divided into four stages, functionally connected so dysfunction in one stage will impact the others. The first two are voluntary and the other two are involuntary [2]. Cognitive and sensory awareness of food presence will stimulate saliva production necessary to swallow. The swallowing phases are the following:

Oral preparatory stage. In this voluntary stage, food is manipulated in the mouth while mixed with saliva till it acquires the right consistency to be swallowed. It involves lip closure, buccal muscle tone, mastication, tongue movement, and anterior approximation of the palate.

The oral activity is dependent on sensory input such as taste, temperature, touch, and proprioception.

No premature spill of food or liquid into the pharynx should occur in this phase.

Oral stage. With lips closed and buccal muscles tensed the tongue propels the bolus posteriorly until the pharyngeal swallow is triggered which occurs when the head of the bolus crosses the lower rim of the mandible. It takes 1–1.5 s. Thanks to sufficient buccal muscle tone no residues should remain in the sulcus between the mandible and the cheeks.

Pharyngeal stage. This phase initiates when the pharyngeal swallow triggers mediated by the glossopharyngeal nerve. Although it is an involuntary reflex a voluntary initiation is necessary as well as the presence of food or saliva. Lesions of the cortex exhibit therefore a delayed triggering of the swallowing reflexes. Other secondary triggering points are the larynx inlet or areas in the pyriform sinuses. The pharyngeal phase is mediated by the lower brainstem in close relationship to the respiratory centre, coordinating a respiration cease by closing the airway for a second while swallowing. Five simultaneous neuromuscular actions occur via brainstem reflexes when the pharyngeal swallow is triggered: closure of the soft palate, tongue base retraction, peristaltic contraction of the pharynx, elevation and closure of the larynx, and cricopharyngeal muscle relaxation. The pharyngeal stage lasts 1 s. Presbyphagic individuals may have a pharyngeal stage that extends to 1.3 s.

The top to bottom contraction wave of the pharyngeal constrictors obliterates the pharynx air space and contributes to bolus propulsion although their main action is helping to clean pharynx residues [3]. Tongue base forceful retraction and the negative pressure in the laryngopharynx work together with the constrictors to move food through the pharynx [4].

The cricopharyngeal (CP) muscle, the main active component of the upper esophageal sphincter (UES), has a tonic contraction and relaxes when swallowing, belching, or vomiting, but for normal swallowing is kept open by the combined action of larynx forward and upward movement, pharyngeal shorteners widening, and bolus pressure. There are five phases in the relaxation of the UES:

1. Inhibition of the tonic contraction of the CP (0.1 s).
2. UES opening by the biomechanics of hyolaryngeal anterosuperior excursion: the hyoid pulls anteriorly and superiorly the larynx and the contraction of the thyrohyoid pull forward the larynx, and the UES open.
3. Distension of UES by the superior and lateral traction force of the muscles shortening the pharynx (stylopharyngeus, palatopharyngeus, and salpingopharyngeus).
4. Distension of the UES by pressure applied by the bolus. Therefore weight and volume will help the opening.
5. Passive collapse of the distended UES as the bolus passes.
6. Closure of UES by contraction of the CP muscle.

Esophageal stage. A peristaltic wave motion drives the bolus to the stomach. This phase lasts from 3 to 20 s with an average of 8 s.

Efficient swallowing requires cooperation and coordination of the cranial nerves involved (V, VII, IX, X, and XII). Table 17.1 display the nerves involved and the actions determined.

Table 17.1 Nerves and muscles implied in swallowing and their actions

<u>*Trigeminal nerve (CN V)*</u> **Motor innervation** *Mastication*—temporalis, masseter, medial and lateral pterygoid *Hypolaryngeal excursion*—Mylohyoid, anterior belly digastric *Tensing velum*—Tensor veli palatini **Sensory innervation** *Bolus manipulation*—sensation from mouth, cheeks, and anterior 2/3 of the tongue (not taste)	<u>*Facial nerve (CN VII)*</u> **Motor innervation** *Lip closure*: orbicularis oris, Zygomaticus *Buccal tone*: buccinator *Hypolaryngeal excursion*—posterior belly digastric, stylohyoid **Sensory and autonomic innervation** *Taste*—taste from the anterior 2/3 of the tongue. *Salivation*—parasympathetic fibers to the submandibular and sublingual salivary glands	<u>*Glossopharyngeal nerve (CN IX)*</u> **Motor innervation** *Pharyngeal constriction*—upper pharyngeal constrictor *Pharyngeal shortening*—stylopharyngeus **Sensory and autonomic innervation** *Taste and sensation*—sensation from the posterior 1/3 of the tongue (including taste), the velum, the fauces and the superior portion of the pharynx *Salivation*—parasympathetic fibers to the parotid salivary glands
<u>*Vagus nerve (CN X)*</u> **Motor innervation** *Velopharyngeal closure*—levator veli palatini *Tongue base retraction*—palatoglossus *Pharyngeal squeeze*—pharyngeal constrictors *Airway closure*—all intrinsic laryngeal muscles *UES closure and opening*—cricopharyngeus *Esophageal motility*—esophageal musculature, both striated in proximal 1/3 and smooth muscle in distal 2/3 of esophagus **Sensory innervation** *Sensation*—sensory information from the velum, posterior and inferior portions of the pharynx, all sensation in the larynx, esophagus		<u>*Hypoglossal nerve (CN XII)*</u> **Motor innervation** *Tongue mobility*—all extrinsic and intrinsic tongue muscles *Hypolaryngeal elevation*—thyrohyoid approximation through thyrohyoid and hyoid protraction through geniohyoid

Modelling of swallowing. Of the many models used to describe the oropharyngeal swallowing, McConnel's "Piston Model," proposed in 1988, remains the most widely used around the world. The "Piston Model" is based on the following assumption: the primary function of the oropharynx is to generate a pressure gradient for swallowing without aspiration.

Citing McConnel: "*the tongue base acts like a plunger or a 'Piston' to develop a propulsive bolus-driving force*" [3, 5]. According to this model the bolus-driving force will depend on two somewhat interdependent elements: (1) the propulsion forces (PF) and (2) the flow resistance forces (FRF). The PF is largely dependent on two elements: (a) the tongue appearing as the major pressure-generator and (b) the resistance of the pharyngeal walls acting as a dynamic chamber for the tongue. In contrast the FRF is mainly determined by the upper esophageal sphincter (UES) behavior (hypo-relaxed, hyper-contracted, lack of passive opening, etc.) [6].

17.3 Neural Control of Swallowing

The swallowing reflex can be triggered voluntarily or involuntarily by the sensory impulses in the posterior oropharynx, larynx, and hypopharynx [7]. The swallowing reflex response is controlled by the brain stem but modulated by cortical input. Sensory feedback can modify the intensity of the pharyngeal reflex as it synapses in both the brain stem and the cortex, in particular when related to the volume of the bolus ingested. Once the bolus enters the pharynx, the afferent fibers trigger a region of the nucleus tractus solitarius that sets up a sequence of cranial motor nuclei activation.

Cognitive awareness, drive for food and nutrition plays an important role. The coordination with apnea is essential. The muscle groups involved in swallowing are represented bilaterally but asymmetrically in the premotor cortex, in a somatotopic fashion, with a dominant hemisphere independent of handedness [8, 9]. The clinical implication is that impairment of swallowing will be more prominent if the hemisphere affected is the dominant one and that there will be a possibility of rehabilitation reorganizing the swallowing areas in the non-dominant hemisphere. The cerebral cortex has an important role in swallowing initiation and strong involvement in the coordination of the normal swallow. Suppression of cortical input makes oral time longer, uncoordinated and with a prolonged triggering time of the reflexive swallow. The sensory motor cortex receives afferent information of the oral, pharyngeal, and laryngeal areas modulating the brain stem response according to the type of information received. The brainstem is responsible for the involuntary phases. Brainstem representation is both sided and they are interconnected. That means a unilateral lesion can result in bilateral pharyngeal motor and sensory dysfunction.

The brainstem swallowing center, called the central pattern generator (CPG), is formed by two groups of interneurons: one located in the nucleus tractus solitarius (NTS), called the dorsal swallowing group (DSG), which is a primary sensory nucleus from the afferent stimuli and the other one located in the ventrolateral medulla (VLM), called ventral swallowing group (VSG), adjacent to the nucleus ambiguus (Fig. 17.1). The interneurons in the DSG are involved in the triggering, shaping, and timing of swallowing, and modulate the VSG premotor neurons which distribute the swallowing drive to the motorneurons of the different cranial nerves involved in swallowing [10]. The CPG is activated by either peripheral afferent input such as the ones conducted by the superior laryngeal nerve (SNL) or by supramedullary inputs, conducted by the cerebral cortex in the case of a voluntary swallow [11]. Sinclair et al. [12] demonstrated that electric stimulation of SLN elicits swallowing more readily than stimulation of the IX cranial nerve alone. SLN impairment greatly affects deglutition specially related to aspiration risk.

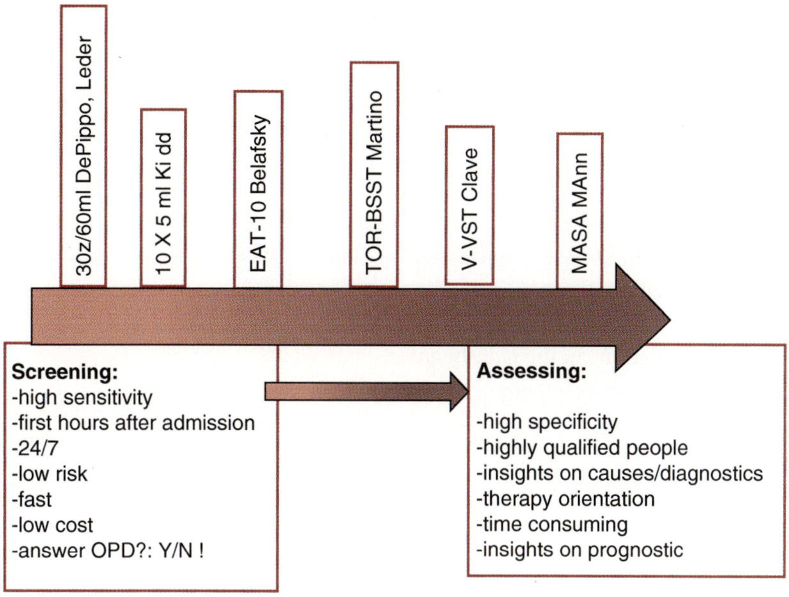

Fig. 17.1 Nonexhaustive list of different screening/assessments tests

17.3.1 Neurophysiology of the Protective Function of the Larynx

The most basic action of the larynx is to provide sphincteric protection of the lower airway. Protective vocal fold adduction is mainly due to thyroarytenoid (TA) contraction and is elicited by stimulation of the internal branch of the superior laryngeal nerve. Therefore, if the larynx is locally anesthetized the adductor response is not elicited.

Anesthesia dependency of the contralateral adductor reflex:

In humans under general anesthesia, response to the internal branch of the SLN stimulation elicits two types of responses, one with a short latency of 10–18 msec that produces the adduction of the ipsilateral VF and a second one, with a longer latency of 50 to 80 msec that produces a bilateral vocal fold adduction. In anesthetized cats this bilateral cross reflex reaction is already present at the short latency response. Sasaki et al. [13] suggested that "*whereas the contralateral short latency response in humans is supported by central facilitation in the awake state, anesthesia suppression of facilitative mechanisms restricts the response to an only ipsilateral one.*" These findings could explain the greater incidence of aspiration in sedated patients.

In other words, awake patient would benefit of a short lasting internal branch of the SLN mediated bilateral closure of their laryngeal sphincter whereas anesthetized patients would only benefit of a unilateral reflex of this kind.

17.4 The Effect of Aging in Swallowing

Changes associated with aging can impact swallowing and have to be differentiated from dysphagia from other neurolaryngological causes.

There is evidence that suggests that the aging larynx suffers structural and functional changes [14–16]. Saliva production is decreased. Oral time is longer as muscles are weaker. The pharynx becomes larger and more dilated. The UES relaxation is altered due to neurologic impairment and to decreased hyolaryngeal elevation. The incidence of CP bar is higher. Pooling in pyriform sinuses is common, although aspiration does not seem to occur. Increased effort is necessary to swallow and pharyngeal transit becomes longer. This exposes the airway to the risk of aspiration. The laryngeal adductor reflex decreases with age in relationship to decreases in SLN sensitivity. The decline in the rest of sensory end organs capabilities and cortical function further impair normal swallowing ongoing adaptations in the elderly are necessary to accommodate these changes.

17.5 Signs and Symptoms of Abnormal Swallow

Dysphagia is defined as a sensation of difficulty with swallowing that can occur anywhere from the mouth to the stomach. Dysphagia symptoms are summarized in Table 17.2.

As compensation mechanisms may have taken place, detailed questioning about dietary behaviors is necessary: chewing more, liquid ingestion after solids, cutting food in smaller pieces, double swallowing, etc. to find asymptomatic dysphagia patients.

Based on McConnel's modelization mentioned above, one can infer from it, some clinical signs and diagnostic hints. Table 17.3 summarizes the link between McConnel's postulated swallowing issues, clinical signs, and a non-exhaustive list of diagnostic possibilities.

17.6 Evaluation of Swallowing

Dysphagia screening and repeat objective testing in patients with NM diseases are essential to reduce the risk of aspiration pneumonia, malnutrition, or dehydration. There are two groups of diagnostic methods: (1) screening tests and bedside assessment tests and (2) the instrumental tests: Flexible endoscopic examination of swallowing (FEES), Videofluoroscopy or modified barium swallow (MBS), manometry and electrophysiological studies in between others.

Table 17.2. Symptoms of dysphagia

Dysphagia symptoms
Difficulty chewing
Drooling
Difficulty initiating swallowing
Food retained between the cheeks and teeth
Coughing, laryngospasm
Choking with liquid or solid food, before, during or after swallowing
Increased saliva
Frequent throat clearing
Wet voice after eating
Sensation of food stuck in the throat
Pain when swallowing
Regurgitation of food or liquids

17.6.1 Screening Tests and Bedside Assessment Tests

Multiple screening and bedside assessment tests have been published these last decades [17–26]. By definition a screening test should have a high sensibility, be rapid and easily performed. They are mainly used in short length-of-stay institutions such as acute care hospitals. On the other hand, bedside assessment tests have a high specificity and can be time and effort consuming in order to orient a treatment plan or assess the degree of impairment. These are more likely to be used in long length-of-stay institutions such as speciality department, rehabilitation centers, or nursing homes.

Figure 17.1 shows a non-exhaustive list of different screening/assessments tests that are available in the recent literature. They are classified on an analogical scale regarding their screening or assessment characteristics, Fig. 17.1.

Bedside assessment tests consist of a quick medical history and clinical observation of how the patient manages oral intake and saliva swallowing.

17.6.2 Dysphagia ENT Assessment

The objective is to find the alterations that lead to the dysphagia encountered in the previous tests, assess the type of diet to follow, and plan an initial treatment.

Table 17.3 Types of swallowing issues

Type of swallowing issues	Clinical signs	Example of diagnostic related to clinical signs
Orality issues	1. Improper bolus conditioning 2. Defect of mouth water tightness (a) Anterior: drooling (b) Posterior: posterior spillage/ anticipated pharyngeal phase triggering 3. Absence of pharyngeal phase triggering	1. Edentate/masticator muscle issues/xerostomy 2.a Facial palsy 2.b Velar incompetence/myasthenia gravis/ skull base tumor (IX) 3. Dementia
Propulsive issues	1. Pressure leaks (a) Soft velar leaks (b) Pharyngeal hypotonia dilatation, pouching (c) UES pouching 2. Tongue plunger issues (a) Weakness (b) Stiffness 3. Pharyngeal weakness	1.a Lesion of the IX/myasthenia gravis 1.b Post stroke 1.c Zenker's diverticulum 2.a Myasthenia/myositis 2.b Parkinson's disease 3. Post-stroke/oculo-pharyngeal dystrophy/myasthenia/ post-stroke/post-radiotherapy
Resistive issues	Lack of UES opening 1. Stiffness 2. Impaired neuromuscular control of EUS tone/ lack of UES relaxation 3. Lack of anterosuperior excursion of the larynx 4. EUS tone setting reflex conflict	1. Post-radiotherapy 2. Post-stroke/recurrent/superior laryngeal nerve injury 3. Myasthenia/myositis/dystrophies/frailty syndrome/ tracheostomy 4. GERD/hiatal hernia
Mixed issues (resistive & propulsive	1. Global defect and/or incoordination of neuromuscular inhibitory and excitatory control 2. Global muscular weakness impeaching pharyngeal contraction and superior laryngeal anterior–superior excursion	1. Post-stroke 2. Myotonic dystrophy/post radiotherapy
Esophageal issue	1. Mechanical 2. Lack of esophageal motility	1.a Tumor 1.b Nutcracker esophagus 1.c Eosinophilic esophagitis 2. Achalasia

17.6.2.1 Clinical Examination

Detailed directed medical history will focus on neurological impairments, dietary restrictions, pneumonia suffering, nutritional state, and the presence of tracheostomy or feeding tubes. As compensation mechanisms may have taken place detailed questioning about dietary behavior is necessary.

Observe mental state, general appearance, posture, conversation, affective response, intellectual ability, temporospatial orientation, and possibility of cooperation in the rehabilitation.

General ENT examination will include facial mobility, lip sealing, dental health, tongue movement and strength, pharyngolaryngeal sensation, phono-respiratory coordination, and patient ability to follow directions. Sensory motor assessment of the cranial nerves involved in swallowing: V, VII, IX, X, and XII [27] will follow.

17.6.2.2 Instrumental Dysphagia Assessment

The two gold standards of oropharyngeal instrumental examination are FEES and MBS. They are complementary tests that yield different information and both can detect silent aspiration. Patient complaints and test availability will dictate the choice of test. They both assess the effect of therapeutic strategies: postural changes, sensory or dietary modifications, or therapeutic maneuvers. Comparison between FEES and MBS is shown in Table 17.4.

Flexible Endoscopic Evaluation of Swallowing and FEES with Sensory Testing FEEST

Introduced by Langmore and colleagues in 1988 [28–30], FEES combines the everyday fibrolaryngoscopy giving detailed insight into the *anatomic and physiologic* issues implicated in deglutition and a *functional* test with the aid of ingesting colored consistencies in different volumes, followed by performing specific head posture modifications or swallowing maneuvers that can improve swallowing. In 1993, Aviv introduced the sensory testing of the SLN with pulses of air in the aryepiglottic folds, FEEST [31].

The anatomic-physiologic assessment should note: velopharyngeal closure, appearance and symmetry of the larynx and pharynx at rest, base of tongue, pharyngeal constrictors function, pooling, handling of secretions, and swallow frequency, [30]. The location of the secretion should be noted: vallecula, pharynx, pyriform sinuses, larynx vestibule, or trachea. The ability to clear them by cough elicitation is an important indicator of sensory indemnity and a predictor of safety.

We should highlight the importance of the *pharyngeal squeeze maneuver*, a test that gives an insight of the recruitment of the pharyngeal musculature, elicited by producing the highest pitch possible as a formal test of pharyngeal strength. It can compare to the pharyngeal constriction ratio seen on videofluoroscopy. It is also an important predictor of swallowing safety [32–34].

The laryngeal sensory testing examines the *laryngeal adductor reflex (LAR),* a brisk and easy to identify closure of the vocal folds responsive to a stimulus. LAR is elicited even in patients with poor consciousness, incapacitated or in the absence of patient cooperation.

The presence of normal LAR can be seen as a good indicator of swallowing abilities after stroke [11, 35].

Table 17.4 Comparison between FEES and MBS

Fiberoptic endoscopic evaluation of swallowing (FEES)	Modified barium swallow (MBS)
Bedside performed	Not beside performed
Cheap with no specific setting needed	Costly setting
Easily available	Not available everywhere
No radiation	High volume of radiation
Repeated examinations possible	Repeated exposure to radiation not recommended
Blackout when swallowing. Indirect aspiration signs	Clear and quantifiable measures of penetration and aspiration
Limited to pharyngolaryngeal lumen	Explores oral cavity, pharynx, esophagus, and stomach
Cervical spine not seen	Cervical spine perfectly visible
Direct view of anatomy and mucosal status	Indirect view of anatomy and mucosal status
Indirect assessment of laryngohyoidal motion and velopharyngeal closure	Perfect quantifiable assessment of laryngohyoidal motion and velopharyngeal closure
No objective measurements	Objective measures of interrelationship of laryngohyoidal elevation, pharyngeal constriction and UES opening
Assesses sensory and motor integrity	Indirect sensory testing
Can last long enough to evaluate fatigue	Restricted by radiation time
Perfect assessment of vocal fold motion	Poor indirect assessment of vocal fold motion

Videofluoroscopic Swallowing Studies or Modified Barium Swallow

The technique of MBS consists of a radiographic video of the rapid sequences that make a swallow, ingesting different barium consistencies in different volumes and the effect of different maneuvers and positions, usually performed by radiologists and speech language pathologists. The volumes, consistencies, positions, and maneuvers are similar to the ones used in FEES and in rehabilitation.

An anteroposterior and lateral RX projections are taken which can be replayed at very low speed for accurate objective evaluation. A recording acquisition of six images per seconds is required.

Developed by Logeman 93 [36], many standardized protocols have been proposed, although a reduced personalized assessment can be determined in each patient case.

In NM disorders, MBS is specially recommended to assess oral phase, velopharyngeal closure, pooling, speed and time of each phase and the interrelationship between laryngohyoid elevation, pharynx contraction, and UES opening. It identifies and quantifies the presence of aspiration during swallowing and its severity.

The *Penetration aspiration scale by Rosenbeck* [37] and the *Dysphagia severity rating by Waxman* [38, 39] would complete the assessment of food intake safety, and would recommend dietary modifications for the dysphagia severity.

One has to take into account that even though objective examinations are the gold standard to assess aspiration risk, they only examine a discrete moment of deglutition with food that may not taste or feel pleasant. Therefore one has to be cautious when recommending dietary modifications or suppression of oral intake. Barium swallow and thickened water is not palatable and swallowing is highly dependent on cognitive sensory inputs, moreover, during FEES. The endoscope also slightly impairs physiological deglutition and breathing coordination.

The volumes used for testing should not be higher than 15 ml at a time, and we should consider 2.5 ml as a more physiological volume that resembles normal saliva reflex deglutition.

Other instrumental examinations of particular interest in NM diseases are:

Electrophysiological Studies

Electrophysiological studies have not widely been used in dysphagia but they can complement others in the diagnoses and follow-up. They can differentiate between myopathy and neuropathy and they will confirm muscle involvement even if the patient is asymptomatic. They also give an objective insight into the coordination of the different phases. Simultaneous dynamic studies from the different swallowing muscles: superior pharyngeal constrictors (SPC), TA, interarytenoid (IA), and CP can be recorded using hooked wired electrodes. The activity of the submandibular muscles (SM) tends to be recorded with bipolar surface electrodes. The upward and downward laryngeal movement seen on deglutition can be recorded with a piezoelectric sensor attached in the CP membrane. Different combinations of recordings can be done depending on the object of the study. An excellent review can be seen in [40].

The normal swallow starts with the contraction of the SM muscles followed by the SPC and the relaxation of the CP. During the CP relaxation period the TA and interarytenoid (IA) muscles contract. The CP activity reappears before the TA and IA relax again. The time sequence and coordination in between these muscles is essential in understanding the dysphagia events. The SM give important information of the onset and duration of the oropharyngeal swallowing since they elevate the larynx and initiate other reflexive mechanisms of the pharyngeal phase. They also support the tongue propulsion force. In neurologic dysphagic patients the SM EMG is prolonged, postulated to be related to muscle weakness, central effect or to a compensatory maneuver to overcome aspiration [41].

The CP muscle is important to study in neurogenic dysphagia. The approach can be either percutaneous or intraluminal. Percutaneously the electrode is introduced lateral and inferiorly to the posterior cricoid lamina. Intraluminally, the larynx can be topically anesthetized and the electrode is passed through the thyrocricoid membrane and advanced medially and inferiorly to the posterior cricoid lamina under endoscopic vision. The electrodes can also be introduced by direct laryngoscopy in an anesthetized patient. The CP muscle is tonically activated during rest and relaxes when swallowing with opposing phases to the other swallowing muscles [4, 42].

Ertekin has extensively described different electrophysiological tests to assess swallowing and its relationship to NM disorders [4, 41–45] (Table 17.5). Many tests could correlate to FEES or MBS ones but additional information is always obtained. We summarize the following concepts:

Table 17.5 Different electrodiagnostic tests in neuromuscular disorders

	Dysphagia limit	SM-EMG (surface electrodes)	Needle EMG	Laryngeal upward/ downward (piezoelectric transducer on cp membrane)	CP-EMG	Lack of coordination or abnormal opening timing
MG [41]	Decreased	Prolonged and decreased amplitude	Normal	Prolonged	Normal	Yes, due to slow transit, CP closes before
Muscle disorders [41]	Decreased	Prolonged	Myotonic MUAP	Abnormal	Hyperreflexive	Yes, due to slow transit, CP closes before
Corticobulbar: ALS and SBP, Parkinson plus [83]	Decreased	Prolonged	Denervation signs: fibrillation and positive sharp waves	Paretic	Hyperreflexive, abnormal burst in swallowing pause	Opening delayed with premature closure
Parkinson [43]	Decreased	Prolonged	Normal	Normal	Hyperreflexive/ normal	Yes, due to slow oral and pharyngeal transit, CP closes early

1. *Dysphagia limit.* It is the maximum volume of water that you can swallow at once. Any multiplication of the number of swallows called, *piecemeal deglutition,* below 20 ml is considered abnormal. It is tested by placing mechanical sensors in the cricothyroid membrane, and submental surface EMG electrodes taped under the chin. The recording of both sensors indicates the beginning of laryngeal elevation. Subjects are given 3, 5, 10, 15, and 20 ml in a stepwise manner stopping if piecemeal deglutition is observed. This test is very sensitive and specific for the diagnosis of dysphagia even in dysphagic patients unaware of their condition [41, 44].
2. *Laryngeal movement sensors integrated with surface SM-EMG* measures the coordination between the contraction of the SM and the laryngeal upward and downward movement. Different swallowing patterns of abnormalities have been observed in neurologic dysphagic patients.
3. *CP-EMG with simultaneous SM-EMG* analyzes the coordination between end of swallowing and CP relaxation, often abnormal in neurologic disorders such as late CP opening, premature closure, or abnormal bursts.
4. *Tonicity of the CP muscle* is also assessed. In this test, 3 ml of water is swallowed. According to the tonicity, hyperreflexic CP-EMG is the type of EMG abnormality mostly encountered in motor neuron diseases (ALS, suprabulbar palsy) due to corticobulbar involvement. This prevents any inhibitory influence on the UES. Dysphagia in these patients comes from the lack of coordination between the paretic laryngeal elevators and the hyperreflexive CP muscle. The CP-EMG pause tends to be shorter, ending prematurely before the larynx descends. Unexpected bursts of activity can occur during the swallowing pause. Therefore the bolus is retained in the pharyngeal spaces and penetration or aspiration can occur when the larynx finally descends [42].

In muscular disorders, laryngeal elevators are involved but the CP is structurally intact. Coordination though can be abnormal due to the slow pharynx transit that will find the CP closed when it can no longer compensate.

Parkinson patients will have similar findings but the CP muscle will not compensate the slow bolus transport. Debate has been found whereas the CP muscle is abnormal or not in PD. Controversy still surrounds CP tonicity and its meaning.

Manometry: High Resolution Manometry and Videofluoromanometry (VFM)

Manometry consists in recording a pressure inside a lumen. It provides quantitative evaluation of the pressures and relative timing involved between the pharyngeal contraction, UES relaxation, body of the esophagus contraction, and LES opening. It is useful for patients who may benefit from CP myotomy as it sensors the pressure of the UES when contracted, relaxed, and the time it takes. Solid state or sleeve transducers disseminated along a nasogastric catheter make these recordings possible.

High-resolution manometry uses catheters with numerous transducers along them that allow an instantaneous, tridimensional graph representing time, space, and pressure signals represented by a color scale. High-resolution manometry is of particular interest in demonstrating UES relaxation.

VFM consists of simultaneous recording of radiographic images and manometric data. The reasons why pioneers combined these two techniques are rather evident. Manometry alone in the pharyngoesophageal segment is difficult to interpret without concurrent X-ray.

Recently, Rommel et al. [46] integrated data recorded by high resolution VFM associated with impedancemetry in a mathematical formula that would infer the "aspiration risk."

To talk about "aspiration risk" rather than "aspiration events" detected at FEES or MBS is a new concept of utmost interest. Indeed, many aspiration diagnoses are done based on a couple of swallows assessed by FEES or MBS regardless of the circumstances the examination has been done. One can suspect there could be many false diagnoses. This is why talking about aspiration risk is, by far, a more robust way to assess the severity of dysphagia and thus the need for treatment [46, 47].

17.7 Neurolaryngological Diseases that Affect Deglutition

In general swallowing abnormalities are not very specific to a particular NM disorders and tend to affect multiple phases of deglutition in variable degrees and changing over time. Understanding the phase impaired and the detailed structures affected is key in planning for the best multidisciplinary treatment.

Table 17.6 summarizes the signs and symptoms of vocal and swallowing actions in NM disorders. More on the role of vocal fold immobility related to neurolaryngological diseases can be found in Chap. 6.

17.7.1 Stroke

17.7.1.1 Dysphagia in Supratentorial Stroke (Cortical and Subcortical)

Supratentorial Stroke (STS) can potentially impact all phases of swallowing. It can cause (a) *preswallow pooling* mostly produced by sensory deficit, delayed pharyngeal swallow and/or "linguo-pharyngeal discoordination" (called by some authors "apraxia of swallowing"), (b) *post-swallow residue* related to inadequate uplifting and anterior hyoid movement and/or poor pharyngeal motility and/or contralesional side pharyngeal hemiparesis, (c) *nasal redirection,* and (d) *laryngeal penetration/aspiration* as a consequence of the previously mentioned impairments.

17.7.1.2 Dysphagia in Brainstem Stroke (Lateral Medulla and Pontine Area)

The acute symptomatology of these patients is often dramatic. These are completely aphagic patients spitting their saliva into a container due to their inability to swallow.

In cases of sole Brainstem Stroke (BSS) lesions, cognition, language, and oral phase are intact. On the other hand, pure IX, X cranial nerve features such as a vocal fold palsy and/or unilateral pharyngeal hemiparesis are often seen.

Table 17.6 Signs and symptoms of vocal and swallowing signs of neuromuscular disorders

Site of lesion	Neurologic symptoms	Laryngeal findings	Vocal symptoms	Swallowing findings	Swallowing symptoms	Neurologic diseases
Upper motor neuron	Spastic paralysis Hyperreflexia Muscle weakness Slow movements	Spastic vocal fold paresis/paralysis	Strained voice, breathy voice, laryngospasm, breathing incoordination, spastic dysarthria, incoordination, altered prosody, low volume, slow speech, monotony, altered prosodic accent	Poor oral sling Increased time oral phase Reduced bolus propulsion Reduced pharyngeal constriction Insufficient larynx closure CP dysfunction Lack of coordination Decreased amplitude and precision movement	Dysphagia Silent aspiration Slow imprecise swallowing Drooling	Amyotrophic lateral sclerosis, progressive lateral sclerosis, pseudobulbar palsy CVA
Lower motor neuron	Flaccid paralysis Hyporeflexia Muscle atrophy Fasciculations	Flaccid vocal fold paresis/paralysis, glottic insufficiency In some cases, paradoxical vocal fold motion	Weak, breathy voice, rhinolalia, flaccid dysarthria, imprecise articulation	Poor oral sling Poor tongue movement and retraction Reduced pharyngeal constriction	Dysphagia Worse silent aspiration than UMN Nasal regurgitation Drooling	Amyotrophic lateral sclerosis, progressive bulbar palsy, spinal muscle atrophy
Extrapyramidal	Poor movement control, spasticity, tremor	Vocal fold bowing, tremor, dystonia, dysdiadochokinesia	Tremor, laryngeal dystonia, weak, breathy voice, monotone, Hypokinetic dysarthria	All the above Slow oral movements Discoordination	Dysphagia Oral phase discoordination Poor tongue retraction Silent aspiration	Parkinson, Spasmodic dysphonia, Laryngeal tremor

Peripheral nerve	Weakness, atrophy, sensory deficits	Paresis/paralysis	Weak, breathy voice, rhinolalia, dysphagia, aspirations, pitch abnormalities	LMN dysfunction	Aspiration due to glottic closure insufficiency	Vagal nerve, SLN, RLN injury, intensive care polyneuritis, Guillain–Barré syndrome, post poliomyelitis syndrome
Inflammatory myopathies	Weakness affecting some muscular groups	Motion impairment	Breathy voice, impairments largely depending on the muscular groups that are involved	Weakness affecting both larynx elevation musculature and pharynx musculature	Pharyngeal clearance deficit, secondary aspirations	Dermatopolymyositis, polymyositis, inclusion body myositis
Muscular dystrophy	Weakness of muscles affected	Articulation problems in relation to facial and tongue musculature involvement	Open rhinolalia, lack of voice projection, hypotonia	Weakness affecting both larynx elevation musculature and pharynx musculature	Pharyngeal clearance deficit, secondary aspirations	Duchêne's dystrophy, oculopharyngeal dystrophy, facioscapulo humeral dystrophies, myotonic dystrophy (Steinert's disease)
Neuromuscular junction disorder	Fatigability	Fluctuating paresis/paralysis	Weak, breathy voice, dysarthria, vocal fatigue, Open rhinolalia	Poor oral sling Insufficient velar closure Increased oral phase Reduced bolus propulsion Reduced pharyngeal constriction Insufficient larynx closure CP dysfunction Worsens with use	Slow oral phase Pharyngeal propulsion deficit Worsens with use	Myasthenia

This dramatic initial presentation, along with the long recovery that will follow, contrasts with the ease of rehabilitation, as they have: intact sensation and cognition impressive initial presentation along with the long recovery that will follow, contrasts with the ease of rehabilitation with such, sensation intact, cognition intact, full coping cohorts of patients [48–50].

17.7.2 Parkinson Disease (PD)

Parkinson disease (PD) is an α-synuclein protein accumulation disease leading to Lewis corpus accumulation and eventually cell apoptosis within the substantia nigra. The result of this lack of striatal dopamine translates into a combination of somewhat contradictory motion disorders such as tremor and rigidity.

Dysphagia in PD is mostly multifactorial. Orality will be impaired by cognitive impairment, head and neck posture, jaw and lips rigidity leading to drooling and impaired lingual transfer at a late stage.

Review sentence between the two phases a swallowing, hesitation or pause—comparable to the lingual ataxia of dementia patients—can also be seen.

The pharyngoesophageal transfer will be impaired by pharyngeal constrictor muscle rigidity and a lack of upper esophageal sphincter relaxation, combining thus a propulsive and a resistive dysfunction at the same time.

17.7.3 Parkinson Plus: Multiple System Atrophy and Progressive Supranuclear Palsy

Parkinson plus (PD+) diseases mimic the extrapyramidal signs of PD but are completely resistant to dopamine treatments. They are both the consequence of a protein accumulation leading to cell apoptosis. Their symptomatology will depend on the anatomical site where apoptosis occurs. *Parkinsonism*, on the other hand, refers to other diseases such as chronic vascular brain or neuroleptic intoxication that mimics PD symptomatology, by blocking the dopa receptors and not by accumulating protein intracellularly.

17.7.3.1 Multiple System Atrophy (MSA)

Exactly like PD, the protein that is accumulated is the α-synuclein. The accumulation occurs in other nuclei and loci such as the vagus nerve nuclei or the cerebellum. Depending on the location of the apoptosis, some patients will develop Parkinson features (MSA-P) or Cerebellar features (MSA-C) [51].

17.7.3.2 Progressive Supranuclear Palsy (PSP)

Unlike PD, the protein accumulated is the protein TAU (like in Alzheimer's disease). As the name of the disease tells us, the deposit of proteins affects supranuclear loci mainly cortical ones.

Again, symptomatology will depend on the sites that are affected [52].

Table 17.7 summarized the differences between MSA and PSP.

17.7.4 Myasthenia Gravis (MG)

Myasthenia gravis is an autoimmune disease that creates acetylcholine post-synaptic receptor antibodies (AChR Ab) that reduces muscle-activating activity and eventually causes muscular fatigue. It affects bulbar musculature causing dysarthria and dysphagia. Every muscle that comes into play in swallowing can potentially be affected and will determine the clinical presentation. Confirmation diagnosis can be obtained by electrophysiological studies such us repetitive nerve stimulation and single fiber EMG, after ruling out neuropathies and myopathies by EMG. AChR Ab and acetylcholinesterase antibody (AChE Ab) tend to be positive in generalized myasthenia but are less likely to have abnormal results in the pharyngolaryngeal forms. Tensilon test (intravenous injection of the acetylcholinesterase inhibitor, edrophonium chloride) is not specific for myasthenia, but it could support the diagnosis along with the neurophysiological studies [53, 54]. The subjective response considered positive is an improvement in the quality of swallowing because of the immediate increase in muscle strength [55].

Edrophonium is given in a gradually incremental dose starting with 2 mg intravenously. If after 2 min no clear response develops, up to 8 additional mg could be injected. The response will last no longer than 5 min. The test could be started with a placebo of 2 ml of saline. Care must be taken for cholinergic effects, such as bradycardia and atropine has to be available in case they occur.

Table 17.7 Swallowing maneuvers, tested when performing FEEST of MBS or rehabilitation

Postural techniques	Type of dysfunction	Reasoning	Literature
Head back	Inefficient oral transit (reduced posterior propulsion of bolus by tongue)	Utilizes gravity to clear oral cavity	
Chin down The patient approximates the chin to the chest when swallowing. This causes posterior displacement of the tongue and epiglottis and a narrowing in the pharynx, making the space smaller and more difficult to aspirate. Therefore less effort is needed to swallow. Adequate for patients with poor tongue movement and aspiration problems	Delays in triggering the pharyngeal swallow (bolus passed ramus of mandible, but pharyngeal swallow not triggered)	1. Widens vallecula to prevent bolus entering airway: narrows airway entrance; pushes epiglottis posteriorly	Shanahan et al. (1993) [84]
Chin tuck	Reduced posterior motion of tongue base (residue in vallecula)	Pushes tongue base backwards towards pharyngeal wall	
Head rotated to weaker side (with or without chin down for more airway protection) The patient is instructed to turn his head to the paralyzed laryngopharynx before swallowing. This increases the opening of the nonaffected UES	1. Unilateral laryngeal dysfunction (aspiration during swallow) 2. Unilateral pharyngeal paresis (residue on one side of pharynx) 3. Cricopharyngeal dysfunction (residue in pyriform sinus)	1. Places extrinsic pressure on thyroid cartilage, increasing adduction 2. Eliminates damage side from bolus path 3. Pulls cricoid cartilage away from posterior pharyngeal wall, reducing resting pressure in CP sphincter	Logemann et al. (1989) [85] and Tsukamoto (2000) [86]
Head tilt to stronger side The patient tilts his head to the paralyzed pharyngolarynx to help the bolus come down to that side aid by gravity	Unilateral oral and pharyngeal weakness on the same side (residue in mouth and pharynx on the same side)	Directs bolus down to stronger side	Logemann (1983)
Lying down on one side This bypasses laryngeal introitus. It is indicated in aspiration, when bilateral pharyngeal impairment or when reduced laryngeal elevation	Reduces pharyngeal contraction (residue spread throughout pharynx)	Eliminates gravitational effect on pharyngeal residue	

(continued)

Table 17.7 (continued)

Postural techniques	Type of dysfunction	Reasoning	Literature
Compensatory maneuvers			
Supraglottic swallow: The patients are instructed to breathe in voluntarily and hold their breath just before forcefully swallowing and are asked to cough immediately. That produces a Valsalva and closure of the vocal folds. Effortful cough follows. Useful when there is a reduced vocal fold closure due to paresis, paralysis, or late vocal fold closure	Reduced or late vocal fold closure Delayed pharyngeal swallow	1. Voluntary breath hold usually closes vocal folds before and during swallow	Martin et al. (1993) [87], Ohmae et al. (1996) [88], and Hirst et al. (1998) [89]
Super Supraglottic swallow: The patient is instructed to hold his breath after effortful breathing in, before and during swallow. This also tilts arytenoids forward, closing the airway. Effortful cough follows	Reduced closure of airway entrance	Effortful breath pulls arytenoid forward, closing airway entrance before and during swallow	Martin et al. (1993) [87]
Effortful swallow Implies a volitional greater effort when swallowing and greater posterior tongue base movement. Useful for patients with weaker or less organized swallowing function	Reduced posterior movement of tongue base	Effort increased posterior tongue base movement	Pouderoux and Kahrilas (1995) [90], Lazarus et al. (2002) [91], and Huckabee et al. (2005) [92]
Mendelson maneuver Designed to increase the opening duration of the UES by increasing the duration of laryngeal elevation. The patient is instructed to consciously maintain elevated the larynx before swallowing. Indicated for poor hyolaryngeal elevation and poor pharyngeal clearance	1. Reduced laryngeal movement 2. Discoordinated swallow	1. Laryngeal movement opens the upper esophageal sphincter (UES); prolonging laryngeal elevation prolongs UES opening 2. Normalizes timing o pharyngeal swallow events	1. Cook et al. (1989), Jocob et al. (1989), and Bryant (1991) 2. Lazarus, Logemann Gibbons (1993) [93]

17.7.5 Inflammatory Myopathies (IM)

IM are autoimmune diseases that create inflammation and destruction of the striated muscle. There are three different types of IM: Polymyositis, dermatomysositis, and inclusion body myositis.

Polymyositis and dermatomyositis (the latest affecting also the skin causing a bluish-purple rash) tend to develop acute dysphagia crisis that usually respond well to treatment.

Treatment can be tedious and long though, requiring in half of the cases an alternative feeding strategy for a couple of months.

On the other hand, inclusion body myositis is a slow and relentlessly progressive muscle weakness that does not respond to therapy.

17.7.6 Muscular dystrophies

17.7.6.1 Myotonic dystrophy

Type One Myotonic Dystrophy (MD)—the most frequent—or Steiner's disease is an autosomal dominant disease characterized by a CTG triplet repetition on the dystrophia myotonic-protein kinase (DMPK) gene of chromosome 19q. The severity of MD is proportional to the number of CTG repetition in nuclear DNA of the muscular cells. It is important to know that this number of triplet's repetition can vary from one muscle to another.

Myotonia is a consequence of abnormal electrical activity in muscle cells membrane, caused by a dysfunction in ion channel. Myotonia leads to degeneration of muscle cells and replacement by nonmuscular tissue, mainly fat and connective tissue.

MD represents a typical propulsive issue caused by an important weakness of the pharyngeal constrictor and the striated muscle of the upper third of the esophagus. Later on, a resistive issue comes into play by weakness of the suprahyoid musculature reducing the excursion of the hyolaryngeal complex and thus the passive opening of the UES. MD patients due to the cognitive aspects of their disease often underestimate the severity of the OPD, the aspiration in particular.

17.7.6.2 Duchenne's Dystrophy

Duchenne's dystrophy (DM) is a chromosome X-linked recessive disease characterized by a mutation of gene DMD. This genetic modification stops the production of dystrophine and causes proximal limb and respiratory muscle weakness. Dysphagia is more related to decrease of pulmonary function and to inappropriate cephalic posture than to a direct involvement of the swallowing musculature.

17.7.6.3 Oculo-Pharyngeal Dystrophy

Oculo-pharyngeal dystrophy (OPD) is a genetic disease that can be either autosomal (frequent) or recessive (rare), caused by expansion of a GCG triplet of gene PABPN1 on chromosome 14q. The disease characterized by muscular death of (a) the levator palpebrae superioralis causing ptosis and (b) the pharyngeal constrictor and later the tongue muscles causing a lack of bolus propulsion. Later in the natural history of the disease, a UES lack of relaxation can also be seen.

17.7.6.4 Fascioscapulohumeral Dystrophy

Fascioscapulohumeral dystrophy (FSHD) is a slowly progressive autosomal-dominant disease affecting mostly the trapezius muscle and the upper limbs. FSHD patients can also present high frequency deafness. Dysphagia by pharyngeal involvement only concerns approximately 10% of FSHD patients [56, 57].

17.7.7 Motor Neuron Disease: Amyotrophic Lateral Sclerosis (ALS), Progresive Bulbar Palsy (PBP) and Progressive Muscular Atrophy (PMA)

Motor neuron diseases can affect the upper motor neurons (UMN), the lower motor neurons or both (LMN). In case of UMN disease there is a degeneration of motor cortex cells called Betz cells as well as the corticospinal tracts. In case of LMN disease, degeneration concerns the anterior horn cells in the spinal cord for limb symptoms and the brainstem nuclei in the pons and medulla for cranial nerves V, VII, IX, X, and XII for bulbar for swallowing symptoms, Fig. 17.2.

The symptoms of exclusive LMN disease will be muscular weakness, atrophy, fasciculations and diminished reflexes whether the symptoms of exclusive UMN disease will be muscular stiffness and spasticity, slowness of movement, hypertonia, and limb hyperreflexia (Table 17.6).

This is why the clinical expression of motor neuron diseases can be so heterogeneous, mixing coordination, oral stage, propulsive and resistive clinical features.

The classic *ALS* involves both types of motor neurons (UMN and LMN) mixing both symptomatology.

All classical ALS patients will present bulbar signs at the time of their death.

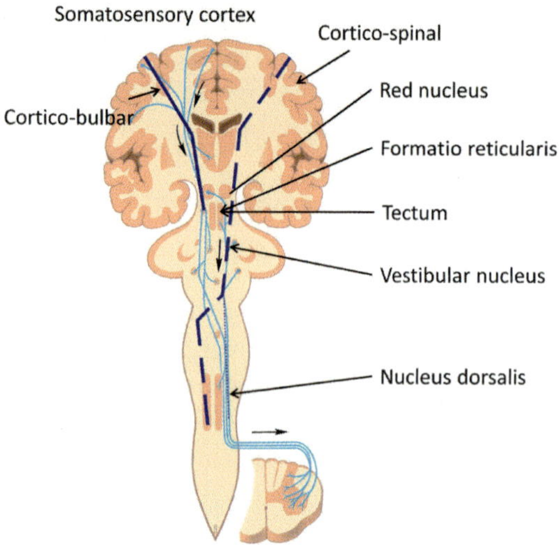

Fig. 17.2 Upper and lower motor neuron pathways

There is a variant of ALS called primary lateral sclerosis (*PLS*) showing exclusively UMN signs, where classical ALS patients have an average survival of about 4 years, PLS patients can survive for decades.

The *PBP* involves mostly UMN and has an exclusive bulbar clinical expression. The median survival of PBP patients is about 2–3 years.

The *PMA* involves LMN and has almost exclusive limb symptoms. Some rare PMA patients may present bulbar features. Their survival rate is somewhere between the ALS and the PLS patients.

17.7.8 Postpolio Syndrome

Poliomyelitis survivors can present a recurrence of dysphagia symptoms decades after being cured. Although the mechanisms of this "reactivation" are still unclear some studies have shown a slowly progressive deterioration of bulbar neurons that may or may not have been involved in the primo-infection.

17.8 Treatments for Dysphagia in Neurolaryngological Diseases

The goals of dysphagia treatment efforts are (a) to improve or to maintain bolus oropharyngeal transfer and (b) to prevent aspiration.

Treatment modalities that have to be considered:

- *Alternative feeding modalities.* The decision of oral or nonoral diet will depend on the amount of time necessary to complete meals, the risk and severity of the aspiration, the nutritional and medical state of the patient, and the possibility of rehabilitation. When efficiency or safety standards are not met, oral intake should be discontinued and replaced by either a nasogastric feeding tube, percutaneous gastrostomy, jejunostomy or central line feeding permanently or temporarily.
- *Volume and viscosity modification of bolus and vigilance (the three Vs).*
  - Vigilance. Meals should be administered during times of maximal attentiveness. Assistance by caretaker is necessary.
  - Volume change. When the volume is small (1–3 ml), oral and pharyngeal phase occur separately, whereas if the bolus is big (10–20 ml) they occur simultaneously [58–60]. Volume should be increased if there are oral sensitivity deficits to stimulate proprioception and facilitate swallowing reflex. Volumes should be decreased if there are manipulation or propulsion issues
  - Viscosity. In general thin liquids are easier to swallow since they offer less resistance to flow, but they are difficult to manage when due to an issue with bolus control, early spillage over tongue base could be aspirated in an unprepared open larynx. In these cases increase in viscosity helps the bolus goes slower allowing the patient to cope with oral and pharyngeal discoordination. Thin liquids would only be advocated in cases of reduced pharyngoesophageal lumen size. Carbonated liquids improve sensation. Thermal or gustatory stimulation facilitates swallow response [27]
- *Rehabilitation techniques* [27]. They require patient collaboration.

1. Specific exercises of the tongue, pharynx, palate, and larynx can improve specific functional impairments.

2. Swallowing maneuvers, delivered by speech-language pathologists. These maneuvers can be tested when performing FEEST of MBA, Table 17.7.
3. McNeill Dysphagia Therapy, [61].

   As mentioned by their discovers G. Carnaby-Mann and M. Crary: "the McNeill Dysphagia therapy Program" focuses on progressive strengthening and coordination of swallowing in the context of functional swallow activities and the development of movement patterns of the coordination of the muscular components of the swallowing process."

   It consists in an intensive "swallowing drill" that increases demands on the system by progressive increasing resistive forces and alterations in velocity of movement. The "load" that increases the swallowing effort consists in volume, texture, and swallow frequencies modifications.

   The benefit of this systematic approach has been clearly demonstrated in one of the few well-conducted case–control studies published in swallowing therapy literature. Physiotherapy (pulmonary, upper limb, and posture)
4. Physiotherapists have a specific role in OPD. Each oral feeding rehabilitation effort presents risk of aspiration. Physiotherapy has three essential goals, (a) improve the global tone and head posture, (b) improve the tolerance of apnea during swallowing and eventually (c) improve cough efficiency.

- *Disease specific medications*
  - L-Dopa for PD

    L-Dopa constitutes a very efficient treatment on extrapyramidal symptoms of PD. On the other hand, oropharyngeal dysfunction responds very little to L Dopa.

    Dopaminergic medication has no action on PD+ diseases.

    Likewise, deep brain stimulation of the nucleus sub-thalamicus not only does not improve OPD but rather aggravates the symptomatology [62].
  - Pyridostygmine (Mestinon®) and other treatments of myasthenia gravis.

    Pyridostygmine (from 30 mg to 120 mg) increases Ach availability and improves neuromuscular conduction. The time to optimal effect varies from 30 to 90 min. The co-stimulation of muscarinic Ach receptors can cause trachea-bronchial hyper-secretions. That represents an important negative side effect in a dysphagic population.

    Prednisone (5–100 mg/day) and Azathioprine (Imuran®)(max 2–3 mg/Kg/day) are also used in cases of Mestinon® inefficacity.

    Cyclosporine (2–3 mg/kg/day) and plasmapheresis can also be tried.

    Immunoglobulin IV treatment will be reserved for refractory cases.
  - Immunomodulatory drugs for myopathies

    Inflammatory myositis has no known cure yet. A lot of medications, under specialized supervision, can help control the symptoms including OPD:

    Prednisone, hydroxychloroquine, azathioprine, immunoglobulin IV, cyclophosphamide, an immunosuppressive drug such as tacrolimus, an α-TNF (anti-α tumor necrosis factor) such as Infliximab®, or a chimeric monoclonal antibody against protein CD-20 such as Rituximab®
  - Botulinum toxin

    Botulinum toxin (Botox®, Dysport®) injections are used in two different situations: (a) to release and UES tension or (b) to paralyze salivary glands muscles. These treatments can be successful but present the disadvantage to worsening OPD in case of involuntary diffusion outside the muscle that was targeted. Besides, to be effective, botulinum toxin injection has to be injected in healthy muscle. In many aged patients the cricopharyngeal muscle is rather fibrotic or affected by the disease itself [63].
  - Specific drugs that could facilitate swallowing

    Substance P

    Substance P is the neurotransmitters of the pharyngeal plexus that facilitates swallowing and protective coughing [64].

    Angiotensin Converting Enzyme inhibitor (ACEi)

    It is hypothesized that the inhibition in the cyclooxygenase pathways results in an increased production of Substance P. ACEi

would through this mechanism enhance the swallow [65, 66].
Capsaicin
This molecule, found in chillies and other vegetables, would enhance the pharyngeal phase triggering and lower the cough reflex threshold [67].

- *Surgeries*
- **Airway protective surgeries**
  - *Tracheotomies*
    It is by far the first step surgery proposed for intractable aspirations. It has the advantage to be reversible. It eases pulmonary function by reducing the upper airways dead space and by offering an easy access to the trachea for intratracheal aspiration.
    Airways sealing and protection is not perfect though, and the puncturing of the anterior wall of the trachea impedes a proper uplifting of the larynx during the pharyngeal phase.
    This is why tracheotomy is not considered as a gold standard permanent treatment for intractable aspirations but rather a provisional one [68, 69].
  - *Injection or solid implants laryngoplasties*
    In case of vocal fold palsy creating a glottis leak, glottis closure can be obtained by paraglottic volume expansion on the palsy side. The procedure will not only enhance airways sealing during swallow but will also largely improve cough efficiency. There is a consensus to prioritize a transoral or transcutaneous implant injection for small leaks (phonatory quotient ≤300 ml/sec) and to conduct a type 1 thyroplasty under sedation for large gaps (phonatory quotient ≥300 ml/sec), [70, 71].
  - *Laryngopexies*
    Laryngopexy is a procedure that tends to put the larynx in a permanent pharyngeal phase position by fixing it cranially and anteriorly to the mandible. Strap muscle inferior section can be necessary in case of (post-radiotherapy) fibrosis.
    A myotomy of the cricopharyngeal muscle is often performed during the same procedure [72].
  - *Salivary glands surgery*
    Bilateral submandibular salivary gland excision may be proposed when excessive drooling and/or dangerous salivary pooling is observed. It can be associated with laryngopexy in case of tedious salivary clearance.
  - *Laryngeal plugs devices*
    Many "plugs" to laryngotracheal lumen in order to seal the airways have been proposed. One can divide them into the "closed-trachea devices" presenting a valve system allowing mouth breathing (Larynxane ST®, Protip ®Strasbourg, France) [73] and the "open-trachea devices" necessitating a tracheostomy and primarily utilized in laryngotracheoplasties (Montgomery T-tube, Monnier's tube, Aboulker tube, etc.)
  - *Glottoplasties/epiglottoplasties*
    These procedures consist in the closure of the laryngeal introitus whether by suturing the vocal folds or fixing the epiglottis edges on the laryngeal vestibule.
    Poor voice outcomes and lack of water tightness of the laryngeal vestibule are the main reasons why these procedures are not performed anymore. Functional laryngectomy associated with vocal prosthesis placement is, by far, the best procedure for tracheal sealing [74].
  - *Tracheal diversion*
    This procedure consists in the section of the subglottic trachea, the upper edge and the lower edge of the section being further connected independently to the skin. Again, the loss of voicing and healing issues outdated a bit this procedure.
  - *Functional laryngectomy*
    As mentioned before functional laryngectomy, whether or not associated with the placement of a vocal prosthesis, represents the gold standard procedure for intractable aspiration. Indication should be balanced

with vital prognosis and patient functional wishes.

- **Resistance release surgeries**
  - *Cricopharyngeal myotomy CPM/UES dilatation*

    Cricopharyngeal myotomy represents the gold standard treatment for UES resistive problems. It can be performed endoscopically with a CO2 laser or by open lateral cervicotomy [75]. Both techniques offer good results. Whether one or the other technique should be promoted is still debated [76–78]. It appears though that the choice of myotomy technique is less important than the two preoperative considerations that will follow:

    There is simply no point to perform myotomy if no residual pharyngeal propulsion is noted at manometry or MBS. Even if the resistive issue is withdrawn, no bolus will go through the UES without any propulsive force. A residual propulsive force in the pharynx seems to be enough according to Kos et al. [79]. Adequate laryngeal/hyoid elevation has to be intact as well. A videofluoroscopic obstruction at the CP level has to be demonstrated as well as elevated UES pressure in manometry. Intact voluntary initiation of swallowing and good neurologic prognosis is necessary.

    Surgeons planning a CPM should pay attention to the lower esophageal compartment. In case of esophageal dysmotility or important hiatal hernia, the UES plays an important role in airways protection by contracting in case of massive bolus reflux.

In that regard, UES dilatation by "bouginage" or balloon dilatation has the great advantage to respect the muscle integrity and thus keeping its airways protective prerogatives.

- *UES protractor*

  P. Belafsky introduced recently a surgical concept of utmost originality. Instead of cutting the CP, he proposed a device, anchored to the cricoid cartilage that allows passive opening of the UES by moving the cricoid anteriorly. This elegant method, respecting the muscular integrity of the UES and mimicking the physiology of swallowing is still experimental. The good cognitive status and limb dexterity that this type of device requires may represent an important hurdle [80].

- *Pharyngeal stimulation and neuroplasticity*

  Hamdy et al. [9] showed in various articles that pharyngeal stimulation could foster cortical neuroplasticity and thus improve swallowing function recovery after stroke [81, 82].The device consists in electric stimulators that are disseminated along a nasogastric tube. A prospective multicentric study is ongoing.

References

1. Reychler G, Roeseler J, Delguste P. Kinésithérapie respiratoire. 3rd ed. Issy-les-Moulineaux: Elsevier Masson; 2014.
2. Massey BT, Shaker R. Oral, pharyngeal and upper esophageal sphincter motility disorders. GI Motil Online. 2006.
3. McConnel FM, Cerenko D, Jackson RT, Guffin TN. Timing of major events of pharyngeal swallowing. Arch Otolaryngol Head Neck Surg. 1988;114:1413–8.
4. Ertekin C, Palmer JB. Physiology and electromyography of swallowing and its disorders. Suppl Clin Neurophysiol. 2000;53:148–54.
5. McConnel FM, Cerenko D, Jackson RT, Hersh T. Clinical application of the manofluorogram. Laryngoscope. 1988;98:705–11.
6. Desuter G, Beguin C, Piessevaux H, Goncette L, Van Parijs V, Van den Bergh P. Physiologic variables for videofluoromanometric assessment of dysphagia: an exploratory study. Acta Gastro-Enterol Belg. 2009;72:312–20.
7. Jean A. Brain stem control of swallowing: neuronal network and cellular mechanisms. Physiol Rev. 2001;81(2):929–69.
8. Hamdy S. The organisation and re-organisation of human swallowing motor cortex. Suppl Clin Neurophysiol. 2003;56:204–10.
9. Hamdy S, Aziz Q, Rothwell JC, Singh KD, Barlow J, Hughes DG, Tallis RC, Thompson DG. The cortical topography of human swallowing musculature in health and disease. Nat Med. 1996;2:1217–24.
10. Ertekin C, Aydogdu I. Neurophysiology of swallowing. Clin Neurophysiol. 2003;114:2226–44.
11. Aviv JE, Martin JH, Kim T, Sacco RL, Thomson JE, Diamond B, Close LG. Laryngopharyngeal sensory

discrimination testing and the laryngeal adductor reflex. Ann Otol Rhinol Laryngol. 1999;108:725–30.
12. Sinclair WJ. Role of the pharyngeal plexus in initiation of swallowing. Am J Phys. 1971;221:1260–3.
13. Kim YH, Sasaki CT. Glottic closing force in an anesthetized, awake pig model: biomechanical effects on the laryngeal closure reflex resulting from altered central facilitation. Acta Otolaryngol. 2001;121:310–4.
14. Leonard R, Kendall K, McKenzie S. UES opening and cricopharyngeal bar in nondysphagic elderly and nonelderly adults. Dysphagia. 2004;19:182–91.
15. Logemann JA, Pauloski BR, Rademaker AW, Colangelo LA, Kahrilas PJ, Smith CH. Temporal and biomechanical characteristics of oropharyngeal swallow in younger and older men. J Speech Lang Hear Res JSLHR. 2000;43:1264–74.
16. Shaker R, Lang IM. Effect of aging on the deglutitive oral, pharyngeal, and esophageal motor function. Dysphagia. 1994;9:221–8.
17. Antonios N, Carnaby-Mann G, Crary M, Miller L, Hubbard H, Hood K, Sambandam R, Xavier A, Silliman S. Analysis of a physician tool for evaluating dysphagia on an inpatient stroke unit: the modified mann assessment of swallowing ability. J Stroke Cerebrovasc Dis. 2010;19:49–57.
18. Belafsky PC, Mouadeb DA, Rees CJ, Pryor JC, Postma GN, Allen J, Leonard RJ. Validity and reliability of the eating assessment tool (EAT-10). Ann Otol Rhinol Laryngol. 2008;117:919–24.
19. Carnaby-Mann G, Lenius K. The bedside examination in dysphagia. Phys Med Rehabil Clin N Am. 2008;19:747–68. viii
20. Clavé P, Arreola V, Romea M, Medina L, Palomera E, Serra-Prat M. Accuracy of the volume-viscosity swallow test for clinical screening of oropharyngeal dysphagia and aspiration. Clin Nutr Edinb Scotl. 2008;27:806–15.
21. Leder SB, Suiter DM, Warner HL, Acton LM, Siegel MD. Safe initiation of oral diets in hospitalized patients based on passing a 3-ounce (90 cc) water swallow challenge protocol. QJM Mon J Assoc Physicians. 2012;105:257–63.
22. Leder SB, Suiter DM, Warner HL, Acton LM, Swainson BA. Success of recommending oral diets in acute stroke patients based on passing a 90-cc water swallow challenge protocol. Top Stroke Rehabil. 2012;19:40–4.
23. Logemann JA. Screening, diagnosis, and management of neurogenic dysphagia. Semin Neurol. 1996;16:319–27.
24. Martino R, Maki E, Diamant N. Identification of dysphagia using the Toronto bedside swallowing screening test (TOR-BSST©): are 10 teaspoons of water necessary? Int J Speech Lang Pathol. 2014;16:193–8.
25. Martino R, Silver F, Teasell R, Bayley M, Nicholson G, Streiner DL, Diamant NE. The Toronto bedside swallowing screening test (TOR-BSST): development and validation of a dysphagia screening tool for patients with stroke. Stroke J Cereb Circ. 2009;40:555–61.
26. Suiter DM, Leder SB, Karas DE. The 3-ounce (90-cc) water swallow challenge: a screening test for children with suspected oropharyngeal dysphagia. Otolaryngol Head Neck Surg. 2009;140:187–90.
27. Logemann JA. Evaluation and treatment of swallowing disorders. 2nd ed. Austin, Tex: Pro-Ed Australia; 1997.
28. Langmore SE. Endoscopic evaluation and treatment of swallowing disorders. New York: Thieme Medical Publishers; 2000.
29. Langmore SE. Endoscopic evaluation of oral and pharyngeal phases of swallowing. GI Motil Online. 2006.
30. Langmore SE, Schatz K, Olsen N. Fiberoptic endoscopic examination of swallowing safety: a new procedure. Dysphagia. 1988;2:216–9.
31. Aviv JE, Martin JH, Keen MS, Debell M, Blitzer A. Air pulse quantification of supraglottic and pharyngeal sensation: a new technique. Ann Otol Rhinol Laryngol. 1993;102:777–80.
32. Bastian RW. Videoendoscopic evaluation of patients with dysphagia: an adjunct to the modified barium swallow. Otolaryngol Head Neck Surg. 1991;104:339–50.
33. Fuller SC, Leonard R, Aminpour S, Belafsky PC. Validation of the pharyngeal squeeze maneuver. Otolaryngol Head Neck Surg. 2009;140:391–4.
34. Leonard R, Belafsky PC, Rees CJ. Relationship between fluoroscopic and manometric measures of pharyngeal constriction: the pharyngeal constriction ratio. Ann Otol Rhinol Laryngol. 2006;115: 897–901.
35. Aviv JE, Murry T, Zschommler A, Cohen M, Gartner C. Flexible endoscopic evaluation of swallowing with sensory testing: patient characteristics and analysis of safety in 1,340 consecutive examinations. Ann Otol Rhinol Laryngol. 2005;114:173–6.
36. Logemann JA. Manual for the videofluorographic study of swallowing. Austin, Tex: Pro-ed; 1993.
37. Rosenbek JC, Robbins JA, Roecker EB, Coyle JL, Wood JL. A penetration-aspiration scale. Dysphagia. 1996;11:93–8.
38. Barbiera F, Condello S, De Palo A, Todaro D, Mandracchia C, De Cicco D. Role of videofluorography swallow study in management of dysphagia in neurologically compromised patients. Radiol Med. 2006;111:818–27.
39. Waxman MJ, Durfee D, Moore M, Morantz RA, Koller W. Nutritional aspects and swallowing function of patients with Parkinson's disease. Nutr Clin Pract. 1990;5:196–9.
40. Perlman AL. Electromyography in oral and pharyngeal motor disorders. GI Motil Online. 2006.
41. Ertekin C, Aydogdu I, Yüceyar N, Tarlaci S, Kiylioglu N, Pehlivan M, Celebi G. Electrodiagnostic methods for neurogenic dysphagia. Electroencephalogr Clin Neurophysiol. 1998;109:331–40.
42. Ertekin C, Aydogdu I. Electromyography of human cricopharyngeal muscle of the upper esophageal sphincter. Muscle Nerve. 2002;26:729–39.

43. Ertekin C. Electrophysiological evaluation of oropharyngeal dysphagia in Parkinson's disease. J Mov Disord. 2014;7:31–56.
44. Ertekin C, Aydoğdu I, Yüceyar N. Piecemeal deglutition and dysphagia limit in normal subjects and in patients with swallowing disorders. J Neurol Neurosurg Psychiatry. 1996;61:491–6.
45. Ertekin C, Pehlivan M, Aydoğdu I, Ertaş M, Uludağ B, Celebi G, Colakoğlu Z, Sağduyu A, Yüceyar N. An electrophysiological investigation of deglutition in man. Muscle Nerve. 1995;18:1177–86.
46. Rommel N, Denys S, Liesenborghs C, Scheerens C, Selleslagh M, Goeleven A, Vanbeckevoort D, Omari T, Tack J, Dejaeger E. Automatische Impedantie Manometrie (AIM): objectieve diagnostiek van oro-faryngale dysfagie. Tijdschr Gerontol Geriatr. 2014;45:290–9.
47. Omari T, Tack J, Rommel N. Impedance as an adjunct to manometric testing to investigate symptoms of dysphagia: what it has failed to do and what it may tell us in the future. United European Gastroenterol J. 2014;2:355–66.
48. Cola MG, Daniels SK, Corey DM, Lemen LC, Romero M, Foundas AL. Relevance of subcortical stroke in dysphagia. Stroke J Cereb Circ. 2010;41:482–6.
49. Daniels SK, Schroeder MF, DeGeorge PC, Corey DM, Foundas AL, Rosenbek JC. Defining and measuring dysphagia following stroke. Am J Speech-Lang Pathol. 2009;18:74–81.
50. González-Fernández M, Daniels SK. Dysphagia in stroke and neurologic disease. Phys Med Rehabil Clin N Am. 2008;19:867–88. x
51. Stefanova N, Bücke P, Duerr S, Wenning GK. Multiple system atrophy: an update. Lancet Neurol. 2009;8:1172–8.
52. Williams DR, Lees AJ. Progressive supranuclear palsy: clinicopathological concepts and diagnostic challenges. Lancet Neurol. 2009;8:270–9.
53. Daroff RB, Mazziotta JC. Neurology in clinical practice. 6th ed. Philadelphia: Saunders; 2012.
54. Pevzner A, Schoser B, Peters K, Cosma N-C, Karakatsani A, Schalke B, Melms A, Kröger S. Anti-LRP4 autoantibodies in AChR- and MuSK-antibody-negative myasthenia gravis. J Neurol. 2012;259:427–35.
55. Sataloff RT, Mandel S, Heman-Ackah YD, Abaza M. Laryngeal electromyography. 2nd ed. San Diego, CA: Plural Publishing, Inc.; 2005.
56. Pilz W, Baijens LWJ, Kremer B. Oropharyngeal dysphagia in myotonic dystrophy type 1: a systematic review. Dysphagia. 2014;29:319–31.
57. Trollet C, Gidaro T, Klein P, Périé S, Butler-Browne G, Lacau St Guily J. Oculopharyngeal muscular dystrophy. In: Pagon RA, Adam MP, Ardinger HH, Bird TD, Dolan CR, Fong C-T, Smith RJ, Stephens K, editors. Genereviews(®). Seattle (WA): University of Washington; 1993.
58. Kahrilas PJ, Lin S, Chen J, Logemann JA. Oropharyngeal accommodation to swallow volume. Gastroenterology. 1996;111:297–306.
59. Kahrilas PJ, Lin S, Logemann JA, Ergun GA, Facchini F. Deglutitive tongue action: volume accommodation and bolus propulsion. Gastroenterology. 1993;104:152–62.
60. Shaker R, Ren J, Podvrsan B, Dodds WJ, Hogan WJ, Kern M, Hoffmann R, Hintz J. Effect of aging and bolus variables on pharyngeal and upper esophageal sphincter motor function. Am J Phys. 1993;264:G427–32.
61. Carnaby-Mann GD, Crary MA. McNeill dysphagia therapy program: a case-control study. Arch Phys Med Rehabil. 2010;91:743–9.
62. Baijens LWJ, Speyer R. Effects of therapy for dysphagia in Parkinson's disease: systematic review. Dysphagia. 2009;24:91–102.
63. Kelly EA, Koszewski IJ, Jaradeh SS, Merati AL, Blumin JH, Bock JM. Botulinum toxin injection for the treatment of upper esophageal sphincter dysfunction. Ann Otol Rhinol Laryngol. 2013;122:100–8.
64. Gerfen CR, McGinty JF, Young WS. Dopamine differentially regulates dynorphin, substance P, and enkephalin expression in striatal neurons: in situ hybridization histochemical analysis. J Neurosci. 1991;11:1016–31.
65. Arai T, Yasuda Y, Takaya T, Toshima S, Kashiki Y, Shibayama M, Yoshimi N, Fujiwara H. Angiotensin-converting enzyme inhibitors, angiotensin-II receptor antagonists, and pneumonia in elderly hypertensive patients with stroke. Chest. 2001;119:660–1.
66. Arai T, Yasuda Y, Takaya T, Toshima S, Kashiki Y, Yoshimi N, Shibayama M, Fujiwara H. ACE inhibitors and reduction of the risk of pneumonia in elderly people. Am J Hypertens. 2000;13:1050–1.
67. Rofes L, Arreola V, Martin A, Clavé P. Natural capsaicinoids improve swallow response in older patients with oropharyngeal dysphagia. Gut. 2013;62:1280–7.
68. Desuter G, Henrard S, Boucquey D, Van Boven M, Gardiner Q, Remacle M. Learning curve of medialization thyroplasty using a montgomeryTM implant. Eur Arch Otorhinolaryngol. 2014;272(2):385–90.
69. Leder SB, Joe JK, Ross DA, Coelho DH, Mendes J. Presence of a tracheotomy tube and aspiration status in early, postsurgical head and neck cancer patients. Head Neck. 2005;27:757–61.
70. Bou-Malhab F, Hans S, Perie S, Laccourreye O, Brasnu D. Swallowing disorders in unilateral recurrent laryngeal nerve paralysis. Ann Otolaryngol. 2000;117:26–33.
71. Young VN, Zullo TG, Rosen CA. Analysis of laryngeal framework surgery: 10-year follow-up to a national survey. Laryngoscope. 2010;120:1602–8.
72. Kos MP, David EFL, Aalders IJ, Smit CF, Mahieu HF. Long-term results of laryngeal suspension and upper esophageal sphincter myotomy as treatment for life-threatening aspiration. Ann Otol Rhinol Laryngol. 2008;117:574–80.
73. Chambres O, Schultz P, Debry C. The Larynxane ST intralaryngeal endoprosthesis for laryngotracheal pathologies. J Laryngol Otol. 2006;120:942–8.

74. Nagano H, Yoshifuku K, Kurono Y. Polymyositis with dysphagia treated with endoscopic balloon dilatation. Auris Nasus Larynx. 2009;36:705–8.
75. Kuhn MA, Belafsky PC. Management of cricopharyngeus muscle dysfunction. Otolaryngol Clin N Am. 2013;46:1087–99.
76. Mason RJ, Bremner CG, DeMeester TR, Crookes PF, Peters JH, Hagen JA, DeMeester SR. Pharyngeal swallowing disorders: selection for and outcome after myotomy. Ann Surg. 1998;228:598–608.
77. Pitman M, Weissbrod P. Endoscopic CO2 laser cricopharyngeal myotomy. Laryngoscope. 2009;119:45–53.
78. Verdonck J, Morton RP. Systematic review on treatment of Zenker's diverticulum. Eur Arch Otorhinolaryngol. 2014;272(11):3095–107.
79. Kos MP, David EF, Klinkenberg-Knol EC, Mahieu HF. Long-term results of external upper esophageal sphincter myotomy for oropharyngeal dysphagia. Dysphagia. 2010;25:169–76.
80. Belafsky PC. Manual control of the upper esophageal sphincter. Laryngoscope. 2010;120(Suppl 1): S1–S16.
81. Michou E, Mistry S, Jefferson S, Tyrrell P, Hamdy S. Characterizing the mechanisms of central and peripheral forms of neurostimulation in chronic dysphagic stroke patients. Brain Stimulat. 2014;7: 66–73.
82. Michou E, Mistry S, Rothwell J, Hamdy S. Priming pharyngeal motor cortex by repeated paired associative stimulation: implications for dysphagia neurorehabilitation. Neurorehabil Neural Repair. 2013;27:355–62.
83. Shipe C, Zivković SA. Electrodiagnostic evaluation of motor neuron disorders. Am J Electroneurodiagnostic Technol. 2004;44(1):30–6.
84. Shanahan TK, Logemann JA, Rademaker AW, Pauloski BR, Kahrilas PJ. Chin-down posture effect on aspiration in dysphagic patients. Arch Phys Med Rehabil. 1993;74(7):736–9.
85. Logemann JA, Kahrilas PJ, Kobara M, Vakil NB. The benefit of head rotation on pharyngoesophageal dysphagia. Arch Phys Med Rehabil. 1989;70(10):767–71.
86. Tsukamoto Y. CT study of closure of the hemipharynx with head rotation in a case of lateral medullary syndrome. Dysphagia. 2000;15(1):17–8.
87. Martin BJ, Logemann JA, Shaker R, Dodds WJ. Normal laryngeal valving patterns during three breath-hold maneuvers: a pilot investigation. Dysphagia. 1993;8(1):11–20.
88. Ohmae Y, Logemann JA, Kaiser P, Hanson DG, Kahrilas PJ. Effects of two breath-holding maneuvers on oropharyngeal swallow. Ann Otol Rhinol Laryngol. 1996;105(2):123–31.
89. Hirst LJ, Sama A, Carding PN, Wilson JA. Is a "safe swallow" really safe? Int J Lang Commun Disord. 1998;33(Suppl):279–80.
90. Pouderoux P, Kahrilas PJ. Deglutitive tongue force modulation by volition, volume, and viscosity in humans. Gastroenterology. 1995;108(5):1418–26.
91. Lazarus C, Logemann JA, Song CW, Rademaker AW, Kahrilas PJ. Effects of voluntary maneuvers on tongue base function for swallowing. Folia Phoniatr Logop Off Organ Int Assoc Logop Phoniatr IALP. 2002;54(4):171–6.
92. Huckabee M-L, Butler SG, Barclay M, Jit S. Submental surface electromyographic measurement and pharyngeal pressures during normal and effortful swallowing. Arch Phys Med Rehabil. 2005;86(11):2144–9.
93. Lazarus CL, Logemann JA, Rademaker AW, Kahrilas PJ, Pajak T, Lazar R, et al. Effects of bolus volume, viscosity, and repeated swallows in nonstroke subjects and stroke patients. Arch Phys Med Rehabil. 1993;74(10):1066–70.

Future of Neurolaryngology

18

Frederik G. Dikkers

Abstract

Neurolaryngology is a discipline which seems to have a promising future. In order to try to see what the future might look like, experts were addressed. The experts were Council members of the European Laryngological Society (ELS).

A questionnaire with four open questions was sent to seven Presidential Council members and all 16 Scientific Council members of the ELS. Questions dealt with field with most expected improvement, new surgical techniques, robotic surgery, and any additional remarks on future neurolaryngology.

Replies to most expected improvement are grouped together in Diagnostics, Nerve reinnervation and regeneration, Electric stimulation, Technical improvements, pacing, laryngeal transplantation, Treatment, and Complications. Answers to the question whether new surgical techniques would develop were provided in three categories: Reinnervation, Pacing, and Endoscopic and minimally invasive surgical techniques. Respondents were quite divergent about the possibilities of robotic surgery. One is positive about the future of neurolaryngology, despite the threat of negative economic influence.

A wide variety of answers was given to our four questions. No firm conclusions can be drawn from the replies. Nerve reinnervation and regeneration are expected to improve. Surgical techniques are expected to improve, neurogenesis might improve, whether or not with the help of stem cell therapy. Little is expected from electric stimulation. Pacing is

F.G. Dikkers
Department of Otorhinolaryngology,
Academic Medical Center, University of Amsterdam,
P.O. box 22660, 1100 DD Amsterdam
The Netherlands
e-mail: f.g.dikkers@amc.nl

C. Sittel, O. Guntinas-Lichius (eds.), *Neurolaryngology*,
https://doi.org/10.1007/978-3-319-61724-4_18

expected to be of great influence of the future. No clear solutions were provided on advancement with surgical techniques. Robotic surgery in neurolaryngology is thought to contribute little. The thought of the future of laryngeal transplantation is indecisive, and again widely divergent. Future laryngologists are expected to work more interdisciplinary.

No clear drawing of neurolaryngology of the future can be made. However, there are contours of increased integration of electronic devices in laryngeal functional rehabilitation.

18.1 Introduction

Neurolaryngology did not exist a decade ago in the way it currently does. This implies that there will be significant changes in the time to come. Nobody is expected to be able to predict the future, and nobody can. The English statesman Winston Churchill (1874–1965) has been quoted as: "It is always wise to look ahead, but difficult to look further than you can see." However, it is necessary for clinicians to be able to have an idea what experts think is imminent. Experts should be involved, as experts perform fundamental work today of developments which come into practice in the close, or more distant, future. Experts can tell in which fields they expect changes.

The European Laryngological Society (ELS, www.elsoc.org) is world's largest laryngological society. As a non-political and non-profit society, it is devoted to the knowledge and developments in all fields of Laryngology. It aims to unite European otorhinolaryngologists in order

- To further the scientific development in the field of laryngology;
- To widen the knowledge and to assess the practical implementation of technical and scientific developments in this field;
- To promote and foster the professional skills of members;
- To further the scientific development in the field of laryngology;
- To encourage continuing education of laryngologists through the organization of conventions, meetings, courses, and workshops.

By the end of 2016 ELS united approximately 350 specialists from more than 50 countries in all continents. The ELS is led by the Presidential Council (PC) and the Scientific Council (SC), the two most important councils of the ELS. The PC deals with daily matters and organization of ELS congresses and workshops. PC members propose the names of members to be candidates for office elections. It consists of eight persons.

The SC unites specialists in the field. SC members have proved their academic merits by either frequent publications, or engagement in scientific discussions at ELS' biannual congresses and workshops, or both. In addition, many SC members are member of one or more Working Committees of the ELS. According to ELS statutes, members of the SC are selected by the PC. Candidates can be suggested by members of the SC, or by laryngologists who have been member of the SC before. The ultimate proposal to become member of the SC is done by the PC. The SC includes all members of the PC. At the time of request, the SC consisted of 24 members, composed of 16 SC, and eight PC members. The question was raised to SC members: What do you think of the future of neurolaryngology?

18.2 Methodology of the Assessment

An e-mail including an open questionnaire was sent to PC and SC members of the ELS as both councils were composed in November 2014. All members of these councils received the letter. As the author is one of the PC members, 23 invitations to contribute to this questionnaire were sent. All addressees received two reminders. The questionnaire had four open questions:

1. On which neurolaryngologic field do you expect most improvement in the next decade?
2. Can you imagine that new surgical techniques develop? If so, could you elaborate on that?
3. Do you see a role for robotic surgery? If so, could you expand on that?
4. Do you have any additional remark on future neurolaryngology?

The time span of this future was undetermined. The author of this chapter did not provide answers to the questionnaire.

18.3 Results of the Assessment

Twelve replies were received. Seven of them did not adhere to the questions raised, but freely philosophized. Five respondents strictly adhered to the questions. Results are displayed per question.

18.3.1 On Which Neurolaryngologic Field Do You Expect Most Improvement in the Next Decade?

Replies were provided in several open categories, inherently created by the respondents. Replies to this question are grouped together in Diagnostics, Nerve reinnervation and regeneration, Electric stimulation, Technical improvements, pacing, laryngeal transplantation, Treatment, and Complications.

18.3.1.1 Diagnostics

Several respondents expected that in the future development and analysis of electromyography (EMG) would be promising. Some elaborated on that: EMG will be much more systematized and will allow better understanding of mobility troubles, for instance modalities of recovery. More than now laryngologists will be able to confirm subtle pareses with EMG. The diagnosis of cricoarytenoid fixation, or interarytenoid synechia will improve, is the prognosis.

Intra-operative nerve monitoring is also expected to improve. This might lead to reduction of incidence of iatrogenic vocal fold palsy.

Better ultrasonography might lead to refinements in diagnosis of laryngeal muscle atrophy leading to increased judgment of modalities of restoration of vocal fold paralysis. Generally, more early diagnosis is expected, because of ubiquitous availability of internet and YouTube.

Concerning diagnosis, there is limited expectation of genetics. There was one reply, however, expecting that genetic basis of spasmodic dysphonia will improve very much.

18.3.1.2 Nerve Reinnervation and Regeneration

Most improvement is expected in the field of nerve reinnervation and nerve regeneration. Nerve reinnervation is expected to enhance: transplant nerves are expected to grow together easily with normal routed laryngeal nerves. Nerve-to-nerve reinnervation will enhance as well, facilitating better outcomes in traumatic nerve defects. It is even expected that under stimulation and application of different substances (possibly obtained using stem cell techniques) neurogenesis can be created, enhancing nerve regeneration. Nerve reinnervation is expected to act as good potential in adding the deselective reinnervation procedure to treatment modalities for unilateral vocal fold paralysis. Nerve reinnervation will act complementary to nerve regeneration, and vice versa. Reinnervation of the larynx for unilateral vocal fold paralysis might even replace traditional procedures.

Stem cell therapy, inducing nerve regeneration, will improve recovery. Two tracks might develop: prevention of nerve degeneration at the time of nerve injury, or prevention of synkinesis.

18.3.1.3 Electric Stimulation

Micro-implants will be created by nanotechnology, is an expectation. These micro-implants will receive their energy from the surrounding tissue and adapt to patients' activity. Micro-implants can be implanted in several areas of the larynx and create a network that coordinates laryngeal stimulation. Normal laryngeal function can thus be restored. This might be of use in elderly, in Parkinson, and in spasmodic dysphonia (SD).

Additional functional gain is expected in the field of aspiration, and even dysphagia. Improvement will have to be made in the field of trigger selection. Advances in technology (medical devices) and the future of stem cells application also give hope for better solutions.

18.3.1.4 Technical Improvements, Pacing, Laryngeal Transplantation

Nerve-to-nerve anastomosis will improve due to a controlled growth factors' role. One might discover a molecular target for neural repair. Probably one will be able to use organic conductive bio-electrodes, or be able to bio-engineer them. All together, there will be technically better trauma handling than today. One expectation is that reinnervation procedures might even be performed on a day-care basis.

One respondent states that currently clinicians have the impression that peripheral nerves have better ability to regenerate after injury compared to regeneration in the central nervous system. This respondent states that regeneration needs several extrinsic and intrinsic factors as well as a suitable environment, e.g. VEGF. Under stimulation and application of different substances this respondent expects to induce neurogenesis. Missprouting might be avoided by an exact understanding of the representation of the muscle in the profile of the superior and inferior laryngeal nerve.

One respondent is very positive about pacing. Pacing will be the treatment of choice for glottic stenosis due to bilateral paralysis as well as for glottic insufficiency due to unilateral paresis. Pacing will also have a role in the treatment of OSAS, either in combination with hypoglossal nerve stimulation or other techniques of preventing upper airway collapse. Philosophizing about remote speculations, pacing might even play a role in voice enhancement in a basically healthy organ with the primary goal of functional and acoustic-aesthetic improvement.

Future object of research might be (and should be) active implants with the ability to mimic some sort of glottic valve mechanism.

Laryngeal transplantation is expected by several respondents to be promising. It will be feasible, either with larynges harvested externally, or with larynges grown from stem cells. Laryngeal transplantation will be a procedure executed faster than it is now, as there will be increased knowledge of reinnervation procedures. It might even be possible to selectively train endolaryngeal muscles with the use of micro-implants for better laryngeal function.

The indication for laryngeal transplantation might be secondary salvage treatment of bilateral vocal fold paralysis in a scarred larynx. Laryngeal transplantation might also be applied to dystonia.

To the contrary, however, the respondent who puts his stakes on laryngeal pacing respondent was very explicit: laryngeal transplantation is a dead-end street.

18.3.1.5 Treatment

Several respondents expect that treatment will be more holistically than it was at the time of the questionnaire. To achieve holistic treatment, more interdisciplinary work is necessary (between laryngology, speech and language pathology, pulmonology, neurologists/clinical physiologists, neurolaryngology, neuroimaging) to enhance knowledge about laryngeal dystonia and conditions like vocal cord dysfunction. For instance, laryngologists should interact and collaborate much more with neurologists who subspecialize in muscles, peripheral nerves, and EMG to get hints about parallel patterns happening somewhere else in the human body. Such work should take place in special institutions like a Communication Disorders Care Center, is one advice.

Another tendency which is felt is that laryngologist's focus should be on conservative therapy. Conservative therapy is explicitly stated not to be the same as "wait and see" strategy, but active management, where voice therapy is only one part of comprehensive rehabilitation. Not the end organ should be treated, is the warning, but the whole body, with the central nervous system as a top priority and the top secret.

One realizes that not all conditions can be treated. Unfortunately, little is expected from surgical techniques on SD. While results might be promising temporarily, the end result is still expected to be disappointing.

18.3.1.6 Complications

Viral and bacterial infections will be more easily detectable by chip diagnosis, implying better treatment. Therefore precise antibiotic treatment can be applied in the case of infection-related nerve damage.

Robotic surgery might induce a lower rate of postoperative infection. Complete function can be restored.

Rejection of a transplanted larynx by the recipient will be more easily controlled, according to a respondent. He probably refers to improved development of immunodepressants.

18.3.2 Can you imagine that new surgical techniques develop? If so, could you elaborate?

Answers to the question whether new surgical techniques would develop were provided in three categories. These are Reinnervation, Pacing, and Endoscopic and minimally invasive surgical techniques.

18.3.2.1 Reinnervation

There are diverging views on reinnervation. One respondent expects that reinnervation will not progress rapidly enough, while another predicts that it will be put into practice gradually. One feels that surgical reinnervation of the larynx should be a spectacular technique, which would induce better results. Maybe it will be possible thanks to the electrical stimulation of the larynx "or some other alternative"—unfortunately this was not specified.

18.3.2.2 Pacing

Several respondents are very hopeful concerning pacing. The general expectation is that modification of laryngeal nerves via electrodes will change our therapeutic spectrum. Laryngologists will become able to influence laryngeal muscles via external stimulation. This might happen sooner, or more gradually.

Pacing will be the treatment of choice for glottic stenosis due to bilateral paralysis as well as for glottic insufficiency due to unilateral paresis. In addition, there might be a role for laryngeal pacing in the treatment of OSAS, either in combination with hypoglossal nerve stimulation or other techniques of preventing upper airway collapse. As a remote speculation one might think of procedures like voice enhancement based on sophisticated neural stimulation in a basically healthy organ with the primary goal of functional and acoustic-aesthetical improvement.

One respondent observed that recurrent laryngeal nerve stimulation today is at the threshold of clinical routine for patients suffering from bilateral vocal fold paralysis of lower motor neuron type. His most likely expectation is that it will become a treatment option for unilateral paralysis, too—the time span of 20 years was mentioned here.

Most likely, replies a respondent, active implants with the ability to mimic some sort of glottic valve mechanism will be future object of research. However, challenges like 24/7 reliability, biological integration, and autonomous functioning will be difficult to solve, if at all. Having overcome these problems active implants will be more reliable, reproducible, and affordable than laryngeal transplantation.

Another way of treatment might be central stimulation (activation or inhibition), which can be obtained by transcranial magnetic stimulation.

18.3.2.3 Endoscopic and Minimally Invasive Surgical Techniques

Endoscopic and minimally invasive surgical techniques might develop further. Endoscopic examination currently has a place in the diagnostic field. This place will expand, as using digitalized microscopes may be developed. Improvement is expected as well in laryngeal suspension techniques as in laryngoplasty. Surgery to improve swallowing outcomes continues to advance, with laryngeal suspension techniques showing promise. However, one respondent raises the question if surgery always offers the best solution in cases where doctors use surgery today. The focus should be on prevention, especially in field of iatrogenic vocal fold paralysis.

One respondent predicted improvement in surgery for complex bulbar palsies, invalidating a patient with dysphonia and dysphagia. No elaboration was provided—it is therefore unclear whether this dealt with an endoscopic or minimally invasive technique, or not.

18.3.3 Do You See a Role for Robotic Surgery? If So, Could You Expand on That?

Respondents were quite divergent about the possibilities of robotic surgery. One stated that it seems to be clear that robotic surgery eliminates the surgeon's physiological tremor allowing the procedure to be much more precise. It also guarantees a comfortable and ergonomic position of the surgeon during the operation.

Some respondents are very enthusiastic about robotic surgery: it is highly likely to develop soon and it may replace contemporary procedures; clinical application of robotic surgery already became a fact; in a not a very distant future robotic surgery will be much more accessible in neurolaryngology.

Some were more reluctant, and ordered laryngologists to follow this development and actively take part to the robotic operations performed in larynx.

However, the answer provided most times was more negative: until robotic equipment is further miniaturized, I see no prospect, or: I do not really see a role for robotic surgery for nerve surgery, or: if miniaturization is achieved, maybe yes.

18.3.4 Do You Have Any Additional Remark on Future Neurolaryngology?

Few answers were provided to the final open question. One's tendency is to be optimistic about the future: Contemporary knowledge and experience in this field of medicine allows us to be optimistic.

One respondent concluded that too much still has to be learned. Even a straightforward answer to what happens if a patient's recurrent laryngeal nerve is cut cannot be predicted: position and degree of immobility can still vary. Synkinesis is an additional problem that still needs to be resolved. Synkinesis seems to be present in most clinical cases.

Several respondents brought forward the topic of economic restrictions. Respondents realize that developments are depending on economic factors. They also realize that there's an increasing gap between innovative power and technical feasibility versus availability of resources in health care systems. For instance, in a not a very distant future robotic surgery will be much more accessible in both medicine and in neurolaryngology, despite the costs. However, respondents warn that evolution of medical possibilities has to be related to improvements for patients, not for industrial developments.

Ultimately economic factors will either prevent innovative ideas to become marketable products, or markedly decrease the number of eligible patients benefiting from sophisticated medical technology, or both.

18.4 Discussion About the Future of Neurolaryngology

In order to try to give contours to the future of neurolaryngology, an open questionnaire was sent to 23 people dedicated to laryngology. Twelve replies were received. A wide variety of answers was given to our four questions. Answers differed from technical advancement to mere speculation, and wishful thinking. No firm conclusions can be drawn from the replies. This might be due to the open character of the questions, or to the fact that predicting the future is an unsecure task.

Respondents provided answers in several categories. Some progress is expected in EMG diagnostics, as well as in pre-operative ultrasonography and in intra-operative nerve monitoring.

Nerve reinnervation and regeneration is expected to improve. Surgical techniques are expected to improve, neurogenesis might improve, whether or not with the help of stem cell therapy. The increase of number of publications found with PubMed search term “stem cells nerve regeneration” reflects this belief. Having less than ten hits annually before 1991, there were 33 hits in 2000, 201 in 2010, and 253 in 2016 (Fig. 18.1). It can thus be expected that nerve reinnervation becomes a much more common procedure than it was in 2016.

Electric stimulation and Pacing were distinguished by the author, while it is unclear if respondents had that intention. No clear definitions of the terms Electric stimulation and Pacing were provided. It might therefore be possible that these two terms were used in an interchangeable fashion. The term Electric stimulation is used where the author had the impression that a respondent meant amplification of an electric impulse. Little is expected from Electric stimulation.

Pacing is defined as selective reinnervation and neurostimulation. It is thus used where spontaneous electric activity is delivered by an implanted device. Literature shows where there is recent experimental interest: Functional electrical stimulation (FES) of the posterior cricoarytenoid muscle (PCA) to restore respiratory function of the larynx may become an option for the treatment of bilateral recurrent laryngeal nerve paralysis (RLNP) in the near future [1]. Laryngeal pacing seems to be on the right path to open up a dynamic rehabilitation of the bilaterally motion-impaired larynx [2, 3, 4]. Pacing is expected to be of great influence in the future—it might change our therapeutic spectrum. Laryngologists should advance further, with development of biologic integration and autonomous functioning.

No clear solutions were provided on advancement with surgical techniques. Ultimately, use of robotic surgery in neurolaryngology is thought to

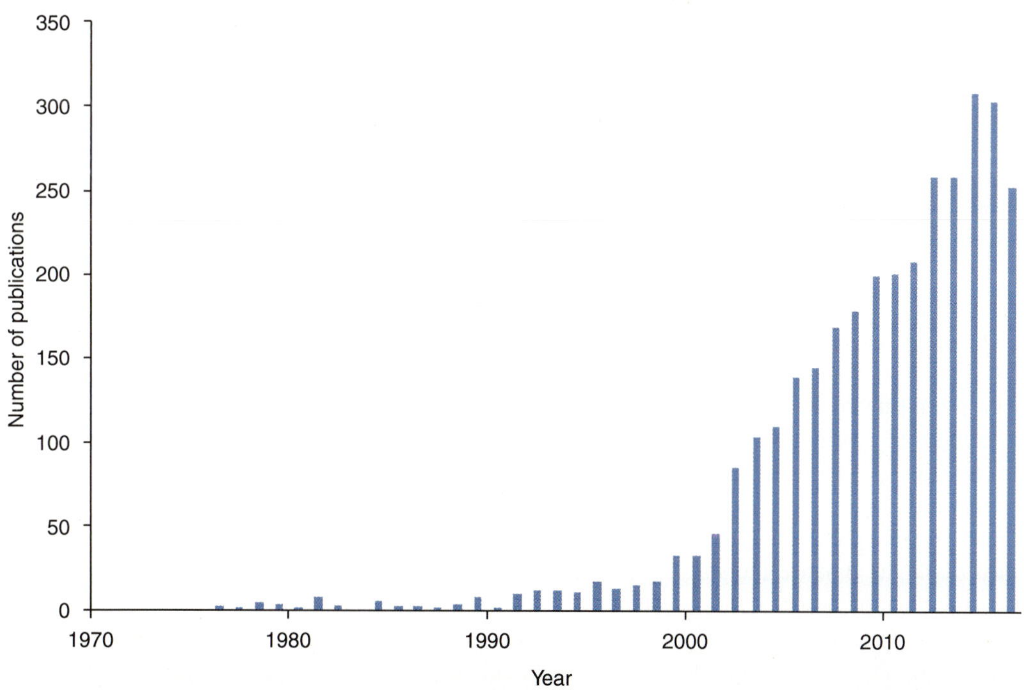

Fig. 18.1 Graphical display of number of publications found per year from 1970 to 2014, with PubMed search term (“stem cells”[MeSH Terms] OR (“stem”[All Fields] AND “cells”[All Fields]) OR “stem cells”[All Fields] OR (“stem”[All Fields] AND “cell”[All Fields]) OR “stem cell”[All Fields]) AND (“nerve regeneration”[MeSH Terms] OR “nerve”[All Fields] AND “regeneration”[All Fields]) OR “nerve regeneration”[All Fields]). Note steep increase as of 1999

contribute little. No creative or alternative thoughts concerning application of robotic surgery emerged from the panel.

The thought of the future of laryngeal transplantation is indecisive, and again widely divergent. Clinical results up to 2015 have quantitatively been disappointing, with less than five patients reported. In 1998, the first successful total laryngeal transplant was performed. After approximately a decade, a slowly progressive, chronic rejection process gradually rendered the organ nonfunctional, and the patient and his providers deemed the larynx appropriate for explantation [5].

Laryngologists are expected (and thus urged!) to work more interdisciplinary. Many respondents shared this view, which seems very logical. Installation of interdisciplinary teams, predominantly with voice specialists and specialists involved in work with the prefix neuro-, should prevail.

Sometimes replies were opposed to each other. Two examples will be provided.

Unilateral vocal fold paralysis will be solved by reinnervation of the larynx; this might even replace traditional procedures. On the other hand, an expectation is that pacing will be the treatment of choice for glottic stenosis due to bilateral paralysis as well as for glottic insufficiency due to unilateral paresis. The first answer clearly implies environmental factors to improve, while the second response discusses pure technical advancements.

The second example deals with laryngeal transplantation. Laryngeal transplantation is expected to be promising by several respondents. Again, environmental conditions might improve, creating larynges grown from stem cells. Selective reinnervation procedures, including selectively trained by micro-implants for better laryngeal function, might enhance the surgical procedure. The indication for laryngeal transplantation might be widely expanded: cancer patients, trauma, but also scarred larynx or dystonia. A respondent who is expecting a lot from pacing expressed a completely different opinion: laryngeal transplantation is a dead-end street.

No clear drawing of neurolaryngology of the future can be made. However, there are contours of increased integration of electronic devices in laryngeal functional rehabilitation.

Acknowledgements The contribution of the following persons (in alphabetical order) is highly appreciated: Leena-Maija Aaltonen, Christoph Arens, Declan Costello, Vojko Djukic, Markus Hess, Jean–Paul Marie, Maciej Misiolek, Giorgio Peretti, Cesare Piazza, Ricard Simo, Christian Sittel, Elisabeth Sjögren. Together these respondents from (alphabetically) England, Finland, France, Germany, Italy, the Netherlands, Poland, Serbia predicted the neurolaryngologic future as they see it.

References

1. Förster G, Arnold D, Bischoff SJ, Schubert H, Scholle HC, Müller AH. Laryngeal pacing in minipigs: in vivo test of a new minimal invasive transcricoidal electrode insertion method for functional electrical stimulation of the PCA. Eur Arch Otorhinolaryngol. 2013;270(1):225–31.
2. Müller AH. Laryngeal pacing for bilateral vocal fold immobility. Curr Opin Otolaryngol Head Neck Surg. 2011;19(6):439–43.
3. Müller AH, Hagen R, Förster G, Grossmann W, Baumbusch K, Pototschnig C. Laryngeal pacing via an implantable stimulator for the rehabilitation of subjects suffering from bilateral vocal fold paralysis: A prospective first-in-human study. Laryngoscope. 2016;126(8):1810–6.
4. Müller AH, Hagen R, Pototschnig C, Förster G, Grossmann W, Baumbusch K, Gugatschka M, Nawka T. Laryngeal pacing for bilateral vocal fold paralysis: Voice and respiratory aspects. Laryngoscope. 2017;127(8):1838–44.
5. Lorenz RR, Strome M. Total laryngeal transplant explanted: 14 years of lessons learned. Otolaryngol Head Neck Surg. 2014;150(4):509–11.

Printed by Printforce, the Netherlands